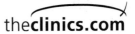

GASTROENTEROLOGY CLINICS OF NORTH AMERICA

Colon Cancer Screening, Surveillance, Prevention, and Therapy

GUEST EDITOR
Mitchell S. Cappell, MD, PhD

March 2008 • Volume 37 • Number 1

SAUNDERS

An Imprint of Elsevier, Inc.
PHILADELPHIA   LONDON   TORONTO   MONTREAL   SYDNEY   TOKYO

W.B. SAUNDERS COMPANY
A Division of Elsevier Inc.

Elsevier Inc. • 1600 John F. Kennedy Blvd., Suite 1800 • Philadelphia, Pennsylvania 19103-2899

http://www.theclinics.com

**GASTROENTEROLOGY CLINICS
OF NORTH AMERICA**
March 2008
Editor: Kerry Holland

Volume 37, Number 1
ISSN 0889-8553
ISBN-13: 978-1-4160-5839-7
ISBN-10: 1-4160-5839-7

The ideas and opinions expressed in *Gastroenterology Clinics of North America* do not necessarily reflect those of the Publisher. The Publisher does not assume any responsibility for any injury and/or damage to persons or property arising out of or related to any use of the material contained in this periodical. The reader is advised to check the appropriate medical literature and the product information currently provided by the manufacturer of each drug to be administered to verify the dosage, the method and duration of administration, or contraindications. It is the responsibility of the treating physician or other health care professional, relying on independent experience and knowledge of the patient, to determine drug dosages and the best treatment for the patient. Mention of any product in this issue should not be construed as endorsement by the contributors, editors, or the Publisher of the product or manufacturers' claims.

Gastroenterology Clinics of North America (ISSN 0889-8553) is published quarterly by Elsevier Inc., 360 Park Avenue South, New York, NY 10010-1710. Months of issue are March, June, September, and December. Business and Editorial Offices: 1600 John F. Kennedy Blvd., Suite 1800, Philadelphia, PA 19103-2899. Customer Service Office: 6277 Sea Harbor Drive, Orlando, FL 32887-4800. Periodicals postage paid at New York, NY and additional mailing offices. Subscription prices are $237.00 per year (US individuals), $121.00 per year (US students), $344.00 per year (US institutions), $261.00 per year (Canadian individuals), $410.00 per year (Canadian institutions), $309.00 per year (international individuals), $157.00 per year (international students), and $426.00 per year (international institutions). Foreign air speed delivery is included in all *Clinics* subscription prices. All prices are subject to change without notice. POSTMASTER: Send address changes to *Gastroenterology Clinics of North America*, Elsevier Periodicals Customer Service 6277 Sea Harbor Drive, Orlando, FL 32887-4800. **Customer Service: 1-800-654-2452 (US). From outside the United States, call 1-407-563-6020. Fax: 1-407-563-8521. E-mail: JournalsCustomerService-usa@elsevier.com.**

Gastroenterology Clinics of North America is also published in Italian by Il Pensiero Scientifico Editore, Rome, Italy; and in Portuguese by Interlivros Edicoes Ltda., Rua Commandante Coelho 1085, 21250 Cordovil, Rio de Janeiro, Brazil.

Gastroenterology Clinics of North America is covered in *Index Medicus, Excerpta Medica, Current Contents/Clinical Medicine, Science Citation Index, ISI/BIOMED,* and *BIOSIS.*

Printed in the United States of America.

GASTROENTEROLOGY CLINICS
OF NORTH AMERICA

Colon Cancer Screening, Surveillance, Prevention, and Therapy

GUEST EDITOR

MITCHELL S. CAPPELL, MD, PhD, Chief, Division of Gastroenterology, William Beaumont Hospital, Royal Oak, Michigan

CONTRIBUTORS

TIMOTHY R. ASMIS, MD, Gastrointestinal Oncology Fellow, Gastrointestinal Oncology, Memorial Sloan Kettering Cancer Center, New York, New York

DONALD BARKEL, MD, Department of Surgery, William Beaumont Hospital, Royal Oak, Michigan

MANOOP S. BHUTANI, MD, FASGE, FACG, FACP, Professor of Medicine, Department of Gastroenterology, Hepatology, and Nutrition, Unit 436, UT MD Anderson Cancer Center, Houston, Texas

MITCHELL S. CAPPELL, MD, PhD, Chief, Division of Gastroenterology, William Beaumont Hospital, Royal Oak, Michigan

TUSAR K. DESAI, MD, Division of Gastroenterology, Department of Medicine, William Beaumont Hospital, Royal Oak, Michigan

MICHAEL C. DUFFY, MD, Division of Gastroenterology, William Beaumont Hospital, Royal Oak, Michigan

JAMES E. EAST, MRCP, Endoscopy Research Fellow, Wolfson Unit for Endoscopy, St. Mark's Hospital, Harrow, Middlesex, United Kingdom

JEREMY R. JASS, MD, FRCPath, Professor, Clinical Chair in Gastrointestinal Pathology, Department of Cellular Pathology, St. Mark's Hospital, Harrow, Middlesex, United Kingdom

AMULYA KONDA, MD, Gastroenterology Fellow, Division of Gastroenterology, Department of Medicine, William Beaumont Hospital, Royal Oak, Michigan

ELIZABETH LITTLE, MD, Radiology Resident, Department of Radiology, Albert Einstein Medical Center, Philadelphia, Pennsylvania

JACK S. MANDEL, PhD, MPH, Rollins Professor and Chair, Georgia Cancer Coalition Distinguished Cancer Scholar, Department of Epidemiology, Rollins School of Public Health, Emory University, Atlanta, Georgia

JAMES R. MARSHALL, PhD, Professor of Oncology, Roswell Park Cancer Institute, Buffalo, New York

SUSAN L. MIHALKO, BAS, CGRN, RN, Administrative Manager, Endoscopy Center, William Beaumont Hospital, Royal Oak, Michigan

ANTHONY B. MILLER, MD, Professor Emeritus, Department of Public Health Sciences, University of Toronto, Oakville, Ontario, Canada

DOUGLAS K. REX, MD, Division of Gastroenterology, Department of Medicine, Indiana University School of Medicine, Indiana University Hospital, Indianapolis, Indiana

JOHN M. ROBERTSON, MD, Vice-Chief, Department of Radiation Oncology, William Beaumont Hospital, Royal Oak, Michigan

LEONARD SALTZ, MD, Attending Physician, Gastrointestinal Oncology, Memorial Sloan Kettering Cancer Center, New York; and Professor of Medicine, Weill Medical College of Cornell University, New York

BRIAN P. SAUNDERS, MD, FRCP, Director, Wolfson Unit for Endoscopy, St. Mark's Hospital, Harrow, Middlesex, United Kingdom

CAROL E.H. SCOTT-CONNER, MD, PhD, Professor of Surgery, Department of Surgery, University of Iowa Carver College of Medicine, Iowa City, Iowa

SUSAN SUMMERTON, MD, Section Chief of GI Radiology, Department of Radiology, Albert Einstein Medical Center; and Assistant Professor of Radiology, Jefferson Medical College, Thomas Jefferson University, Philadelphia, Pennsylvania

KEVIN A. TOLLIVER, MD, Division of Gastroenterology, Department of Medicine, Indiana University School of Medicine, Indiana University Hospital, Indianapolis, Indiana

NEAL WILKINSON, MD, Clinical Assistant Professor of Surgery, Department of Surgery, University of Iowa Carver College of Medicine, Iowa City, Iowa

GASTROENTEROLOGY CLINICS
OF NORTH AMERICA

Colon Cancer Screening, Surveillance, Prevention, and Therapy

CONTENTS   VOLUME 37 • NUMBER 1 • MARCH 2008

Colon cancer is believed to arise from two types of precursor polyps via two distinct pathways: conventional adenomas by the conventional adenoma-to-carcinoma sequence and serrated adenomas according to the serrated adenoma-to-carcinoma theory. Conventional adenomas arise from mutation of the *APC* gene; progression to colon cancer is a multistep process. The fundamental genetic defect in serrated adenomas is unknown. Environmental factors can increase the risk for colon cancer. Advanced colon cancer often presents with symptoms, but early colon cancer and premalignant adenomatous polyps commonly are asymptomatic, rendering them difficult to detect and providing the rationale for mass screening of adults over age 50.

There is now strong evidence for an alternative pathway of colorectal carcinogenesis implicating hyperplastic polyps and serrated adenomas. This article briefly reviews the evidence for this serrated pathway, provides diagnostic criteria for clinically significant hyperplastic polyps and allied serrated polyps, and suggests how this information may be translated into safe, effective guidelines for colonoscopy-based colon cancer prevention. Consideration also is given to the definition and management of hyperplastic polyposis syndrome. The currently proposed management plan for serrated polyps is tentative because of incomplete knowledge of the nature and behavior of these polyps. This article highlights key areas warranting further research.

Screening for Colorectal Cancer 97
Jack S. Mandel

Although there are several methods available for colon cancer screening, none is optimal. This article reviews methods for screening, including fecal occult blood tests, flexible sigmoidoscopy, colonoscopy, CT colonography, capsule endoscopy, and double contrast barium enema. A simple, inexpensive, noninvasive, and relatively sensitive screening test is needed to identify people at risk for developing advanced adenomas or colorectal cancer who would benefit from colonoscopy. It is hoped that new markers will be identified that perform better. Until then we fortunately have a variety of screening strategies that do work.

Implementation of Colonoscopy for Mass Screening for Colon Cancer and Colonic Polyps: Efficiency with High Quality of Care 117
Susan L. Mihalko

As awareness of colon cancer by the public continues to increase, screening colonoscopy procedures will proportionately increase. There is much written on the design of new ambulatory gastroenterology clinics, but little practical information about high-volume, mass colonoscopic screening of patients in the hospital outpatient setting. Many institutions struggle with inefficient endoscopy units that cannot always meet the dual needs of high quality and efficient performance of screening endoscopy. The patient undergoing screening colonoscopy seeks an efficient unit with state-of-the-art equipment, highly skilled physicians, highly competent staff, accurate case documentation, comfortable surroundings, and consumer-friendly follow-through of care. Optimizing these factors in existing spaces may require revision of an endoscopy unit's operations and, possibly, renovation of the endoscopy suite.

Reducing the Incidence and Mortality of Colon Cancer: Mass Screening and Colonoscopic Polypectomy 129
Mitchell S. Cappell

Most colon cancers arise from conventional adenomatous polyps (conventional adenoma-to-carcinoma sequence), while some colon cancers appear to arise from the recently recognized serrated adenomatous polyp (serrated adenoma-to-carcinoma theory). Because conventional adenomas and serrated adenomas are usually asymptomatic, mass screening of asymptomatic patients has become the cornerstone for detecting and eliminating these precursor lesions to reduce the risk of colon cancer. Colonoscopy has become the primary screening test because of its high sensitivity and specificity, and the ability to perform polypectomy. Other screening tests include guaiac tests or fecal immunochemical tests (FIT) for fecal occult blood, and flexible sigmoidoscopy. A minimal colonoscopic withdrawal time of 6 minutes is important to maximize polyp detection at colonoscopy. Chromoendoscopy is an experimental technique used to highlight abnormal colonic areas to identify neoplastic tissue and to potentially determine the histology of colonic polyps at colonoscopy based on superficial pit anatomy.

CT colonography (CTC) is an innovative technology that entails CT examination of the entire colon and computerized processing of the raw data after colon cleansing and colonic distention. CTC could potentially increase the screening rate for colon cancer because of its relative safety, relatively low expense, and greater patient acceptance, but its role in mass colon cancer screening is controversial because of its highly variable sensitivity, the inability to sample polyps for histologic analysis, and lack of therapeutic capabilities. This article reviews the CTC literature, including imaging and adjunctive techniques, radiologic interpretation, procedure indications, contraindications, risks, sensitivity, interpretation pitfalls, and controversies.

Colorectal cancer (CRC) is the second most common cause of cancer-related mortality in the United States. Colonoscopic screening with removal of adenomatous polyps in individuals at average risk is known to decrease the incidence and associated mortality from colon cancer. Certain conditions, notably inflammatory bowel disease involving the colon, a family history of polyps or cancer, a personal history of colon cancer or polyps, and other conditions such as acromegaly, ureterosigmoidostomy, and *Streptococcus bovis* bacteremia are associated with an increased risk of colonic neoplasia. This article reviews the CRC risks associated with these conditions and the currently recommended surveillance strategies.

Endoscopic ultrasound (EUS) has evolved as a useful technique for imaging and intervention in the colon and rectum. This article reviews the clinical applications of EUS for imaging and intervention in colorectal cancer, with an emphasis on the most recent clinical studies.

GASTROENTEROLOGY CLINICS
OF NORTH AMERICA

ELSEVIER
SAUNDERS

GASTROENTEROLOGY CLINICS
OF NORTH AMERICA

SEVIER
UNDERS

Preface

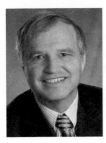

Mitchell S. Cappell, MD, PhD
Guest Editor

Consider the war on colon cancer. Every year more than 150,000 Americans develop colon cancer, with more than 50,000 fatalities [1]. This number of fatalities per year is comparable to all the American fatalities in the decade-long Vietnam War and is more than 12 fold the number of American fatalities in the current 5 years of war in Iraq. Throughout the world more than 1 million people develop colon cancer every year, about half of whom succumb to this disease [2]. The mortality from this cancer since World War II exceeds by several fold the mortality among all the armed forces in World War II, the bloodiest war in history. In the approximately 8 minutes that it takes to read this preface, another American on average will die from colon cancer, and 10 individuals will die worldwide. Incredibly, about 1 in 18 of you, the readers of this article, will develop colon cancer within your lifetime, a risk that I, likewise, share [3].

This war aims to save lives, hundreds of thousands per year worldwide, rather than extinguish them as in conventional warfare. The armed forces in this war are colonoscopists, epidemiologists, bureaucrats, and endoscopy nurses; their guns are colonoscopes; and their ammunition is polypectomy snares. Consider the "body count" since the declaration of war. During the last 30 years the incidence of this cancer has decreased by about 20% and the mortality has declined by 40% [4]. These declines have recently accelerated, with an incredible 5% decrease in mortality in 2004 [5]. These cumulative effects have reduced American fatalities by 20,000 per year.

Although impressive, these reductions are insufficient. Fifty thousand too many Americans still die from colon cancer per year. Victory in this war is predicated on prevention by appropriate screening and polypectomy of precancerous lesions. Half of the eligible population fails to undergo any form of

0889-8553/08/$ – see front matter
doi:10.1016/j.gtc.2007.12.004

colon cancer screening [6,7]. Screening cannot save the lives of unscreened patients. Further reductions require redoubled efforts. The residual patients become harder to recruit for colon cancer screening as the more compliant patients have already undergone screening [8].

Much of the inefficiency in screening stems from insufficient knowledge by clinicians, who in turn fail to educate or refer their patients for screening. Education is thus critical for clinicians—whether internists, family practitioners, or other nongastroenterologists—to appropriately refer their patients for colonoscopic screening and surveillance. This issue is dedicated to educating the internist and general practitioner about this cancer and further educating the gastroenterologist and colon cancer researcher. I hope that this monograph functions on multiple levels—to provide the basic clinical knowledge, to comprehensively review the data, and to analyze the latest discoveries—to be useful to all these constituencies to benefit our patients.

I am delighted to offer the readers a distinguished assembly of researchers and authorities as authors. As we eliminate the straightforward, easily identifiable conventional adenomas, the more clinically obscure and less colonoscopically evident serrated adenomas assume greater importance in preventing the residual interval colon cancers after an apparent clearing colonoscopy. Jeremy Jass, the internationally renowned authority on serrated adenomas, and James East provide an important review of this rapidly evolving subject. Tusar Desai and Donald Barkel provide the perspective of academic clinicians in private practice to the complex field of syndromic colon cancer. There is much that is new and highly relevant in this review of this fast-evolving subject. Although much of the current focus on colon cancer prevention centers on removal of premalignant colonic polyps, more work is needed to prevent carcinogenesis at the earliest stages by reducing risk factors and by intervening in the molecular pathways of carcinogenesis. James Marshall comprehensively reviews the subject of colon cancer prevention through diet, drugs, and lifestyle. Anthony Miller has devoted his professional career to clinical epidemiology, especially disease prevention. He provides a terrific compilation of the complexities in applying the theory of mass screening to colon cancer.

Jack Mandel provides a thorough and timely review of the different modalities of colon cancer screening, including reviews of all the major trials of these modalities. Nurse Sue Mihalko provides a unique perspective and novel information on screening from her vast experience over 2 decades as administrator of the endoscopy unit at William Beaumont Hospital, the second largest endoscopy unit in the United States. This unit is highly efficient and is recognized for its high quality of care, user friendliness, and patient safety. She describes the principles of running an efficient, high-quality endoscopy unit and divulges many of her secrets.

CT colonography is the most controversial subject in colon cancer screening because of variable data about sensitivity, specificity, and efficacy; it is also one of the fastest-evolving areas because of rapid advances in computer technology. Susan Summerton and colleagues thoroughly review this subject to provide the clinician and researcher the information to critically review the literature and to rationally judge its role in colon cancer screening.

Two highly academic clinicians, my colleague Mike Duffy and a second-year gastroenterology fellow, Amulya Konda, thoroughly review the complex and important subject of surveillance of patients at increased risk for colon cancer to properly refer these patients for surveillance colonoscopy. Manoop Bhutani has played a leading role in the development of endoscopic ultrasound through important clinical and research contributions during nearly 2 decades. I am delighted to present his comprehensive clinical review on endoscopic ultrasound for cancer staging.

Douglas Rex is an internationally acclaimed clinical-academic gastroenterologist who has made major contributions in improving the sensitivity of colonoscopy for polyp detection, in critically evaluating CT colonography, in the use of anesthetics for colonoscopy, and in techniques of colonoscopic polypectomy. His article is an important reference on polypectomy techniques and is essential reading for the colonoscopist.

The article by Carol Scott-Conner, an international authority on minimally invasive colon cancer surgery, and Neal Wilkinson is of great interest to the surgeon and other physicians treating patients who have colon cancer. Despite all efforts at colon cancer prevention or early diagnosis, significant numbers of patients still present with advanced cancer that requires radiotherapy or chemotherapy. John Robertson, a terrific colon cancer specialist, reviews the important clinical trials on radiotherapy for advanced colon cancer. Timothy Asmis and Leonard Saltz, dedicated oncologic researchers, comprehensively review chemotherapy for colon cancer, with a special focus on large cooperative trials.

I thank my supervisors Drs. Ananias Diokno, Leslie Rocher, Mike Maddens, and John Musich, for their encouragement and support for this academic endeavor. I thank my secretary, Mary Fronczak, for help in typing. I thank the librarians at William Beaumont Hospital, including Janet Zimmerman, Andrea Rogers, Ken Nelson, Janet West, and Chris Smiatacz, for their help in literature searches and procuring journal articles from other libraries. I thank Kerry Holland, the editor of the *Gastroenterology Clinics of North America*, for her extremely helpful advice and friendly collaboration in this project, and the folks at Saunders for an ongoing relationship that has included my editorship of nine volumes in the *Clinics of North America* series. Finally, I thank my wife for tolerating my not being home at night or on weekends while working on this issue, and my children, Adina, David, Miriam, and Daniel, for their support.

On a personal note, I have participated in this war from the perspective of both a practicing clinician and researcher on colon cancer. As a clinical gastroenterologist I was drafted early in this war. Ed Goldberg and I published a paper in 1992 demonstrating preliminary evidence of a decline in colon cancer mortality in America [9], findings that have been confirmed and greatly extended in the ensuing 15 years. Let us rededicate our commitment and redouble our efforts to eradicate colon cancer entirely, like the old scourges of yore, such as small pox or bubonic plague!

Mitchell S. Cappell, MD, PhD
Division of Gastroenterology
William Beaumont Hospital, MOB 233
3601 West Thirteen Mile Road
Royal Oak, MI 48073, USA

References

[1] Jemal A, Siegel R, Ward E, et al. Cancer statistics, 2007. CA Cancer J Clin 2007;57:43–66.
[2] Shibuya K, Mathers CD, Boschi-Pinto C, et al. Global and regional estimates of cancer mortality and incidence by site: II. Results for the global burden of disease 2000. BMC Cancer 2002;2:26.
[3] Cappell MS. The pathophysiology, clinical presentation, and diagnosis of colon cancer and adenomatous polyps. Med Clin N Am 2005;89:1–42.
[4] National Center for Health Statistics, Division of Vital Statistics, Centers for Disease Control. Available at: www.cdc.gov. Accessed October 24, 2007.
[5] Espey DK, Wu XC, Swan J, et al. Annual report to the nation on the status of cancer, 1975–2004, featuring cancer in American Indians and Alaska Natives. Cancer 2007; 110:2119–52.
[6] Khankari K, Eder M, Osborn CY, et al. Improving colorectal cancer screening among the medically underserved: a pilot study within a federally qualified health center. J Gen Intern Med 2007;22:1410–4.
[7] Anonymous. Surveillance for certain behaviors among selected local areas: United States. Behavioral risk factor surveillance system. Morb Mort Wkly Rep 2004;53: SSS05.
[8] Wolf MS, Satterlee M, Calhoun EA, et al. Colorectal cancer screening among the medically underserved. J Healthcare Poor Underserved 2006;17:46–54.
[9] Cappell MS, Goldberg ES. The relationship between the clinical presentation and spread of colon cancer in 315 consecutive patients: a significant trend of earlier cancer detection from 1982 through 1988 at a university hospital. J Clin Gastroenterol 1992;14:227–35.

Gastroenterol Clin N Am 37 (2008) 1–24

GASTROENTEROLOGY CLINICS
OF NORTH AMERICA

Pathophysiology, Clinical Presentation, and Management of Colon Cancer

Mitchell S. Cappell, MD, PhD

Division of Gastroenterology, William Beaumont Hospital, MOB 233,
3601 West Thirteen Mile Road, Royal Oak, MI 48073, USA

Colorectal cancer afflicts approximately 150,000 Americans annually, approximately one third of whom die [1]. It afflicts approximately 250,000 annually in Europe [2] and approximately 1 million people worldwide [3]. A review of the pathophysiology, clinical presentation, and diagnosis of colon cancer is important and timely. This field is changing rapidly because of breakthroughs in the molecular basis of carcinogenesis and in the technology for colon cancer detection and therapy. This article provides an overview of the pathophysiology, clinical presentation, and management of colon cancer, with a focus on recent advances, to help clinicians and gastroenterologists appropriately screen, diagnose, and manage patients to reduce mortality from this cancer. The other articles in this issue focus on individual aspects of colon cancer in detail.

PATHOPHYSIOLOGY AND MOLECULAR GENETICS
Precursor Lesions

Colon cancer is the best understood complex (multistep) cancer in terms of molecular genetics. The first step in carcinogenesis is the development of specific types of neoplastic polyps in colonic mucosa. Polyp histology is critical for determining malignant potential. The two common histologic types are hyperplastic and adenomatous. Histologically, hyperplastic polyps contain an increased number of glandular cells with decreased cytoplasmic mucus but generally lack nuclear hyperchromatism, stratification, or atypia [4]. Adenomatous nuclei usually are hyperchromatic, enlarged, cigar-shaped, and crowded together in a palisade pattern. Adenomas are classified as tubular or villous. Histologically, tubular adenomas are composed of branched tubules, whereas villous adenomas contain digitiform villi arranged in a frond. Tubulovillous adenomas contain both elements.

Most colon cancers arise from adenomas (adenoma-to-carcinoma sequence) as demonstrated by epidemiologic, clinical, pathologic, and molecular genetic

E-mail address: mscappell@yahoo.com

0889-8553/08/$ – see front matter
doi:10.1016/j.gtc.2007.12.002

findings. First, operative specimens containing colon cancer frequently contain one or more synchronous adenomas. Second, the risk for colon cancer increases markedly with increasing number of adenomatous polyps within the colon [5]. Third, adenomatous tissue frequently is found contiguous to frank carcinoma [6]. Fourth, patients who have familial adenomatous polyposis (FAP), who have hundreds or thousands of adenomatous colonic polyps, inevitably develop colon cancer if colectomy is not performed [7]. Fifth, patients who have adenomatous polyps larger than 1 cm diagnosed by barium enema who do not undergo colonoscopic polypectomy develop colon cancer at a rate of 1% to 1.5% per annum [8].

Although most hyperplastic polyps seem to have little or no association with colon cancer [9], some hyperplastic polyps are associated with colon cancer. Risk factors for malignancy in hyperplastic polyps include large polyp size (>1 cm diameter), location in the right colon, a focus of adenoma within the polyp (mixed hyperplastic-adenomatous polyp), more than 20 hyperplastic polyps in the colon, a family history of hyperplastic polyposis, and a family history of colon cancer [10]. Hyperplastic polyps seem to be linked to colon cancer via the recently reclassified (sessile) serrated adenoma, previously classified as a hyperplastic polyp [11]. A serrated adenoma arises within a hyperplastic polyp but differs from an ordinary hyperplastic polyp by abnormal proliferation of crypt epithelium and by nuclear atypia [12]. In one study, approximately 18% of removed polyp specimens originally classified as hyperplastic were reclassified as serrated adenomas using the revised classification [13].

The serrated adenoma seems to transform into colon cancer via a different pathway from that of conventional adenomas and to result in a recognizably different form of colon cancer (Table 1). Unlike conventional adenomas, serrated adenomas frequently have *BRAF* genetic mutations and exhibit extensive DNA methylation but lack adenomatous polyposis coli (*APC*) gene mutations [14]. The serrated adenoma is a precursor lesion of colorectal carcinoma with high microsatellite instability (MSI-H), which constitutes approximately 15% of sporadic colon cancer [15]. Like serrated adenomas, MSI-H colon cancers exhibit *BRAF* gene mutations and extensive DNA methylation but generally lack mutations of the *APC* gene or the *K-ras* oncogene [16]. DNA methylation at the promoter region can terminate and silence gene expression without DNA mutation [17]. For example, DNA methylation can inactivate DNA mismatch repair genes, such as the *hMLH1* gene, and thereby lead to microsatellite instability (MSI) [18,19]. The specific genetic defects responsible for the serrated adenoma are, however, unknown.

Considerable evidence supports that serrated adenomas can transform to cancer [10]. First, serrated adenomas share the same genetic mutations characteristic of sporadic MSI-H cancers (described previously), suggesting a common molecular pathway. Second, serrated adenomas sometimes are found contiguous to areas of severe dysplasia, suggesting that the dysplasia arose from this precursor lesion [20]. Third, patients who have hyperplastic polyposis and who have 30 or more hyperplastic polyps distributed throughout the colon

Table 1
Differences between the two pathways for sporadic colorectal cancer: adenoma-to-carcinoma sequence and serrated adenoma-to-carcinoma theory

Characteristic	Conventional adenoma to carcinoma sequence	Serrated adenoma to carcinoma theory
Precursor lesion	Conventional adenoma	Serrated adenoma
Location of precursor lesion	Throughout colon	Predilection for right colon
Morphology of precursor lesion	Usually pedunculated (tubular adenoma) Occasionally sessile (eg, villous adenoma)	Often sessile, may be flat
Frequency of dysplasia in a moderate-sized polyp	Uncommon	Common
Likelihood of a small precursor adenoma transforming into cancer	Infrequent	Frequent??
Progression from a medium sized polyp to cancer	Slow (7 or more years)?	Moderate (3–5 years)???
Kudo pit pattern of adenoma	Types III or IV	Type II???
Basic genetic defect	APC mutation	????
Frequently associated genetic mutation	p53 oncogene	BRAF mutation
DNA hypermethylation	Uncommon	Common
Mismatch repair gene malfunction/ inactivation	Uncommon	Common (hMLH1 inactivation)
MSI-H	Rare	Typical
Genetic syndrome exhibiting same pathway	Familial polyposis coli	Hyperplastic polyposis???
Estimated relative frequency in sporadic colon cancer	85%[a]	15%[a]
Evidence for pathway	Well established and well documented	Theory supported by significant evidence
Pathway first proposed	More than 50 years ago	Last 5–7 years

? denotes uncertain data and ??-????? connotes increasing uncertainty.
[a]The molecular mechanism of colon cancer in inflammatory bowel disease is unknown and may be distinct from either of these molecular pathways.

(or at least five hyperplastic polyps proximal to the sigmoid colon, at least two of which are greater than 1 cm in diameter) [21] frequently have serrated adenomas and frequently develop colon cancer. Fourth, in a retrospective pathologic study, 91 MSI-H colorectal cancers developed in the same area of the proximal colon where hyperplastic polyps previously were identified by colonoscopy with pathologic examination of polyp tissue; all the previously removed polyps on re-review were reclassified as serrated adenomas [22].

With separation of the high-risk serrated adenomas from hyperplastic polyps in the reclassified nomenclature, the remaining conventional hyperplastic polyps are believed to harbor a negligible risk for developing colon cancer.

Syndromic Colon Cancer

Discoveries in the pathogenesis of the uncommon genetic cancer syndrome of FAP led to breakthroughs in understanding the molecular basis of the transformation of sporadic adenomas to colon cancer. Patients who have FAP develop hundreds or thousands of adenomatous polyps throughout the colon beginning after puberty and inevitably develop colon cancer [7]. This syndrome is inherited as a classic Mendelian single autosomal dominant gene. During the past 2 decades, FAP was shown to be the result of germline mutation of the *APC* gene located on chromosome 5q. Patients who have FAP carry this germline mutation in one allele in all somatic cells, including colonocytes (Table 2) [23–26]. This mutation underlies the development of hundreds of adenomatous polyps throughout the colon; colonic adenomas form when the second *APC* allele is lost or undergoes mutation in an individual colonocyte.

In hereditary nonpolyposis colon cancer (HNPCC), multiple kindred develop colon cancer. Affected patients typically have only a few colonic polyps. Colon cancer typically occurs in the right colon beginning as sessile polyps in middle age. The Amsterdam II criteria, used to clinically diagnose HNPCC, include all the following: three or more relations with colon cancer, one of whom is a first-degree relative of the other two; colon cancer involving at least two generations in the family; and at least one colon cancer diagnosed before age 50 [27]. During the past 15 years, HNPCC was shown to be the result of

Table 2
Milestones in the molecular genetics of syndromic colon cancer

First author (reference)	Discovery/finding
A. APC	
Veale [23]	Determined by pedigree analysis that FAP resulting from a single dominant mutation
Herrera [24]	Reported a de novo *APC* mutation associated with a large deletion in chromosome 5
Bodmer [25]	Applied restriction length polymorphism to localize the *APC* mutation to the long arm of chromosome 5
Kinzler [26]	Identified the *APC* gene on chromosome 5 by positional cloning
B. HNPCC	
Peltomaki [28]	Described MSI in HNPCC
Fishel [29]	Identified and cloned the first human mismatch repair gene *hMSH2* (*hMLH2*)
Bronner [30] and Papadopoulos [31]	Identified the second mismatch repair gene, *hMLH1*, and localized it to chromosome 3p
Kolodner [32]	Showed patients who have Muir-Torre syndrome (HNPCC associated with sebaceous gland and skin tumors) have *hMSH2* mutations or other mutations that cause MSI.

mutations of one of the mismatch repair genes, such as *hMLH1*, *hMSH2*, and *hMSH6* (see Table 2) [28–33]. Germline mutations of the *hMLH1* or *hMSH2* gene account for most cases. Mismatch repair enzymes, encoded by the mismatch repair genes, normally recognize errors in nucleotide matching of complementary chromosome strands and initiate segmental excision of the newly synthesized strand to ensure faithful strand replication [27]. Cells with mismatch repair gene mutations cannot repair spontaneous DNA errors and progressively accumulate mutations with succeeding DNA replications throughout the genome, resulting in genetic hypermutability and chaos. Accumulation of mutations in oncogenes and tumor suppressor genes can result in colon cancer. Mismatch repair gene mutation is detected as MSI, in which errors occur in simple DNA repetitive sequences, such as poly-A (ie, AAAA...) or CA-tandem repeating (ie, CACACACA...) nucleotide sequences [27]. The molecular genetics of variants of FAP and HNPCC are described in Table 3. The history of

Table 3
Molecular genetics of syndromic colon cancer

Gene mutations	Clinical syndromes	Manifestations
APC	FAP	Development of hundreds of colonic adenomas and inevitably of colon cancer, without colon resection
	Attenuated FAP	Mutations at specific sites (both terminals or exon 9) of APC gene can cause attenuated polyposis syndrome with development of dozens of colonic adenomas
	Gardner's syndrome	Variant of FAP with prominent extracolonic growths, such as osteomas
	Turcot syndrome	Variant of FAP with typical colonic manifestations and medulloblastomas or other tumors of the central nervous systerm, often the result of mutations of the APC gene
MYH		Mutation of the MYH gene causes an attenuated adenomatous polyposis syndrome phenotypically resembling attenuated adenomatous polyposis from APC mutation. It is characterized by the presence of 10 or more adenomatous polyps in the colon and a high risk for developing colon cancer.
Mismatch repair	HNPCC	Develop several adenomatous colonic neoplasms, primarily in the right colon, with rapid malignant transformation
	Turcot syndrome	Variant of HNPCC with typical colonic findings of few colonic neoplasms and glioblastoma multiforme tumors of the central nervous system, sometimes due to mutations of mismatch repair genes

molecular genetic discoveries in other intestinal polyposis syndromes is described in Table 4 [34–37]. Genetic factors in the pathogenesis of syndromic colon cancer are reviewed in the article by Desai and Barkel elsewhere in this issue.

Sporadic Cancer

These breakthroughs not only provided the molecular basis of syndromic hereditary colon cancer but also contributed to understanding sporadic colon cancer. Colon cancer is believed the result of a cascade of genetic mutations leading to progressively disordered local DNA replication and accelerated colonocyte mitosis. Progressive accumulation of multiple genetic mutations results in the transition from normal mucosa to benign adenoma to severe dysplasia to frank carcinoma (Table 5). Malfunction of the mismatch repair genes may account for approximately 15% of sporadic colon cancers [38]. In the HNPCC syndrome, the mismatch repair genes malfunction because of genetic mutation. In sporadic serrated adenomas, the mismatch repair gene *hMLH1* often malfunctions because of DNA hypermethylation. *APC* mutation is believed to account for approximately 80% to 85% of sporadic colon cancers [38]. Colon cancer may arise in inflammatory bowel disease from a different but so far uncharacterized pathway. Spontaneous somatic *APC* mutation in colonocytes is believed to underlie the development of sporadic adenomatous polyps. *APC* gene mutations occur early in adenoma development and often are found in aberrant crypt foci, the earliest identifiable dysplastic crypts [39]. *APC* mutations are found in approximately 50% of sporadic adenomas [40]. Adenomas usually remain benign. Malignant transformation requires further genetic alterations.

The *k-ras* gene encodes for a protein involved in signal transduction from the cell membrane to the nucleus. Specific mutations of this gene activate this signal

Table 4
History of molecular genetics of other intestinal polyposis syndromes

First author (reference)	Discovery/finding
Zigman [34]	Showed the Ruvalcaba-Myhre-Smith syndrome (hamartomatous, lipomatous hemangiomatous, and lymphangiomatous gastrointestinal polyps) results from an autosomal dominant mutation of the *PTEN* gene on chromosome 10q
Nelen [35]	Showed Cowden's disease (gastric and colonic hamartomatous polyps) results from an autosomal dominant mutation of the *PTEN* gene on chromosome 10q
Howe [36]	Showed familial juvenile polyposis (more than 10 juvenile intestinal polyps) results from an autosomal dominant mutation in the *SMAD4* (*DRC4*) gene on chromosome 10q
Jenne [37]	Showed Peutz-Jeghers syndrome (small number of intestinal polyps associated with mucocutaneous pigmentation) results from an autosomal dominant mutation in the *STK11* gene on chromosome 19p

Table 5
Molecular genetics of sporadic colon cancer

Gene	Chromosome location	Normal physiologic function of encoded protein	Clinical manifestations of mutation
APC gene	5q	Regulates cell growth and apoptosis	Homozygous somatic mutation associated with colonic adenomas.
K-ras gene family	Various chromosomes	Encodes a small guanosine triphosphate binding protein on cell membrane involved in transduction of mitogenic signals across cell membrane	Mutated in approximately 50% of colon cancers. May act in an intermediate stage of carcinogenesis. Mutation common in hyperplastic polyps.
P53 gene	17p	Regulates G1 cell cycle and apoptosis	Critical in transition from late adenoma to early cancer.
DCC gene	18q	Encodes a neural cell adhesion molecule; facilitates apoptosis, tumor suppressor	Believed to promote progression to frank carcinoma.
Mismatch repair genes	Located on several chromosomes	Recognize errors in nucleotide matching on complementary chromosome strand and initiate excision of erroneous strand	Progressive accumulation of mutations throughout the genome in affected cells leading to hypermutability and genetic chaos. Mutations of oncogenes or tumor suppressor genes can lead to colon cancer.

pathway and promote colonocyte replication. These mutations are associated with exophytic growth of adenomas in the transition to carcinoma [27]. Approximately 50% of colon cancers have k-ras mutations [41].

The normal p53 gene product arrests the cell cycle after DNA injury to permit DNA repair, if the damage is mild and correctable, or apoptosis, if the damage is severe and irreversible. The wild-type p53 protein product is upregulated after cell stress from radiation exposure, or other noxious events, to prevent new DNA synthesis and halt cell division. Loss of p53 function can promote genomic instability as genetic errors are replicated without check, resulting in loss of heterozygosity (LOH). Mutation of the p53 gene is believed important in the transition from advanced adenoma to frank carcinoma. Approximately 50% of colonic lesions with high-grade dysplasia and approximately 75% of frank cancers exhibit p53 mutations [27].

Accumulation of genetic mutations leads to genetic instability, manifested by LOH [42]. LOH accelerates carcinogenesis. Cells with LOH have one, instead of the normal two, alleles of some genes because of choromosomal loss. A tumor suppressor gene is more likely to lose normal function when only one allele is present after LOH. Only one, rather than two, allelic mutations then are required for loss of its function.

This molecular mechanism is important in loss of function of the deleted in colon cancer (*DCC*) gene. The *DCC* gene encodes for a neural cell adhesion molecule receptor that normally promotes apoptosis and suppresses tumors. Loss of the normal *DCC* gene is believed important in the transition from an intermediate to an advanced adenoma [41].

DNA methylation can inactivate suppressor genes, thereby promoting cancer (described previously for *hMLH1*) [43]. Approximately 25% of colon cancers are associated with methylation and inactivation of p14, normally an upstream inducer of the p53 tumor suppressor pathway [44]. The inactivation produces the same cancer phenotype as *p53* mutation [43]. Methylation of the tumor suppressor gene p16, designated *CDKN2A*, occurs in approximately 35% of colon cancers [45].

PATHOLOGY OF COLON CANCER
Histology
Colon cancers are classified as well differentiated, moderately well differentiated, or poorly differentiated based on the degree of preservation of normal glandular architecture and cytologic features. Poor differentiation presumably is a histologic marker of severe underlying genetic mutations, but the mutations associated with poor differentiation currently are unknown. Approximately 20% of colon cancers are poorly differentiated. They have a poor prognosis [46]. Approximately 15% of colon cancers are classified as mucinous, or colloid, because of prominent intracellular accumulation of mucin. In the signet-ring variety of mucinous colon cancer, cancerous cells contain so much mucin that the nuclei are displaced peripherally. This cancer variant is very aggressive and has a poor prognosis [47]. This biologic behavior may be the result of extracellular mucin dissecting beyond the tumor wall, thereby promoting local extension [48].

Colon cancer associated with HNPCC has unusual histopathologic features, such as mucinous differentiation, prominent lymphocytic reaction, and a medullary growth pattern [49]. The medullary form of colon cancer, previously classified as an undifferentiated carcinoma, is characterized by sheets of eosinophilic and polygonal cells heavily infiltrated with small lymphocytes and devoid of glandular elements. This form of cancer also is associated with high MSI [50].

Other cancers of the colon are rare. Kaposi's sarcoma can involve the colon as part of disseminated disease with the acquired immunodeficiency syndrome [51]. Lymphoma of the colon is rare. It is a non-Hodgkin's lymphoma. It may be associated with the acquired immunodeficiency syndrome [52]. Carcinoid usually occurs in the lower gastrointestinal tract in the rectum or appendix but rarely can present in the rest of the colon.

Gross Pathology
Colon cancer can occur in a pedunculated polyp, sessile polyp, mass, or stricture. Small polyps rarely contain cancer. Only approximately 1% of diminutive

polyps contain cancer [53]. Cancer in a sessile polyp may metastasize earlier than cancer in a pedunculated polyp because of closer proximity to the lymphatic drainage [54]. Also, a flat lesion may be biologically more aggressive than a pedunculated polyp because of cellular growth into the colonic wall rather than the colonic lumen. The relative frequency of right-sided colon cancer has increased gradually during the past several decades, and now approximately one half of colon cancers are right sided [55]. This effect is attributed to a decreased frequency of left-sided cancer resulting from polypectomy of premalignant left-sided polyps at flexible sigmoidoscopy [56]. Flexible sigmoidoscopy results in substantial reduction of the incidence of left-sided colon cancer but negligibly reduces the incidence of right-sided colon cancer [57].

Stage

Colon cancer spreads by local invasion to contiguous organs or by lymphatic or hematogenous invasion. Carcinoma in situ, or high-grade dysplasia, denotes cancer that is confined to the mucosa without penetration of the muscularis mucosa. This cancer is highly unlikely to produce metastases because the lymphatic and vascular channels are below the muscularis mucosa. Invasive colon cancer most commonly is staged from A through D according to the Dukes' classification, with stage A penetrating beyond the muscularis mucosa into the submucosa. Stage B1 extends beyond the submucosa into the muscularis propria; stage B2 extends through the muscularis propria into the serosa; stage C has regional lymph node metastases; and stage D has distant metastases.

Colon cancer recently is staged according to the tumor, node, metastases (TNM) classification by mural depth of the primary tumor (T), by presence of local lymph node metastases (N), and by presence of distant metastases (M). This classification is helpful particularly in endosonographic staging of colon cancer (described later) [58]. In the TNM classification, invasive colon cancer is classified from stage I to IV. Stage I in the TNM classification corresponds to Dukes' A or B1 lesions, stage II corresponds to Dukes' B2 lesion, stage III corresponds to Dukes' C lesion, and stage IV corresponds to Dukes' D lesion. Pathologic stage, as classified by either scheme, correlates highly with cancer prognosis [59].

Approximately 20% of patients initially present with Dukes' D colon cancer, with identified metastases [60]. Perhaps another 30% of patients have no metastases detected preoperatively or intraoperatively but eventually succumb to colon cancer after apparently curative surgery because of gross cancer recurrence presumably from initially undetected micrometastases. The most common sites of gross metastases are the regional lymph nodes and liver. Colon cancer metastasizes early to the liver because of venous drainage of the colon via the portal system. Other sites, including the lungs, peritoneum, pelvis, and adrenals, typically become involved only after hepatic or lymphatic metastases occur. Rectal cancers, which are below the peritoneal reflection, lack a serosa and, therefore, penetrate early into adjacent pelvic structures.

EPIDEMIOLOGY

The incidence of colon cancer exhibits a striking geographic variation: the age-adjusted incidence varies by up to 12-fold among different countries [54]. Industrialized nations have the highest incidence, whereas South American countries and China have a low incidence. The wide international variation is attributed largely to national differences in diet and other environmental factors [61]. The rate in Japan used to be much lower than that in America but recently has increased with industrialization and adaptation of a Western diet. Moreover, descendants of Japanese immigrants to America, like other Americans, have a high incidence of colon cancer attributed to dietary and other environmental adaptations [61].

The lifetime risk for colon cancer in America is approximately 1 in 17 [54]. It is responsible for approximately 10% of all cancer mortality in the United States [1]. The incidence of colon cancer has decreased by approximately 20% in the United States, whereas the mortality has decreased by approximately 30% in the past 25 years [62]. American blacks have a small increased risk for colon cancer compared with whites [63]. American Indians have a significantly lower risk [64]. The incidence is slightly higher in American men than women [54]. The incidence of colon cancer rises sharply with age, beginning at age 50, attributed to accumulation of random somatic mutations with age. Ninety percent of cases occur after age 50, and only 4% of cases occur before age 40 [65].

CLINICAL PRESENTATION

Symptoms

Symptoms are common and prominent late in colon cancer when the prognosis is poor but are less common and less obvious early in the disease. Common symptoms are listed in Table 6 [54,66–68]. Less common symptoms include nausea and vomiting, malaise, anorexia, and abdominal distention [66]. Although colon cancer can present with diarrhea or constipation, a recent change in bowel habits more likely is from colon cancer than chronically abnormal bowel habits.

Symptoms depend on cancer location, cancer size, and presence of metastases. Left colon cancers are more likely than right colon cancers to cause partial

Table 6	
Symptoms associated with colon cancer	
Symptom	Frequency
Abdominal pain	44%
Change in bowel habits	43%
Hematochezia or melena	40%
Weakness or malaise	20%
Involuntary weight loss	6%

Data from Refs. [66–68].

or complete intestinal obstruction because the left colonic lumen is narrower and tends to contain better formed stool due to reabsorption of water in the proximal colon [6]. Large exophytic cancers also are more likely to obstruct the colonic lumen. Partial obstruction produces constipation, nausea, abdominal distention, and abdominal pain. Partial obstruction occasionally and paradoxically produces intermittent diarrhea as stool moves beyond the obstruction.

Distal cancers sometimes cause gross rectal bleeding, but proximal cancers rarely produce this symptom because the blood becomes mixed with stool and chemically degraded during colonic transit. Bleeding from proximal cancers tends to be occult, and patients may present with iron deficiency anemia without gross rectal bleeding. The anemia may produce weakness, fatigue, dyspnea, or palpitations. Advanced cancer, particularly when metastatic, can cause cancer cachexia [6], characterized by a symptomatic tetrad of involuntary weight loss, anorexia, muscle weakness, and a feeling of poor health.

Signs

Colon cancer also tends not to produce signs until advanced [66]. Anemia from gastrointestinal bleeding may produce pallor. Iron deficiency anemia can cause koilonychia manifested by brittle, longitudinally furrowed, and spooned nails; glossitis manifested by lingual erythema and papillae loss; and chelitis manifested by scaling or fissuring of the lips. Hypoalbuminemia may manifest clinically as peripheral edema, ascites, or anasarca. Hypoactive or high-pitched bowel sounds suggest gastrointestinal obstruction. A palpable abdominal mass is a rare finding that suggests advanced disease. Rectal cancer may be palpable by digital rectal examination. Although colon cancer previously was believed to frequently cause fecal occult blood as detected by guaiac tests [69], a recent prospective trial reported that only a minority of patients who had colon cancer had fecal occult blood detected by a single guaiac test [70]. Fecal immunochemical testing for occult blood seems to have a much higher sensitivity for detecting occult blood from colon cancer. For example, in a colonoscopic study of 2512 patients, the fecal immunochemical test detected 87.5% of colon cancers [71]. Other physical findings, although rare, should be searched for systematically, including a palpable Virchow's lymph node in the left supraclavicular space, hepatomegaly from hepatic metastases, and temporal or intercostal muscle wasting from cancer cachexia [54].

Laboratory Abnormalities

Patients who have suspected colon cancer should have routine blood tests, including a hemogram with platelet count determination, serum electrolytes and glucose determination, evaluation of routine serum biochemical parameters of liver function, and a routine coagulation profile. Approximately half of patients who have colon cancer are anemic [66]. Anemia, however, is common, so only a small minority of patients who have anemia have colon cancer. Iron deficiency anemia of undetermined cause, however, warrants evaluation for colon cancer, particularly in the elderly [72]. Advanced colon cancer may result in hypoalbuminemia from malnutrition [6]. Routine serum biochemical parameters of liver function usually are within normal limits in patients who have colon cancer. The serum alkaline phosphatase and the serum lactate dehydrogenase levels may increase, however, with hepatic metastases [6].

The serum carcinoembryonic antigen level is not useful to screen for colon cancer because of insufficient sensitivity, especially for patients who have early and highly curable colon cancer [73]. Preoperative testing, however, is useful for cancer prognosis and as a baseline for comparison with postoperative levels. An elevated serum level preoperatively is a poor prognostic indicator: the higher the serum level the more likely the cancer is extensive and will recur postoperatively [73]. After apparently complete colon cancer resection, the serum level almost always normalizes; failure to normalize postoperatively suggests incomplete resection. A sustained and progressive rise after postoperative normalization strongly suggests cancer recurrence [54]. Patients who have this finding require prompt surveillance colonoscopy to exclude colonic recurrence and abdominal imaging to exclude metastases.

Unusual Clinical Presentations

Colon cancer can cause acute colonic obstruction, most commonly from exophytic intraluminal growth and uncommonly from intussusception or volvulus. Patients present with abdominal pain, nausea and vomiting, obstipation, abdominal tenderness, abdominal distention, and hypoactive bowel sounds. Colon cancer rarely causes ischemic colitis due to colonic dilatation proximal to malignant obstruction or malignant infiltration of blood vessels. Colon cancer rarely can perforate acutely through the colonic wall and cause acute generalized peritonitis and rarely can perforate slowly to form a walled-off inflammatory mass or abscess with localized peritoneal signs. Colon cancer also can penetrate and create fistulas into adjacent organs, such as the bladder or small bowel. Factors promoting colonic perforation include disruption of mucosal integrity resulting from transmural malignant extension or colonic ischemia and increased intraluminal pressure resulting from colonic obstruction. Colonic obstruction or perforation is a poor prognostic indicator. Colon cancer occasionally causes gross rectal bleeding because of cancerous mucosal ulceration. Approximately 6% of metastatic adenocarcinomas with an unknown primary eventually are shown to arise from the colon [74].

COLONOSCOPY

Colonoscopy is a highly specific test for colon cancer. At colonoscopy, polyps are removed and masses are biopsied for a pathologic diagnosis. Early colon cancer may occur in an adenomatous polyp and, therefore, may be difficult to distinguish by colonoscopy from a nonmalignant adenomatous polyp. For example, a 2-cm–wide villous adenoma has an approximately 40% chance of harboring cancer [72]. Polyp risk factors for malignancy include villous rather than tubular histology, large size, sessile morphology, and increasing number of colonic polyps [72]. Advanced colon cancer typically appears as a large, exophytic mass because of intraluminal growth or as a colonic stricture because of circumferential growth.

A colonic stricture, however, may be benign. Malignancy is suggested when a colonic stricture is ulcerated, indurated, asymmetric, and friable and has irregular or overhanging margins. The colonoscopic appearance is suggestive but not definitive. Pathologic examination of multiple colonic biopsies and cytologic analysis of stricture brushings usually are diagnostic.

TESTS FOR INTRAMURAL PENETRATION AND EXTRACOLONIC SPREAD OF COLON CANCER

CT

CT has been the standard modality to image the abdomen in patients who have colorectal cancer. CT is relatively accurate at detecting liver metastases, with an accuracy of approximately 85% [75]. CT is much more sensitive at detecting large than small hepatic lesions. CT is only moderately accurate at T staging. For example, the accuracy for T staging was only 74% in a large multicenter study [75]. CT errors typically occur from underestimating the T stage. CT is approximately only 50% to 70% accurate in N staging of rectal cancer [75].

MRI

MRI is more accurate than CT in detecting focal liver metastases, particularly small metastases, from colon cancer because of the typically sharp contrast between metastatic lesions and the normal liver on MRI [76]. Administration of contrast agents, such as superparamagnetic iron oxide, improves test sensitivity further. MRI also is more specific for hepatic metastases than CT. Hepatic metastases have a much shorter T2 sequence than hepatic hemangiomas or cysts. Hepatic metastases typically demonstrate rapid and strong enhancement with intravascular contrast due to enhanced vascularity but may enhance inhomogeneously due to hypovascular areas within metastases. Despite these advantages, CT is the standard test because of lower cost, greater machine availability, and more widely available expertise in image interpretation [6]. MRI traditionally is reserved for characterizing ambiguous hepatic lesions detected by abdominal ultrasound or CT.

Transrectal and Colonic Ultrasonography

Endosonography has been used for T and N staging of rectal cancer because of the relative inaccuracy of CT for this staging. Preoperative evaluation of the T stage and the N stage has a great impact on the therapy for rectal cancer. Patients who have superficial cancer (T1N0) can be treated by local endoscopic or transanal resection without wide excision. Patients who have T2N0 lesions are treated surgically without preoperative adjuvant therapy. Patients who have deep intramural involvement (T3 or T4) or who have nodal involvement (N1 or N2) receive radiation and possibly chemotherapy before surgery. Patients who do not have rectal sphincter involvement may avoid a colostomy.

Endoscopic ultrasound (EUS) is more accurate than CT or MRI for T staging. In a study of 80 patients who had rectal cancer, the accuracy of T staging by endosonography was 91% compared with 71% for CT ($P = .02$) [77]. Other studies report that rectal endosonography has an approximately 85% accuracy for T staging [78,79]. This accuracy compares favorably to that of MRI for T staging, which ranges from 70% to 80% [80]. Tumors generally appear as homogeneous hypoechoic masses that disrupt the normal five-layer ultrasonographic structure of the rectal wall [81]. Errors in endosonographic T staging may be the result of distortion of the ultrasound image by inflammation in tissue adjacent to cancer. Endosonography is more accurate for staging T1, T3, and T4 lesions than T2 lesions because of difficulty in assessing cancer invasion through the muscularis propria [58]. Endosonography has zn approximately 75% accuracy for N staging [58,77]. This accuracy is greater than the reported accuracy of 55% to 65% for CT and 60% to 65% for MRI [80]. At endosonography, malignant lymph nodes tend to be large (>1 cm), to be hypoechoic, to have sharply demarcated borders, and to be round rather than ovoid or flat [81]. Inflamed lymph nodes, however, occasionally mimic these sonographic features.

Rectal ultrasound has become the standard preoperative imaging modality for local T and N staging of rectal cancer because of relatively high accuracy but has not yet been shown to prolong survival. The rectum easily is accessible via an ultrasound probe using a rigid probe inserted blindly or an echoendoscope inserted under endoscopic guidance. The procedure is safe. Endosonographic findings frequently modify a treatment plan. For example, in a study of 80 patients, endosonographic findings resulted in the addition of preoperative neoadjuvant therapy in 25 patients [77]. The accuracy of endoscopic ultrasound is operator dependent. Other factors affecting accuracy include the ultrasound frequency, with higher frequency improving the resolution but decreasing the depth of penetration; the tumor location, with reduced accuracy for tumors low in the rectum; and prior radiotherapy because of increased wall echogenicity after radiation.

There is scant data on the impact of EUS-guided fine needle aspiration (FNA) in rectal cancer staging [58]. In one study of 41 patients, EUS-guided FNA of a lymph node upgraded the N stage in one patient and downgraded the N stage in eight patients [77]. Unfortunately, these changes were incorrect in three of the nine cases. Although a FNA diagnosis of cancer in a lymph node is secure, a finding of benignity may be erroneous because of sampling error. A recent prospective study, so far published only in abstract form, reported that EUS with FNA demonstrated malignant lymph nodes in 15 patients who had rectal cancer as compared with a yield of only eight patients who had suspicious nodes on CT [82]. Current data are insufficient to recommend standard use of FNA in N staging of rectal cancer [58].

Locally recurrent rectal cancer potentially is important to detect early so that patients can undergo salvage surgery for possible cure. EUS currently is the most reliable imaging study for detecting recurrence. In a study of 62 patients undergoing surveillance after rectal cancer surgery, EUS detected all 11 recurrent cancers [83]. The clinical benefit of early detection of rectal cancer recurrence, however, is limited by the low cure rate of salvage surgery.

Data on endosonography for colon cancer beyond the rectum are limited. Colonic endosonography technically is more demanding and time consuming than rectal endosonography. Most patients who have colon cancer without distant metastases undergo colonic resection, regardless of T or N stage. In a study of 50 small colon cancers, endosonography was 92% accurate in T staging compared with 63% for magnifying colonoscopy [84]. This difference was statistically significant. Endosonography, however, was only 24% accurate for N staging in this study. In a study of 86 patients who had colon cancer, endosonography, using a balloon-sheathed miniprobe inserted during colonoscopy, was 85% accurate for T staging and 73% accurate for N staging [85].

Conventional endosonography produces a 2-D image. The recently developed 3-D endosonography may provide better spatial information that improves diagnostic accuracy. For example, in a study of 86 patients who had rectal cancer, the accuracy of 2-D endosonography was 69%, whereas the accuracy of 3-D endosonography was 78% [86]. 3-D endosonography also was superior to conventional 2-D endosonography in a study of 35 patients who had rectal cancer [87].

PROGNOSTIC FACTORS

Clinicopathologic characteristics and molecular markers of colon cancer greatly help to determine prognosis. Many adverse warning signs and risk factors have been identified (Table 7) [88–98]. Currently, these sometimes are helpful in guiding treatment, including use of neoadjuvant therapy before cancer surgery, as discussed in the article by Robertson elsewhere in this issue. It is hoped that the currently identified molecular risk factors may be a prelude to therapy targeted according to molecular markers. In particular, targeted therapy could block the abnormal molecular pathways involved in specific molecular forms of colon cancer.

Table 7
Prognostic factors associated with a poor outcome from colon cancer

Prognostic factor	First author (reference)
Intramural depth of colon cancer	Tominaga [88]
Regional nodal involvement	Greene [89]
Nodal micrometastases	Yasuda [90]
Vascular invasion	Newland [91]
Residual cancer after definitive therapy	Compton [92]
Elevated serum carcinoembryonic antigen level	Slentz [93]
Histologic grade (degree of differentiation)	Wiggers [94]
Cancer involvement at surgical margins	de Haas-Kock [95]
Liver metastases at clinical presentation	Tsai [96]
18q genetic deletions (especially of DCC gene)	Watanabe [97]
Aneuploidy	Bazan [98]

PREVENTION
Dietary Modifications
Despite the importance of genetic mutations in colon cancer pathogenesis, environmental factors also play an important etiologic role in colon cancer. Colon cancer has many proven environmental and demographic risk factors (Table 8) [99,100]. Other risk factors are suspected but unproven (Table 9). The most prominent of these risk factors for colon cancer are obesity, physical inactivity, alcoholism, smoking, and a diet that is high in fats or low in fruits and vegetables [101]. Environmental factors presumably modulate the risk for genetic mutations responsible for colon cancer, although the precise molecular mechanisms currently are unknown.

Dietary fiber may reduce the risk for colon cancer [99], but this effect is somewhat controversial [102]. Proposed mechanisms include decreased mucosal exposure to intraluminal carcinogens resulting from stimulated intestinal transit, decreased concentration of carcinogens in stool due to increased stool bulk, increased concentrations of anticarcinogenic short-chain fatty acids, and stabilization of insulin levels due to delayed starch absorption that otherwise might promote colonic carcinogenesis [100].

The identification of environmental risk factors is potentially important clinically because modification or elimination of an identified risk factor could lower the cancer risk. Environmental risk factors, however, are believed to exert their effects after long-term (chronic) exposure for decades. This may explain the weak protective effects of most reported experimental environmental interventions, such as dietary modifications, that last only several years. This topic is considered in detail in the article by Marshall elsewhere in this issue.

Chemoprevention
Nonsteroidal anti-inflammatory drugs (NSAIDs) reduce cellular proliferation, slow cell cycle progression, and stimulate apoptosis [100]. NSAIDs are believed to reduce adenoma formation and inhibit colon cancer development by inhibiting the cyclooxygenase enzymes required for the synthesis of prostaglandin E2; prostaglandin E2 promotes tissue inflammation, cellular proliferation, and tumor growth [103]. NSAIDs also may retard carcinogenesis by effects on cell adhesion and apoptosis. Various NSAIDs prevent carcinogen-induced colon cancer in rodents and inhibit adenoma formation in the Min mouse model of human FAP. Case-control and cohort epidemiologic studies also provide evidence of decreased adenoma incidence or decreased colon cancer mortality with chronic NSAID use, particularly use of aspirin. In a prospective study of more than 600,000 adults over a 6-year period, the relative mortality from colon cancer was approximately 0.6 in men and 0.58 in women who used aspirin 16 or more times per month compared with nonusers of the same gender [104]. In the Nurses' Health Study, women who took aspirin for at least 20 years had a relative risk of 0.56 for developing colon cancer compared with nonusers [105]. In a double-blind, placebo-controlled, prospective trial of 635 patients who had prior colon cancer, chronic aspirin use was associated with

Table 8
Recognized risk factors for colon cancer

Parameters	Proposed mechanism
Epidemiology	
Old age	Acquired colonocyte mutations accumulate with age
Living in United States and other highly industrialized nations	Dietary and environmental carcinogens
Diet	
Low fruit and vegetable consumption	Anticarcinogenic substances in fruits and vegetables (eg, folic acid)
Obesity	Carcinogens in an unhealthy diet or role of abnormal insulin levels in carcinogenesis?
Social habits	
Smoking cigarettes	Carcinogens present in tobacco
Alcohol	May promote cell proliferation and inhibit DNA repair
Genetics/family history	
FAP	Develops hundreds of adenomatous colonic polyps. Inevitably develops colon cancer resulting from small but significant risk for malignant transformation in each adenoma.
Gardner's syndrome	Variant of FAP
HNPCC (Lynch syndrome)	Mutant mismatch repair gene leads to accumulation of genetic mutations, including mutations of tumor suppressor genes
Peutz-Jeghers syndrome	Syndromic hamartomatous polyps occasionally may transform to adenomas
Juvenile polyposis	Syndromic juvenile polyps can transform to adenomas and then cancers over time
Family history of nonsyndromic colon cancer	Postulated shared genetic factors leading to mild susceptibility to colon cancer and possibly shared environmental factors
Hyperplastic polyposis	Genetic mutation in hyperplastic polyposis seems to predispose to colon cancer
Inflammatory bowel disease	
Chronic ulcerative colitis	Dysplasia and genetic mutations associated with mucosal injury and repair
Chronic Crohn's colitis	Dysplasia and genetic mutations associated with cell injury and repair
History of prior neoplasia	
Colonic adenomatous polyps	Precursor lesions of colon cancer
Prior colon cancer	Genetic predisposition or environmental factors
Other	
Pelvic radiation	Carcinogenic effects resulting from radiation-induced mutations
Streptococcus bovis bacteremia	May promote colonocyte proliferation
Ureterosigmoidostomy	Carcinogens excreted in urine or colonic mucosal proliferation during repair after urine-induced mucosal injury
Acromegaly	Growth hormone promotes proliferation of preexisting colonic adenomas and cancers

Table 9
Questionable or controversial risk factors for colon cancer

Parameter	Proposed mechanism
Physical inactivity	Physical activity may stimulate immunosurveillance and stimulate intestinal peristalsis to decrease mucosal contact with fecal carcinogens
Low calcium	Calcium binds to bile acids that otherwise are potentially colonotoxic
High fat	Various theories (eg, increased bile secretion)
High red meat	Animal fat in red meat or carcinogens (eg, nitrosamines) in cooked meat
Low selenium	Selenium can help neutralize toxic free radicals due to antioxidant effects
Low folate	Folate needed for DNA synthesis and repair
Low carotenoid diet	Carotenoids can help neutralize free radicals resulting from antioxidant effects
Low fiber diet	Dilution of carcinogens in stool due to increased stool bulk and stool water with a high fiber diet
Breast cancer	Shared reproductive hormonal or environmental factors
Diabetes mellitus	Insulin may modulate colonocyte proliferation
Prior cholecystectomy	Continuous colonic exposure to potentially carcinogenic bile acids after cholecystectomy

a one-third reduction of the risk for adenomas compared with controls detected at follow-up colonoscopy at a mean of 12.8 months [106]. In a large, double-blind, placebo-controlled prospective trial of patients who had prior adenomas, chronic low-dose aspirin therapy was associated with a smaller, but still statistically significant, reduction in the incidence of recurrent adenomas at colonoscopy performed 1 or more years later compared with the controls [107]. Other NSAIDs, such as sulindac, seem to cause similar reductions in colon cancer or colon polyp incidence [108], although the effects are less well analyzed.

Cyclooxygenase has two isoforms, COX-1 and COX-2. Although nonselective NSAIDs inhibit both isoforms, several COX-2 selective inhibitors recently have been developed. COX-2 is believed to mediate cell proliferation and tumor growth. Hence, selective COX-2 inhibitors may block adenoma formation and cancer development. Celecoxib, a selective COX-2 inhibitor, was effective in preventing and treating adenomas in the Min mouse model of FAP [109]. Celecoxib shows some promise in causing regression of colonic adenomas in patients who have FAP. In a study of 77 patients who had FAP, patients receiving celecoxib (400 mg twice daily) had a 28% reduction in the mean number of rectal polyps compared with a 4.5% reduction in the placebo-treated group [110].

The effects of NSAIDs on sporadic adenomas generally are less dramatic. Although data support that NSAIDs inhibit colonic carcinogenesis, the optimal specific NSAID, NSAID dosage, and duration of treatment are unknown. The role of COX-2 selective inhibitors versus nonselective COX inhibitors needs to be analyzed and defined better.

NEW AND EVOLVING TECHNOLOGY

Colon cancer incidence and survival has improved only moderately during the past 2 decades despite the manifest efficacy of colonoscopic polypectomy at cancer prevention [56]. This failure is caused by insufficient implementation of colonoscopy screening partly because of the expense, invasiveness, discomfort, and risks for colonoscopy. New simpler, less invasive, and safer tests are being designed to overcome these barriers to universal screening for colon cancer. Potentially exciting screening or diagnostic tests still in the experimental stage include stool genetic markers [111] and videocapsule endoscopy of the colon [112]. The role of CT colonography (virtual colonoscopy) in the screening of colon cancer currently is unclear and may be clarified by further studies as the technology matures [113].

SUMMARY

With improved education of physicians resulting in effective and appropriate implementation of screening colonoscopy guidelines, and with improved technology, equipment, and training, this preventable, lethal disease should be virtually eradicated, as were cholera and other infectious scourges of yore.

References
[1] Jamal A, Siegel R, Ward E, et al. Cancer statistics, 2007. CA Cancer J Clin 2007;57: 43–66.
[2] Hassan C, Zullo A, Laghi A, et al. Colon cancer prevention in Italy: cost-effectiveness analysis with CT colonography and endoscopy. Dig Liver Dis 2007;39:242–50.
[3] Shibuya K, Mathers CD, Boschi-Pinto C, et al. Global and regional estimates of cancer mortality and incidence by site: II. Results for the global burden of disease 2000. BMC Cancer 2002;2:37.
[4] Tsai CJ, Lu DK. Small colorectal polyps: histopathology and clinical significance. Am J Gastroenterol 1995;90:988–94.
[5] Heald RJ, Bussey HJ. Clinical experiences at St. Mark's Hospital with multiple synchronous cancers of the colon and rectum. Dis Colon Rectum 1975;18:6–10.
[6] Cappell MS. From colonic polyps to colon cancer: pathophysiology, clinical presentation, and diagnosis. Clin Lab Med 2005;25:135–77.
[7] Bussey HJR. Familial polyposis coli: family studies, histopathology, differential diagnosis and results of treatment. Baltimore (MD): Johns Hopkins University Press; 1975.
[8] Stryker SJ, Wolff BG, Culp CE, et al. Natural history of untreated colonic polyps. Gastroenterology 1987;93:1009–13.
[9] Winawer SJ, Zauber AG, Fletcher RH, et al. Guidelines for colonoscopy surveillance after polypectomy: a consensus update by the US Multi-Society Task Force on Colorectal Cancer and the American Cancer Society. Gastroenterology 2006;130:1872–85.
[10] Jass JR. Hyperplastic polyps and colorectal cancer: is there a link? Clin Gastroenterol Hepatol 2004;2:1–8.
[11] Higuchi T, Jass JR. My approach to serrated polyps of the colorectum. J Clin Pathol 2004;57:682–6.
[12] Chulmska A, Boudova L, Zamecnik M. Sessile serrated adenomas of the large bowel: clinicopathologic and immunohistochemical study including comparison with common hyperplastic polyps and adenomas. Cesk Patol 2006;42:133–8.
[13] Torlakovic E, Skovlund E, Snover DC, et al. Morphologic reappraisal of serrated colorectal polyps. Am J Surg Pathol 2003;27:65–81.

[14] Spring KJ, Zhao ZZ, Karamatic R, et al. High prevalence of sessile serrated adenomas with BRAF mutations: a prospective study of patients undergoing colonoscopy. Gastroenterology 2006;131:1400–7.

[15] Thibodeau SN, Bren G, Schaid D. Microsatellite instability in cancer of the proximal colon. Science 1993;260:816–9.

[16] Huang J, Papadopoulos N, McKinley AJ, et al. APC mutations in colorectal tumors with mismatch repair deficiency. Proc Natl Acad Sci U S A 1996;93:9049–54.

[17] Brenner DA, editors. Gastroenterology. Gastrointestinal basic science 2002–2003: the year in review. Clin Gastroenterol Hepatol 2004;2:9–13.

[18] Kane MF, Loda M, Gaida GM, et al. Methylation of the hMLH1 promotor correlates with lack of expression of hMLH1 in sporadic colon tumors and mismatch repair-defective human tumor cell lines. Cancer Res 1997;57:808–11.

[19] Kambara T, Simms LA, Whitehall VL, et al. BRAF mutation is associated with DNA methylation in serrated polyps and cancers of the colorectum. Gut 2004;53:1137–44.

[20] Longacre TA, Fenoglio-Preiser CM. Mixed hyperplastic adenomatous polyps/serrated adenomas: a distinct form of colorectal neoplasia. Am J Surg Pathol 1990;14:524–37.

[21] Jeevaratnam P, Cottier DS, Browett PJ, et al. Familial giant hyperplastic polyposis predisposing to colon cancer: a new hereditary bowel cancer syndrome. J Pathol 1996;179:20–5.

[22] Goldstein NS, Bhanot P, Odish E, et al. Hyperplastic-like colon polyps that preceded microsatellite-unstable adenocarcinomas. Am J Clin Pathol 2003;119:778–96.

[23] Veale AMO. Intestinal polyposis. Eugenis Laboratory Memoirs Series 40. New York: Cambridge University Press; 1965.

[24] Herrera L, Kataki S, Gibas L, et al. Gardner syndrome in a man with an interstitial deletion of 5q. Am J Med Genet 1986;25:473–6.

[25] Bodmer WF, Bailey CJ, Bodmer J, et al. Localization of the gene for familial adenomatous polyposis on chromosome 5. Nature 1987;328:614–6.

[26] Kinzler KW, Nilbert MC, Su LK, et al. Identification of FAP locus genes from chromosome 5q21. Science 1991;253:661–5.

[27] Robbins DH, Itzkowitz SH. The molecular and genetic basis of colon cancer. Med Clin North Am 2002;86:1467–95.

[28] Peltomaki P, Aaltonen LA, Sistonen P, et al. Genetic mapping of a locus predisposing to human colorectal cancer. Science 1993;260:810–2.

[29] Fishel R, Lescoe MK, Rao MR, et al. The human mutator gene homolog MSH2 and its association with hereditary nonpolyposis colon cancer. Cell 1993;75:1027–38.

[30] Bronner CE, Baker SM, Morrison PT, et al. Mutation in the DNA mismatch repair gene homologue hMLH1 is associated with hereditary non-polyposis colon cancer. Nature 1994;368:258–61.

[31] Papadopoulos N, Nicolaides NC, Wei YF, et al. Mutation of a mutL homolog in hereditary colon cancer. Science 1994;263:1625–9.

[32] Kolodner RD, Hall NR, Lipford J, et al. Structure of the human MSH2 locus and analysis of the two Muir-Torre kindreds for MSH2 mutations. Genomics 1994;24:516–26.

[33] Ivanovich JL, Read TE, Ciske DJ, et al. A practical approach to familial and hereditary colon cancer. Am J Med 1999;107:68–77.

[34] Zigman AF, Lavine JE, Jones MC, et al. Localization of the Bannayan-Riley-Ruvalcaba syndrome to chromosome 10q23. Gastroenterology 1997;113:1433–7.

[35] Nelen MR, Padberg GW, Peeters EA, et al. Localization of the gene for Cowden disease to chromosome 10q22–23. Nat Genet 1996;13:114–6.

[36] Howe JR, Roth S, Ringold JC, et al. Mutations in the SMAD4/DPC4 gene in juvenile polyposis. Science 1998;280:1086–8.

[37] Jenne DE, Reimann H, Nezu J, et al. Peutz-Jeghers syndrome is caused by mutations in a novel serine threonine kinase. Nat Genet 1998;18:38–43.

[38] Suraweera N, Duval A, Reperant M, et al. Evaluation of tumor microsatellite instability using five quasimonomorphic repeats and pentaplex PCR. Gastroenterology 2002;123: 1804–11.

[39] Jen J, Powell SM, Papadopoulos N, et al. Molecular determinants of dysplasia in colorectal lesions. Cancer Res 1994;54:5523–6.

[40] Miyaki M, Konishi M, Kikuchi-Yanoshita R, et al. Characteristics of somatic mutation of the adenomatous polyposis coli gene in colorectal tumors. Cancer Res 1994;54:3011–20.

[41] Vogelstein B, Fearon ER, Hamilton SR, et al. Genetic alterations during colorectal-tumor development. N Engl J Med 1988;319:525–32.

[42] Kern SE, Fearon ER, Tersmette KW, et al. Clinical and pathological associations with allelic loss in colorectal carcinoma. JAMA 1989;261:3099–103.

[43] Myohanen SK, Baylin SB, Herman JG. Hypermethylation can selectively silence individual p16ink4A alleles in neoplasia. Cancer Res 1998;58:591–3.

[44] Burri N, Shaw P, Bouzourene H, et al. Methylation silencing and mutations of the p14ARF and p16NK4A genes in colon cancer. Lab Invest 2001;81:217–29.

[45] Shannon BA, Iacopetta BJ. Methylation of the hMLH1, p16, and MDR1 genes in colorectal carcinoma: associations with clinicopathological features. Cancer Lett 2001;167:91–7.

[46] Hassan C, Zullo A, Risio M, et al. Histologic risk factors and clinical outcome in colorectal malignant polyp: a pooled-data analysis. Dis Colon Rectum 2005;48:1588–96.

[47] Kang H, O'Connell JB, Maggard MA, et al. A 10-year outcomes evaluation of mucinous and signet-ring cell carcinoma of the colon and rectum. Dis Colon Rectum 2005;48: 1161–8.

[48] Green JB, Timmcke AE, Mitchell WT, et al. Mucinous carcinoma: just another colon cancer? Dis Colon Rectum 1993;36:49–54.

[49] Gryfe R. Clinical implications of our advancing knowledge of colorectal cancer genetics: inherited syndromes, prognosis, prevention, screening and therapeutics. Surg Clin North Am 2006;86:787–817.

[50] Gutalica Z, Torlakovic E. Pathology of the hereditary colorectal carcinoma. Fam Cancer 2007; [epub June 13].

[51] Janier M, Couderic LJ, Morel P, et al. Kaposi's disease in AIDS: 31 cases. Ann Dermatol Venereol 1987;114:185–202 [in French].

[52] Cappell MS, Botros N. Predominantly gastrointestinal symptoms and signs in 11 consecutive AIDS patients with gastrointestinal lymphoma: a multicenter, multiyear study of 763 HIV-seropositive patients. Am J Gastroenterol 1994;89:545–9.

[53] Church JM. Clinical significance of small colorectal polyps. Dis Colon Rectum 2004;47: 481–5.

[54] Cappell MS. The pathophysiology, clinical presentation, and diagnosis of colon cancer and adenomatous polyps. Med Clin North Am 2005;89:1–42.

[55] Jessup JM, McGinnis LS, Steele GD Jr, et al. The National Cancer Data Base: report on colon cancer. Cancer 1996;78:918–26.

[56] Cress RD, Morris CR, Wolfe BM. Cancer of the colon and rectum in California: trends in incidence by race/ethnicity, stage, and subsite. Prev Med 2000;31:447–53.

[57] Newcomb PA, Norfleet RG, Storer BE, et al. Screening sigmoidoscopy and colorectal cancer mortality. J Natl Cancer Inst 1992;84:1572–5.

[58] Sandhu IS, Bhutani MS. Gastrointestinal endoscopic ultrasonography. Med Clin North Am 2002;86:1289–317.

[59] Fisher ER, Sass R, Palekar A, et al. Dukes' classification revisited: findings from the National Surgical Adjuvant Breast and Bowel Projects (Protocol R-01). Cancer 1989;64: 2354–60.

[60] Boland CR, et al. Malignant tumors of the colon. In: Yamada T, Alpers D, Kaplowitz N, editors. Textbook of Gastroenterology. 4th edition. Philadelphia: Lippincott Williams & Wilkins; 2003. p. 1940–90.

[61] Tamura K, Ishiguro S, Munakata A, et al. Annual changes in colorectal carcinoma incidence in Japan: analysis of survey data on incidence in Aomori Prefecture. Cancer 1996;78:1187–94.

[62] Howe HL, Wu X, Ries LA, et al. Annual report to the nation on the status of cancer, 1975–2003, featuring cancer among U.S. Hispanic/Latino populations. Cancer 2006;107:1711–42.

[63] Satia-Abouta J, Galanko JA, Martin CF, et al. Food groups and colon cancer risk in African-Americans and Caucasians. Int J Cancer 2004;109:728–36.

[64] Ries LAG, Eisner MP, Kosary CL, et al. SEER cancer statistics review, 1973–1998. Bethesda (MD): National Cancer Institute; 2001. p. 1–22.

[65] Cappell MS. Colon cancer during pregnancy. Gastroenterol Clin North Am 2003;32:341–83.

[66] Cappell MS, Goldberg ES. The relationship between the clinical presentation and spread of colon cancer in 315 consecutive patients: a significant trend of earlier cancer detection from 1982 through 1988 at a university hospital. J Clin Gastroenterol 1992;14:227–35.

[67] Speights VO, Johnson MW, Stoltenberg PH, et al. Colorectal cancer: current trends in initial clinical manifestations. South Med J 1991;84:575–8.

[68] Steinberg SM, Barkin JS, Kaplan RS, et al. Prognostic indicators of colon tumors: the Gastrointestinal Tumor Study Group experience. Cancer 1986;57:1866–70.

[69] Church TR, Ederer F, Mandel JS. Fecal occult blood screening in the Minnesota study: sensitivity of the screening test. J Natl Cancer Inst 1997;89:1440–8.

[70] Imperiale TF, Ransohoff DF, Itzkowitz SH, et al. Fecal DNA versus fecal occult blood for colorectal-cancer screening in an average-risk population. N Engl J Med 2004;351:2704–14.

[71] Smith A, Young GP, Cole SR, et al. Comparison of a brush-sampling fecal immunochemical test for hemoglobin with a sensitive guaiac-based fecal occult blood test in detection of colorectal neoplasia. Cancer 2006;107:2152–9.

[72] Cappell MS, Friedel D. The role of sigmoidoscopy and colonoscopy in the diagnosis and management of lower gastrointestinal disorders: endoscopic findings, therapy, and complications. Med Clin North Am 2002;86:1253–88.

[73] Grem JL, Steinberg SM, Chen AP, et al. The utility of monitoring carcinoembryonic antigen during systemic therapy for advanced colorectal disease. Oncol Rep 1998;5:559–67.

[74] Nystrom JS, Weiner JM, Heffelfinger-Juttner J, et al. Metastatic and histologic presentations in unknown primary cancer. Semin Oncol 1977;4:53–8.

[75] Zerhouni EA, Rutter C, Hamilton SR, et al. CT and MR imaging in the staging of colorectal carcinoma: report of the Radiology Diagnostic Oncology Group II. Radiology 1996;200:443–51.

[76] Kinkel K, Lu Y, Both M, et al. Detection of hepatic metastases from cancers of the gastrointestinal tract by using noninvasive imaging methods (US, CT, MR imaging, PET): a meta-analysis. Radiology 2002;224:748–56.

[77] Harewood GC, Wiersma MJ, Nelson H, et al. A prospective, blinded assessment of the impact of preoperative staging on the management of rectal cancer. Gastroenterology 2002;123:24–32.

[78] Siddiqui AA, Fayiga Y, Huerta S. The role of endoscopic ultrasound in the evaluation of rectal cancer. Int Semin Surg Oncol 2006;3:36.

[79] Tamerisa R, Irisawa A, Bhutani MS. Endoscopic ultrasound in the diagnosis, staging, and management of gastrointestinal and adjacent malignancies. Med Clin North Am 2005;89:139–58.

[80] Harewood GC. Assessment of publication bias in the reporting of EUS performance in staging rectal cancer. Am J Gastroenterol 2005;100:808–16.

[81] Ahmad NA, Kochman ML, Ginsberg GG. Endoscopic ultrasound and endoscopic mucosal resection for rectal cancers and villous adenomas. Hematol Oncol Clin North Am 2002;16:897–906.

[82] Levy MJ, Clain JE, Gleeson F, et al. Endoscopic ultrasound guided fine needle aspiration (EUS FNA) detection of malignant iliac lymph nodes in rectal cancer [abstract]. Gastrointest Endosc 2006;63(5 Suppl):AB97.

[83] Rotondano G, Esposito P, Pellecchia L, et al. Early detection of locally recurrent rectal cancer by endosonography. Br J Radiol 1997;70:567–71.

[84] Matsumoto T, Hizawa K, Esaki M, et al. Comparison of EUS and magnifying colonoscopy for assessment of small colorectal cancers. Gastrointest Endosc 2002;56:354–60.

[85] Tseng LJ, Jao YT, Mo LR. Preoperative staging of colorectal cancer with a balloon-sheathed miniprobe. Endoscopy 2002;34:564–8.

[86] Kim JC, Kim HC, Yu CS, et al. Efficacy of 3-dimensional endorectal ultrasonography compared with conventional ultrasonography and computed tomography in preoperative rectal cancer staging. Am J Surg 2006;192:89–97.

[87] Giovaninoi M, Bories E, Presenti C, et al. Three-dimensional endorectal ultrasound using a new freehand software program: results in 35 patients with rectal cancer. Endoscopy 2006;38:339–43.

[88] Tominaga T, Sakabe T, Koyama Y, et al. Prognostic factors for patients with colon or rectal carcinoma treated with resection only: five-year follow-up report. Cancer 1996;78:403–8.

[89] Greene FL, Stewart AK, Norton HJ. A new TNM staging strategy for node-positive (stage III) colon cancer: an analysis of 50,042 patients. Ann Surg 2002;236:416–21.

[90] Yasuda K, Adachi Y, Shiraishi N, et al. Pattern of lymph node micrometastasis and prognosis of patients with colorectal cancer. Ann Surg Oncol 2001;8:300–4.

[91] Newland RC, Dent OF, Lyttle MN, et al. Pathologic determinants of survival associated with colorectal cancer with lymph node metastases: a multivariate analysis of 579 patients. Cancer 1994;73:2076–82.

[92] Compton CC, Fielding LP, Burgart LJ, et al. Prognostic factors in colorectal cancer: College of American Pathologists Consensus Statement 1999. Arch Pathol Lab Med 2000;124:979–94.

[93] Slentz K, Senagore A, Hibbert I, et al. Can preoperative and postoperative CEA predict survival after colon cancer resection? Am Surg 1994;60:528–31.

[94] Wiggers T, Arends JW, Volovics A. Regression analysis of clinical and pathological factors in colorectal cancer after curative resections. Dis Colon Rectum 1988;31:33–41.

[95] de Haas-Kock DF, Baeten CG, Jager JJ, et al. Prognostic significance of radial margins of clearance in rectal cancer. Br J Surg 1996;83:781–5.

[96] Tsai MS, Su YH, Ho MC, et al. Clinicopathological features and prognosis in resectable synchronous and metachronous colorectal liver metastasis. Ann Surg Oncol 2007;14:786–94.

[97] Watanabe T, Wu TT, Catalano PJ, et al. Molecular predictors of survival after adjuvant chemotherapy for colon cancer. N Engl J Med 2001;344:1196–206.

[98] Bazan V, Migliavacca M, Zanna I, et al. DNA ploidy and S-phase fraction, but not p53 or NM23-H1 expression, predict outcome in colorectal cancer patients: result of a 5-year prospective study. J Cancer Res Clin Oncol 2002;128:650–8.

[99] Howe GR, Benito E, Castelleto R, et al. Dietary intake of fiber and decreased risk of cancers of the colon and rectum: evidence from the combined analysis of 13 case-control studies. J Natl Cancer Inst 1992;84:1887–96.

[100] Hawk ET, Umar A, Richmond E, et al. Prevention and therapy of colorectal cancer. Med Clin North Am 2005;89:85–110.

[101] Levine JS, Ahnen DJ. Adenomatous polyps of the colon. N Engl J Med 2006;355:2551–7.

[102] Fuchs CS, Giovannucci EL, Colditz GA, et al. Dietary fiber and the risk of colorectal cancer and adenoma in women. N Engl J Med 1999;340:169–76.

[103] Clevers H. Colon cancer: understanding how NSAIDs work. N Engl J Med 2006;354:761–3.

[104] Thun MJ, Namboodiri MM, Heath CW Jr. Aspirin use and reduced risk of fatal colon cancer. N Engl J Med 1991;325:1593–6.

[105] Giovannucci E, Egan K, Hunter DJ, et al. Aspirin and the risk of colorectal cancer in women. N Engl J Med 1995;333:609–14.

[106] Sandler RS, Halabi S, Baron JA, et al. A randomized trial of aspirin to prevent colorectal adenomas in patients with previous colorectal cancer. N Engl J Med 2003;348:883–90.

[107] Baron JA, Cole BF, Sandler RS, et al. A randomized trial of aspirin to prevent colorectal adenomas. N Engl J Med 2003;348:891–9.

[108] Wadell WR, Ganser GF, Cerise EJ, et al. Sulindac for prophylaxis of the colon. Am J Surg 1989;157:175–9.

[109] Jacoby RF, Cole CE, Tutsch K, et al. Chemopreventive efficiency of combined piroxicam and difluoromethylornithine treatment of Apc mutant Min mouse adenomas and selective toxicity against Apc mutant embryos. Cancer Res 2000;60:1864–70.

[110] Steinbach G, Lynch PM, Phillips RK, et al. The effect of celecoxib, a cyclooxygenase-2 inhibitor, in familial adenomatous polyposis. N Engl J Med 2000;342:1946–52.

[111] Itzkowitz SH, Jandorf L, Brand R, et al. Improved fecal DNA test for colorectal cancer screening. Clin Gastroenterol Hepatol 2007;5:111–7.

[112] Schoofs N, Deviere J, van Gossum A. PillCam colon capsule endoscopy compared with colonoscopy for colorectal tumor diagnosis: a prospective study. Endoscopy 2006;38: 971–7.

[113] Rex DK, Lieberman D. ACG colorectal cancer prevention action plan: update on CT-colonography. Am J Gastroenterol 2006;101:1410–3.

Gastroenterol Clin N Am 37 (2008) 25–46

GASTROENTEROLOGY CLINICS
OF NORTH AMERICA

Sporadic and Syndromic Hyperplastic Polyps and Serrated Adenomas of the Colon: Classification, Molecular Genetics, Natural History, and Clinical Management

James E. East, MRCP[a],*, Brian P. Saunders, MD, FRCP[a],
Jeremy R. Jass, MD, FRCPath[b]

[a]Wolfson Unit for Endoscopy, St. Mark's Hospital, Watford Road, Harrow,
Middlesex HA1 3UJ, UK
[b]Department of Cellular Pathology, St. Mark's Hospital, Watford Road, Harrow,
Middlesex HA1 3UJ, UK

The traditional understanding of the evolution of colorectal cancer was based on four straightforward propositions. First, most colorectal cancers arise in precancerous polyps. Second, there are two main types of colorectal polyps: hyperplastic polyps and adenomas. Third, the adenoma is fundamentally an epithelial neoplasm, with malignant potential, whereas the hyperplastic polyp is fundamentally a benign epithelial lesion with no malignant potential. Fourth, adenomas progress to carcinomas through a single linear sequence of genetic alterations involving particular tumor suppressor genes (eg, *APC* and *p53*) and oncogenes (eg, *KRAS*). These propositions were easy to comprehend and to translate into clinical management guidelines and were supported by considerable circumstantial evidence. Therefore, although decades of study identified exceptions to these propositions, the contrary data received no attention. In the last few years, however, these exceptions have been organized to demonstrate an alternative pathway of colorectal carcinogenesis: the serrated pathway involving hyperplastic polyps or related lesions. This article briefly presents the evidence for the serrated pathway, provides diagnostic criteria for clinically significant serrated polyps, and suggests how these data can be translated into safe and effective guidelines for cancer prevention. Because of the incomplete understanding of the behavior of serrated polyps, any clinical management plan must be tentative. The authors therefore highlight key areas warranting further research.

*Corresponding author. *E-mail address:* jameseast6@yahoo.com (J.E. East).

0889-8553/08/$ – see front matter
doi:10.1016/j.gtc.2007.12.014

COLORECTAL CANCER: MORE THAN ONE DISEASE

The serrated pathway concept evolved based on (1) identification of a subtype of colorectal cancer that could not be conceived to develop within a pre-existing adenoma and (2) demonstration that hyperplastic polyps and related lesions could fill the gap left by the adenoma. Study of rare forms of hereditary colorectal cancer provided the initial evidence of different molecular mechanisms for the evolution of colorectal cancer. Investigation of familial adenomatous polyposis led to the discovery of the tumor suppressor gene *APC* and illustrated how mutation and loss of both *APC* alleles can initiate the development of the sporadic adenoma [1]. The *APC* gene guards against chromosomal instability, a key step in the progression of adenoma to carcinoma [2]. Investigation of Lynch syndrome or hereditary nonpolyposis colorectal cancer led to the discovery of the DNA mismatch repair gene [3]. Disruption of DNA mismatch repair causes a different type of genetic instability, called "microsatellite instability" (MSI). Genetic instability is fundamental to carcinogenesis; it leads to rapid accumulation of genetic alterations without apoptosis or programmed cell death.

High-level MSI (MSI-H) is not restricted to Lynch syndrome but occurs in 15% of sporadic colorectal cancer [4,5]. Initially it was assumed that sporadic MSI-H cancers are initiated by *APC* inactivation. The advent of MSI-H then would accelerate the mutation rate of key cancer genes, including *KRAS* and *p53* [3]. MSI-H, however, was shown to be a rare event in adenomas, and most such examples occurred in patients who had Lynch syndrome [6]. It therefore was assumed that MSI-H occurs at a late stage, perhaps during the transition from adenoma to carcinoma [7]. The earlier genetic steps of mutation and loss of the tumor suppressor gene *APC* and mutation of the oncogene *KRAS* therefore should have been demonstrable within sporadic MSI-H colorectal cancer. It took many years to accept that this loss and mutation did not occur, because cancer cell lines were primarily used to screen for somatic mutations, and most MSI-H cell lines were derived from patients who had Lynch syndrome [8]. Mutations of *APC* and *KRAS* often occur in Lynch syndrome cancers but are uncommon in sporadic MSI-H colorectal cancer [9,10]. That sporadic MSI-H colorectal cancers might not be counterparts to the Lynch syndrome was suggested strongly by the identification of molecular alterations in sporadic MSI-H colorectal cancers that were not present in Lynch syndrome cancers, including mutation of the oncogene *BRAF* and extensive DNA methylation [11,12]. DNA methylation can silence tumor suppressor genes, including the DNA mismatch repair gene *MLH1* [13].

The characteristic changes of adenomas are not seen in sporadic MSI-H colorectal cancer, and the genetic changes found in MSI-H sporadic cancers (*BRAF* mutation, extensive DNA methylation, and MSI) are rarely seen in conventional adenomas (DNA methylation is more evident in villous adenomas). It is impossible for sporadic MSI-H colorectal cancers to arise from conventional adenomas because cancers carry a genetic record of their early origins. This subtype of colorectal cancer must arise de novo, or it must arise in a different type of polyp that is characterized by somatic mutation of *BRAF*, extensive DNA methylation, and MSI-H. The requisite molecular changes were found to occur in a variant form of hyperplastic polyp [11].

HYPERPLASTIC POLYPS, SERRATED ADENOMAS, AND THE SERRATED PATHWAY TO COLORECTAL CANCER

For half a century colorectal epithelial polyps were assumed to comprise two main and nonoverlapping groups: hyperplastic polyps and adenomas. Reports of mixed or intermediate types of polyp had occasionally appeared in the pathologic literature, but it was not until 1990 that Longacre and Fenoglio-Preiser [14] explored the concept of an intermediate type of polyp in a detailed survey of more than 18,000 colorectal polyps. Among these polyps, 110 (0.6%) were diagnosed as serrated adenomas. In the original pathologic reports most of these polyps had not been identified as having unusual histology: about one third had been classified as hyperplastic polyps, about one third as typical adenomas, and about one third (0.2% of all polyps) as intermediate lesions. This variability in classification indicates the difficulty in the histologic diagnosis of these rare intermediate lesions. Of note, 11% of the serrated adenomas showed severe dysplasia or intramucosal carcinoma, indicating that these lesions are precancerous and may be particularly prone to malignant transformation. Moreover, these serrated adenomas occurred more often in the proximal colon (35.4%) than did either conventional adenomas (23.3%) or hyperplastic polyps (7.5%). This pathologic study concluded that serrated adenomas were fundamentally adenomas that resembled hyperplastic polyps because the crypt epithelium had adopted a serrated or saw-tooth contour similar to that of hyperplastic polyps. This study also highlighted the existence of mixed hyperplastic and adenomatous polyps. Such lesions were interpreted as chance collisions between the two common types of colorectal polyp.

Although seminal, this study did not conclude that hyperplastic polyps could transform into serrated adenomas even though residual foci of a hyperplastic polyp were sometimes identified within serrated adenomas [14]. The concept of a serrated pathway to colorectal cancer was based on two observations concerning mixed polyps that comprise separate nondysplastic (hyperplastic) and dysplastic (adenomatous) components. First, the two components sometimes showed identical mutations in microsatellite markers. Second, the adenomatous component often was a serrated adenoma rather than a conventional adenoma [15]. Chance collision is a highly unlikely explanation for these twin phenomena because (1) mutations are rare events and therefore are unlikely to occur by chance in contiguous lesions, and (2) serrated adenomas are much rarer than conventional adenomas.

Some dysplastic foci had multiple mutations indicative of MSI-H. It therefore was suggested that the serrated pathway could evolve into colorectal cancers with both low-level MSI (MSI-L) and MSI-H [15], but it still was assumed that most MSI-H colorectal cancers arise in conventional adenomas [7]. After the investigation of mixed polyps and cancers occurring in the hyperplastic polyposis syndrome (HPS), it was argued that most, if not all, sporadic MSI-H colorectal cancers arise in hyperplastic polyps.

HYPERPLASTIC POLYPOSIS AND THE SESSILE SERRATED ADENOMA

Hyperplastic polyposis originally was perceived as lacking any cancer risk. Its clinical significance lay only in the potential for misdiagnosis as familial adenomatous polyposis [16]. Occasional descriptions of malignancy were explained by the presence of coexisting adenomas. Case reports then appeared showing transitions from hyperplastic polyps through dysplasia (mixed polyps) to carcinoma [17]. In a small series of hyperplastic polyposis, the dysplastic components of such mixed or progressing polyps were found to show both loss of expression of the DNA mismatch repair protein and the presence of MSI-H in microdissected DNA. Most, but not all, of the associated colorectal cancers showed MSI-H [18]. Based on these and other data, it was argued that sporadic MSI-H colorectal cancers develop from hyperplastic polyps [18].

Based on analysis of a clinical series of hyperplastic polyposis complicated by colorectal cancer, Torlakovic and Snover [19] proposed in 1996 that these polyps were not hyperplastic polyps but instead were a form of serrated adenoma. This was an important development. Torlakovic and Snover [20] introduced the term "sessile serrated adenoma" in a detailed study of sporadic hyperplastic polyps in 2003. They proposed that there are two types of serrated adenoma, the "traditional" serrated adenoma (TSA), as highlighted in 1990, and a sessile serrated adenoma (SSA) that shows a marked predilection for the proximal colon and lacks the cytologic features of adenomatous dysplasia. The term "serrated adenoma" introduced in 1990 by Longacre and Fenoglio-Preiser [14], however, probably was being applied to the two main types of serrated adenoma as surmised from (1) the original classification of one third of the serrated adenomas as hyperplastic polyps, and (2) the marked predilection for serrated adenomas to be in the proximal colon. The term "TSA" therefore may be inappropriate. The work of Torlakovic and Snover [20] greatly expanded the diagnostic limits of "hyperplastic-like" serrated adenomas by including in this category lesions with architectural, but not cytologic, atypia. A subset of SSAs (or hyperplastic-like serrated adenomas), however, is sufficiently atypical with respect to both architecture and cytology to warrant a label of dysplasia but is distinguishable from TSA.

There are important reasons for distinguishing two types of serrated adenoma. The TSA is more adenoma-like macroscopically and microscopically. It typically is pedunculated with a tubulovillous or villous architecture, and it occurs mainly in the distal colorectum [21]. By contrast, the SSA is usually sessile (as implied by its name), has a tubular architecture, is the typical lesion in hyperplastic polyposis, and shows a strong predilection for the cecum and proximal ascending colon when it occurs sporadically [20]. The distinction between the two types of serrated adenoma is well documented in the Japanese literature. Using dye-spray and magnification of the surface epithelial topography, some serrated adenomas were indistinguishable from hyperplastic polyps (type I serrated adenomas), whereas others had the cerebriform surface typical of tubulovillous or villous adenomas (type II serrated adenomas) [22]. At the molecular level, most SSAs have mutation of *BRAF* and exhibit extensive DNA methylation [11,23]. A subset may show MSI, particularly those with foci of dysplasia [15,24]. By contrast, the molecular signature of TSA is more varied: some have mutation of *BRAF*, others have mutation of *KRAS*, and some have neither mutation [25–27]. TSAs also show infrequent mutation of *APC* or *p53*, or loss of heterozygosity; have no aberrant expression of beta-catenin; and rarely exhibit chromosomal instability and MSI [28–31].

Hyperplastic polyposis may be heterogeneous. It may have two phenotypes: (1) the presence of at least 30 (but not necessarily large) hyperplastic polyps in a pancolonic distribution, and (2) five hyperplastic polyps proximal to the sigmoid colon with at least two being 1 cm in diameter or larger [32]. Some examples can meet both definitions. The proximal and large polyps occurring in the second type of hyperplastic polyposis are likely to be SSAs. Conceivably, the risks of cancer and the molecular pathway of carcinogenesis may differ, with MSI-H cancers linked more closely to the second category. More research is required into the phenotypic and genotypic diversity of hyperplastic polyposis [33,34].

MULTIPLE SERRATED PATHWAYS TO COLORECTAL CANCER

The existence of distinct types of serrated adenoma (SSA and TSA) raises the question of multiple pathways to what has been termed "serrated adenocarcinoma" [35]. The SSA has been associated with proximal colorectal cancers, *BRAF* mutation, and extensive DNA methylation. These cancers include a subset of sporadic MSI-H colorectal cancer with methylation and inactivation of the DNA mismatch repair gene *MLH1*. These colorectal cancers are more common in women [35]. Contrariwise, TSA has been associated with mainly left-sided colorectal cancer that is more common in men and is characterized by low-level DNA methylation, MSI-L, mutation of *KRAS*, and methylation of the direct DNA repair gene *O-6-methylguanine DNA methyltransferase* [35–37].

At least 20% of colorectal cancers have molecular signatures that fit with an origin from either SSA or TSA. Although SSA and TSA have been largely ignored in polypectomy guidelines, circumstantial evidence now suggests that this omission may have led to the development of preventable cancers. In a large retrospective review, 91 MSI-H colorectal cancers were identified in patients who had an earlier diagnosis of a hyperplastic polyp within the same area of the proximal colon [38]. Among 106 proximal hyperplastic polyps in this group of patients, all the polyps showed the features of SSA. Colonoscopic surveillance and polypectomy reduces but does not eliminate the risk of developing colorectal cancer, possibly because of cancer arising from small and/or flat adenomas, missed adenomas, or even de novo initiation of cancer [39]. Interval colorectal cancers are three times more likely than noninterval cancers to occur in the proximal colon [40] and are 3.7 times more likely than noninterval cancers to be MSI-H [41]. These observations may be explained by missed cancers arising from failure to detect or remove prior SSAs. The management problem is less critical for TSAs because these typically present like and are managed like adenomas. SSAs, however, are relatively inconspicuous and often is overlooked by the pathologist, endoscopist, and virtual colonographer.

DIAGNOSIS OF SESSILE SERRATED ADENOMA: RECOGNITION AND NOMENCLATURE

As previously noted, SSAs originally were labeled as "hyperplastic polyps." Based on systematic analysis of histologic features in sporadic hyperplastic polyps, Torlakovic and Snover [20] showed that 18% of "hyperplastic polyps" satisfied the criteria for SSA as described in hyperplastic polyposis. Development of a universally acceptable nomenclature for SSA has been problematic because these lesions have subtle differences from hyperplastic polyps and do not display the features of conventional adenomas. SSAs are characterized by more exaggerated crypt serration, serration throughout the crypt length, hypermucinous epithelium, crypt dilatation, crypt branching, horizontal crypt extensions at the crypt base, and aberrant proliferation. They often exhibit slight cytologic changes and lack the nuclear changes that characterize adenomatous dysplasia [20]. The term "SSA" dominates the literature, but the terms "sessile serrated polyp" [42], and "serrated polyp with abnormal proliferation" are also used [23]. Many pathologists probably still label such lesions merely as "unusually large" or "atypical" hyperplastic polyps.

Hyperplastic polyps exhibit morphologic and molecular heterogeneity. Goblet cell hyperplastic polyps (GCHPs) typically are very small, show minimal deviation from normal, and most often occur in the distal colorectum [20]. Most GCHPs have *KRAS* mutation and little DNA methylation [43]. Microvesicular hyperplastic polyps (MVHPs) are characterized by columnar cells containing mucin-filled microvesicles with inconspicuous goblet cells, larger polyp size, and frequent proximal location [20]. MVHPs usually have mutation of *BRAF*, and those occurring in the proximal colon are likely to show extensive DNA methylation [43]. SSAs and GCHPs are relatively distinctive, but overlaps between SSAs and MVHPs suggest that these lesions represent a continuum. Although a proportion of SSAs and MVHPs are highly characteristic histologically, with high levels of diagnostic agreement among pathologists, some lesions exhibit intermediate features. Pragmatically, all proximal serrated polyps 1 cm in diameter or larger should be deemed clinically significant, but SSAs can be smaller than 1 cm and can occur in the distal colon [20,38]. As precancerous lesions, SSAs need to be recognized and distinguished from clinically insignificant serrated polyps. Further research is required to determine diagnostic features that predict progression to dysplasia and cancer. It is important to develop uniformly accepted terminology and diagnostic criteria for SSA. The histologic spectrum of "serrated polyps" including GCHP, MVHP, SSA, and TSA is illustrated in Fig. 1A–D.

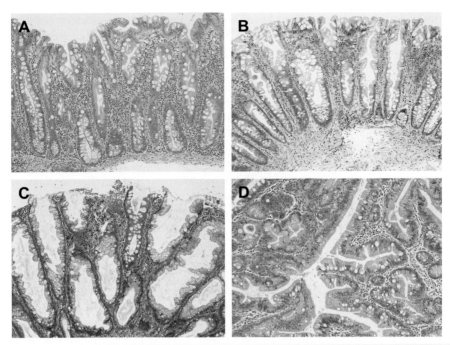

Fig. 1. The histologic spectrum of serrated polyps of colorectum. (A) Goblet cell variant of hyperplastic polyp (GCHP). There is mild and relatively superficial crypt serration. Goblet cells are clearly distinguished from the eosinophilic columnar cells. KRAS is frequently mutated. (B) Microvesicular variant of hyperplastic polyp (MVHP). There is more serration than in GCHP, and columnar cells contain mucin-filled microvesicles. BRAF is frequently mutated. (C) Sessile serrated adenoma (SSA). The crypts are dilated, the lumen is filled with secretory mucin, and the epithelial lining is hypermucinous. There is prominent dilatation of the crypt base with early horizontal spread by crypt epithelium. The crypt:stroma ratio is relatively high (compare with panel B). A single normal crypt is included. BRAF is frequently mutated. (D) Traditional serrated adenoma (TSA). This lesion combines crypt serration with unequivocal adenomatous dysplasia, and the architecture is more complex than SSA (see panel C). Either KRAS or BRAF may be mutated. (All photomicrographs: hematoxylin and eosin staining, original magnification ×10.)

SESSILE SERRATED ADENOMA AND RISK OF COLORECTAL CANCER

Stratification of "hyperplastic polyps" into GCHP, MVHP, and SSA has occurred recently [44]. Without this stratification, the increased risk associated with SSA would be diluted by the negligible risk associated with small, distal hyperplastic polyps [45–47]. Most right-sided hyperplastic polyps (or SSAs) do not become malignant. In an autopsy study conducted in New Zealand, 43 right-sided hyperplastic polyps (12.9% prevalence) were detected among 333 subjects [48]. Many of these lesions probably would be reclassified now as SSAs. The lifetime risk of developing colorectal cancer is approximately 5%, but only about 15% of sporadic colorectal cancers show MSI-H, the molecular characteristic of proximal serrated polyps, for an incidence of 1 in 132 of colorectal cancer with MSI-H (.15 × .05). If the incidence of right-sided hyperplastic polyps (or SSAs) is 1 per 8 patients, only 1 in 17 right-sided hyperplastic polyps develop into colorectal cancers with MSI-H (132/8).

There is confusion regarding the rapidity of malignant change in serrated polyps. SSAs rarely contain unequivocal foci of dysplasia [49]. One of the mechanisms driving this transformation is methylation and the loss of expression of the DNA mismatch repair gene *MLH1* [50]. Once this rare but critical step has occurred, progression from dysplasia to malignancy may occur rapidly. This scenario fits with the important role of genetic instability in tumorigenesis. It is consistent with the concept of aggressive adenomas in Lynch syndrome [51]. It explains the observed excess of interval cancers with MSI-H [41]. It explains the rarity of SSAs caught in the act of malignant transformation [52]. Until this or a similar transformation occurs, SSAs typically remain stable and benign.

DETECTION OF HYPERPLASTIC POLYPS AND SESSILE SERRATED ADENOMAS

Detection of hyperplastic polyps has been little analyzed because these lesions were considered to confer negligible risk of advanced colorectal neoplasia [53,54]. Screening techniques to detect adenomas and early cancers include fecal tests (occult blood and DNA testing), endoscopic tests (flexible sigmoidoscopy and colonoscopy), and radiologic tests (barium enema and CT colonography ["virtual colonoscopy"]). Consideration of size, morphology, anatomic distribution, and pathologic and genetic characteristics of hyperplastic lesions narrows the choices. Hyperplastic polyps are much less likely than adenomas or carcinomas to show evidence of hemorrhage, rendering fecal occult blood testing unlikely to be effective, and some genetic markers used in fecal DNA tests (eg, *KRAS*) are common in adenomas but rare in SSAs [55–58]. Alternate genetic markers more specific to SSAs (eg, *BRAF* mutations) might overcome this limitation. The pilot data seem to be promising [59]. CT colonography has superseded barium enema for colonic polyp detection [60]. Flat lesions are more difficult to detect than polypoid lesions at CT colonography (see the article by Summerton and colleagues in this issue). Most hyperplastic polyps are minimally elevated, flat lesions [61–63]. Flat hyperplastic polyps are more difficult to detect with CT colonography than flat adenomas [64], possibly because the use of air or carbon dioxide to distend bowel renders many hyperplastic polyps almost completely flat and impossible to detect with this imaging modality. No study has directly examined the ability of CT colonography to detect hyperplastic polyps and SSAs, but it seems likely that sensitivity for these polyps would be inferior to optical colonoscopy because of the limitations of CT technology [61,65]. Flexible endoscopy is likely to be the most effective way to detect these lesions, but these lesions, because of their flat morphology and lack of hypervascularity, may be difficult to detect even under direct endoscopic vision (Fig. 2A, B). Many large and flat hyperplastic polyps

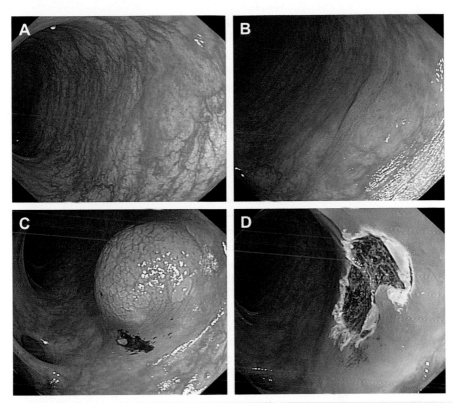

Fig. 2. (A) A 15-mm hyperplastic polyp detected in the transverse colon is highlighted by a coating of brown mucus. (B) The lesion becomes less conspicuous after vigorous irrigation to remove the mucus. (C) The 15-mm hyperplastic polyp is lifted with saline before piecemeal endoscopic mucosal resection. (D) Piecemeal endoscopic resection is performed. Methylene blue in the lifting solution helps define the lesion margins before resection and stains the submucosal plane during resection. (*Courtesy of* Dr. Noriko Suzuki, St. Mark's Hospital, Harrow, Middlesex, UK).

are proximal and beyond the reach of a flexible sigmoidoscope [56]. Colonoscopy supplemented by chromoendoscopy (see later discussion) is the diagnostic method of choice to detect these lesions, particularly SSAs.

Optimizing Colonoscopic Detection

Detection of hyperplastic polyps is difficult at colonoscopy, in part because, with the focus on pedunculated lesions, the importance of flat lesions has been appreciated only recently [66]. The colonoscopic challenge is to detect a minimally elevated, mostly transparent lesion containing a meager, aberrant, spider-like superficial vascular meshwork in contrast to the hypervascular network of adenomas (see Fig. 2B). The miss rate for all polyps in back-to-back studies of colonoscopy is 21% (95% confidence interval [CI], 14%–30%), but the miss rate for non-adenomatous polyps is higher, at 27% (95% CI, 19%–37%). In Harrison and colleagues' [67] study, the miss rate for hyperplastic polyps was 13 of 22 (59%). High-quality bowel preparation and adequate luminal distension is essential, as is slow colonoscopic withdrawal [68–70]. A prominent coating of brown mucus that is difficult to wash off (see Fig. 2A) can be a clue to a large underlying SSA because SSAs produce excessive mucus [56]. Colonoscopists should be particularly vigilant for flat or inconspicuous polyps that may represent SSAs in high-risk groups such as elderly women, patients who have a family history of hyperplastic polyps or a personal history of SSA, and in regions such as the proximal colon [56,71].

In chromoendoscopy a contrast agent is sprayed onto the colonic surface during endoscopy. The most commonly used agent is indigocarmine, which accumulates in the pits (crypt openings) and innominate grooves of the colonic surface, highlighting the superficial topography, particularly flat lesions. It significantly improves polyp detection, particularly of small proximal hyperplastic polyps (Table 1). A summary of four randomized trials indicates that chromoendoscopy roughly doubles the detection rate of hyperplastic polyps in the whole colon and in the proximal colon (see Table 1). These trials, however, did not report hyperplastic polyp size or histologic subtype, such as SSA [72–75]. In a large series of asymptomatic American patients undergoing screening colonoscopy, 4% had a hyperplastic polyp removed in the proximal colon during colonoscopy without chromoendoscopy. This rate compared with rates of 9% in predominantly symptomatic patients undergoing colonoscopy without chromoendoscopy and 16% in symptomatic patients undergoing colonoscopy with chromoendoscopy in the summary of the four randomized trials. In a chromoscopic prospective hospital-based series, Spring and colleagues [56] reported similar mean detection rates of hyperplastic polyps overall (0.81 versus 0.83) and in the proximal colon (0.23 versus 0.33). The chromoscopic detection rate of hyperplastic polyps in the entire colon also was similar in an autopsy study of New Zealanders of European origin, in which the mean rate was 0.83 per patient; in the same study however, the rates of hyperplastic polyps were significantly lower, 0.03 per patient, in the Maori/Polynesian population [48]. An autopsy study of patients in Singapore also reported a lower rate of hyperplastic polyps than that reported in pancolonic chromoendoscopy studies conducted in predominantly European patients (7% versus 45%) [76]. It seems, therefore, that the Spring and colleagues' [56] reports of the detection rate of a single, Japanese-trained endoscopist may be generalizable to Western endoscopists and populations. The indications for colonoscopy, as well as geographic location and racial distribution, affect the incidence, however.

Case series using pancolonic chromoendoscopy have stratified hyperplastic polyps according to location and size [56,71,77]. Mean pancolonic detection rates have ranged from 0.83 to 11.6 per patient compared with 0.81 per patient in the summary of the four randomized trials. Yano and colleagues [71] reported the highest rate; they used pit pattern rather than histology to define hyperplastic polyps and detected many diminutive polyps in the left colon. In

Table 1
Hyperplastic polyp detection in four randomized trials of pancolonic chromoendoscopy

Author [reference]	Year	No. of patients (polyps)	Entire colon				Proximal colon			
			≥1 HP SC	≥1 HP CC	Mean HP/patient at SC	Mean HP/patient at CC	≥1 HP SC	≥1 HP CC	Mean HP/patient at SC	Mean HP/patient at CC
Lapalus [74]	2006	252 (385)	25% (37/146)	40% (59/146)a	0.46 (67/146)	0.75 (110/146)a	7% (10/146)	12% (18/146)	0.09 (13/146)	0.15 (22/146)
Le Rhun [75]	2006	198 (276)	26% (26/99)	48% (48/99)a	0.5 (50/99)	1.1 (109/99)a	-	-	-	-
Hurlstone [73]	2004	260 (289)	15% (20/132)	52% (67/128)a	0.34 (45/132)	0.56 (72/128)	-	-	0.05 (7/132)	0.18 (23/128)
Brooker[b] [72]	2002	259 (365)	25% (34/135)	41% (51/124)a	0.42 (57/135)	0.91 (113/124)a	10% (14/135)	21% (26/124)a	0.15 (20/135)	0.38 (47/124)
Summary	-	969 (1315)	23% (117/512) P < .0001c	45% (225/497)	0.43 (219/512)	0.81 (404/497)	9% (24/281) P = .008c	16% (44/270)	0.10 (40/413)	0.23 (92/398)

Abbreviations: CC, chromoscopic colonoscopy; HP, hyperplastic polyp; SC, standard colonoscopy.
[a] P < .05 chromoscopic colonoscopy (CC) versus standard colonoscopy (SC).
[b] Non-neoplastic polyps.
[c] Compared with examination without pancolonic chromoendoscopy (chi-square test).

the proximal colon the range in the case series was 0.33 to 0.64 compared with 0.23 per patient in the randomized trials. In summary, hyperplastic polyps in the proximal colon can be detected by colonoscopy with chromoendoscopy in from one in five to one in two patients. Almost half of these polyps may be SSAs [56]. Large hyperplastic polyps, three quarters of which were SSAs in Spring and colleagues' [56] series, are detected at a rate of 0.01 to 0.1 per patient, with an average rate of 0.048 (36/752) per patient (Table 2). Thus many, if not most, proximal SSAs are smaller than 10 mm in size.

Chromoendoscopy requires a specially designed spray catheter to ensure complete and even mucosal coverage. It requires additional training by endoscopists and nursing staff. It greatly increases the time needed for colonoscope withdrawal. Several Western commentators have suggested that this technique is impractical and too costly for routine clinical application [78]. Some investigators apply this technique only to the proximal colon, the area at highest risk, to minimize additional procedure time. In one study, an endoscopist unfamiliar with chromoendoscopy rapidly learned the technique and achieved performance levels close to those of a Japanese expert, particularly in the detection of large hyperplastic polyps [77]. New endoscopic technologies such as narrow-band imaging ("electronic chromoendoscopy") may offer similar benefits with less additional time, but the data are limited [79]. High-definition endoscopy may improve detection by providing higher resolution of fine vascular changes, but no data are available so far. Of concern, autofluorescence endoscopy, which can highlight adenomas, does not seem, in the authors' experience, to highlight hyperplastic polyps. Future colonoscopic polyp detection studies should include SSAs with adenomas, as determined by expert pathologic interpretation, as outcome measures.

Table 2

Summary of case series reporting mean hyperplastic polyp detection rate by pancolonic chromoendoscopy according to polyp size and distribution

Study	Year(s) published	≤ 5 mm	6–9 mm	≥ 10 mm	Entire colon	Proximal colon
Total of randomized studies [72–75]	2002–2006	–	–	–	404/497 0.81	92/398 0.23
Spring [56]	2006	116/189 0.61	32/189 0.17	8/189 0.04	156/189 0.83	62/189 0.33
Yano[b] [71]	2005	3020/263 11.5	38/263 0.14	2/263 0.01	3060/263 11.6	168/263 0.64
Togashi[c] [77]	2005	–	–	7/100– 19/200 0.07–0.10	1.27–1.31[a]	–

[a] Non-neoplastic polyps.
[b] Polyps defined as hyperplastic on basis of pit pattern, not histopathology.
[c] Abstract, two endoscopists.

Lesion Characterization

Polyps are characterized at endoscopy as hyperplastic or adenomatous by endoscopic characteristics. Lesions that are sessile or flat, are small, pale, and glistening, and have few very fine vessels within the polyp are likely to be hyperplastic. The accuracy of endoscopic classification is improved by the use of dye-spray and magnified observation of the pit pattern and the size and shape of the colonic crypt openings on the polyp's surface. The Kudo type I (normal) or type II ("stellate" or "papillary") pattern is typical of hyperplastic polyps (Fig. 3) [80]. This technique is highly sensitive and specific for differentiating hyperplastic polyps from adenomas, with an accuracy exceeding 90% by experts. Current endoscopic techniques do not differentiate hyperplastic polyps from SSAs accurately in vivo. Although in theory confocal endomicroscopy could achieve this differentiation, the relatively narrow field of view and horizontal sections may make it difficult to appreciate the global architectural distortions within SSAs. The presence of mucus adherent to the polyp, purely stellate (type II) pits, hemispherical (in small size) or minimally elevated (in large size) morphology, and a smooth surface are anecdotally associated with SSA histology (personal communication, Dr. Kazutomo Togashi, Jichi Medical University, Japan, 2007).

Endoscopic characterization of a proximal colonic lesion may be clinically unnecessary, because any proximal lesion should be removed. In the distal (rectosigmoid) colon this practice is not realistic because of the large numbers of diminutive ($\leq$ 5-mm) hyperplastic polyps often found in this area. Detecting and resecting hyperplastic polyps larger than 5 mm probably is appropriate because of the increased risk that these lesions represent SSAs.

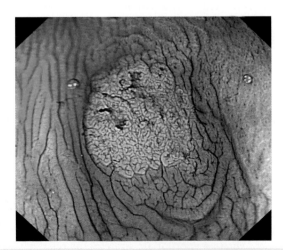

Fig. 3. Small, flat polyp showing Kudo type II (stellate "star-shaped" or papillary) pit pattern during magnification chromoendoscopy, suggesting that this is a hyperplastic polyp. This histology was confirmed by microscopic analysis of the resected polyp.

ENDOSCOPIC MANAGEMENT OF HYPERPLASTIC POLYPS AND SESSILE SERRATED ADENOMAS

Small and diminutive hyperplastic polyps can be dealt with by standard polypectomy techniques used for adenomas; however a single large ($\geq$10-mm) hyperplastic polyp requires careful consideration of the available management strategies. The colonoscopist needs to weigh the risks and benefits of immediate polypectomy versus observation with biopsy to confirm SSA and/or resection at a later date. There are almost no data on therapy for large hyperplastic polyps or SSAs, as opposed to conventional adenomas. Although adenomatous or malignant transformation usually can be detected with the endoscopic techniques described previously, simple hyperplastic polyps cannot be distinguished from SSAs by these techniques. Small case series, however, report direct transformation of SSAs into adenocarcinoma [49]. Endoscopic mucosal resection (EMR) is safe and effective. It is the method of choice. It involves lifting the lesion on a submucosal cushion of saline and then snare resecting the lesion either en toto or as multiple pieces. This technique can be challenging for very flat and large hyperplastic polyps, particularly in the thin-walled right colon where most of these lesions occur. Use of targeted dye-spray or dye in the submucosal cushion to help define the lesion margin is helpful (Fig. 2C, D). The rates of SSA recurrence after EMR are unknown, but it may be wise to apply argon plasma coagulation to lesion edges, as done for adenomas, to ensure destruction of residual tissue and reduce the risk of recurrence [81]. One large series reported a high rate of MSI-H cancers in colonic regions where hyperplastic polyps were biopsied or resected; this series suggests that care must be taken to ensure complete tissue ablation [38].

Complications of EMR include postpolypectomy bleeding, postpolypectomy syndrome, polyp recurrence, and colonic perforation. The existing data predominantly relate to adenomas, which are more vascular, more frequently polypoid, and more often located in the left colon where the risk of perforation may be less. No prospective data currently exist specifically for hyperplastic polyps. Large hyperplastic lesions often occur proximally, and such lesions have an increased risk of delayed bleeding and perforation, particularly when adjacent to the ileocecal valve. Decisions regarding polyp biopsy and colonoscopic surveillance versus immediate polypectomy should balance the potentially higher risks of EMR with the unknown rate of progression. After confirmation of a lesion as an SSA, a formal discussion of the risks and benefits of proceeding to resection versus surveillance may be appropriate, particularly in elderly patients. How often and how quickly these lesions progress and the risk of developing carcinoma if these lesions are not immediately resected are unclear [49]. Following biopsy, such lesions can be difficult to relocate. A mucosal tattoo adjacent to the lesion facilitates lesion reidentification at colonoscopy or surgery. EMR is an appropriate strategy for relatively healthy patients with relatively few lesions that are 1 to 3 cm in diameter. Older patients who have significant comorbidity or very large lesions may be better served by periodic surveillance. Because of the technical skill required to perform

EMR in the right colon safely, removal of large lesions generally should be undertaken by experienced therapeutic endoscopists at a tertiary center. EMR provides the pathologist a much larger specimen, compared with biopsy, for better histologic classification. The newly developed technique of endoscopic submucosal dissection carries a higher risk of perforation than EMR and requires considerable technical skill. This technique has not yet been applied to remove large hyperplastic polyps. This technique should probably be confined to experts at tertiary centers as part of clinical trials. This technique could help detect invasion in a dysplastic polyp by providing an en bloc specimen.

MANAGEMENT OF HYPERPLASTIC POLYPOSIS SYNDROME

Management of HPS involves the removal of premalignant lesions, subsequent surveillance, and counseling of the patient and other family members regarding genetic risk. If the initial presenting lesion is a carcinoma, then, as in the management of colon cancer associated with hereditary nonpolyposis colorectal cancer or attenuated familial adenomatous polyposis, an ileorectal anastomosis is the operation of choice to remove the at-risk colon together with the cancer [82]. This therapy eliminates the need for lifelong colonoscopic surveillance but still requires flexible sigmoidoscopy every 6 to 12 months to survey the rectal remnant [82]. This approach depends on HPS being diagnosed when diagnosing the colorectal cancer. A high index of suspicion therefore is required by the colonoscopist who encounters, for example, a right-sided cancer in a young patient with a strong family history of colorectal cancer. More commonly, the presenting lesions will be multiple precancerous, large, right sided hyperplastic polyps. Depending on patient age and comorbidity and lesion size and location, the following therapeutic options are available:

1. If the lesions seem to be endoscopically resectable (even if requiring multiple endoscopic sessions), resection with the intent to remove all lesions larger than 5 mm, preferably at a tertiary center, followed by surveillance, is recommended. Surgery is reserved when patients want to avoid lifelong colonoscopy or when suitable endoscopic expertise is unavailable.
2. If the lesions are not endoscopically resectable because of size or multiplicity, and the patient is a good surgical candidate, colectomy with ileorectal anastomosis is generally recommended. This strategy avoids future colonoscopy but still requires periodic flexible sigmoidoscopy for surveillance of the rectal remnant.
3. If lesions are not endoscopically resectable, and the patient is a poor surgical candidate or refuses surgery, colonoscopic surveillance with biopsy to detect malignant transformation may be performed, or selective polypectomy of adenomatous appearing lesions may be performed.

Patients and their first-degree relatives should be counseled regarding risk of colorectal cancer and the risk of transmission to offspring and should be offered colonoscopic surveillance with dye-spray. Precise risk estimates are not possible based on current data. Parents and siblings should be offered colonoscopy at the time of index case diagnosis. Children of the index case should have a screening colonoscopy at an age 10 years younger than the age of diagnosis of the index case. Counseling on genetic factors and future colorectal cancer risk in hyperplastic polyposis is best performed by an experienced team, and referral to a specialist group may be appropriate. Referral of such patients to academic centers should promote much-needed research. No germline mutation has been found for HPS, although genetic analysis of polyps for *KRAS* and *BRAF* mutation may assist in the diagnosis [83].

SURVEILLANCE OF SESSILE SERRATED ADENOMAS AND HYPERPLASTIC POLYPOSIS SYNDROME

There are limited data on the natural history and rate of progression of hyperplastic polyps and SSAs to advanced lesions. SSAs that are too few or too small to qualify as HPS may be treated like adenomas in terms of their premalignant risk and as predictors of future colorectal cancer risk. Thus, removal of an SSA 10 mm or larger would trigger colonoscopy at 3 years, as would an adenoma of similar size [84,85]. Whether the risk of SSA and adenomas are additive, so that two SSAs smaller than 10 mm and one adenoma smaller than 10 mm would lead to a colonoscopy every 3 years (as would three adenomas smaller than 10 mm) is unclear but reasonable [85]. Part of the reason for more frequent colonoscopic surveillance when increasing numbers of adenomas are detected at the index examination relates to an increasing rate of missed adenomas [86]. For hyperplastic polyps and SSAs, miss rates are likely to be higher, and therefore the threshold for early surveillance perhaps should be set lower. Similarly, because an SSA has been detected, the use of dye-spray to ensure comprehensive detection on subsequent colonoscopies should be considered, as for ulcerative colitis, or even could be initiated during an index colonoscopy when a large presumptive hyperplastic polyp is detected [87]. Dye-spray may detect additional lesions, leading to a diagnosis of HPS with significant management consequences. The diagnosis of attenuated familial adenomatous polyposis has been missed because of the failure to dye-spray [88]. Surveillance recommendations are summarized in Box 1. New technologies such as narrow-band imaging may help make this approach more practical clinically. There are as yet no head-to-head trials of narrow-band imaging versus chromoendoscopy for detection of hyperplastic polyps. The original definition of hyperplastic polyposis did not consider the effect of time on lesion development; this effect may need to be clarified to account for cumulative polyp burden. If multiple proximal hyperplastic polyps are detected at serial colonoscopies, the cumulative burden of hyperplastic polyps probably should be incorporated into the diagnostic criteria for HPS.

PREVENTIVE STRATEGIES

If 20% of colorectal cancer arises from hyperplastic polyps and SSAs, colonoscopic surveillance and removal of these lesions is likely to help prevent colon cancer. Hyperplastic polyp prevention may be particularly important because

Box 1: Colonoscopic surveillance recommendations

Based on current data, consensus, and expert opinion, the authors propose

1. SSA without cytologic dysplasia have a risk equivalent to adenomas with low-grade dysplasia and after complete resection should have follow-up per the current guidelines for adenomas, stratified according to polyp size and multiplicity.

2. For hyperplastic lesions proximal to the rectosigmoid that are not SSAs, repeat colonoscopy is recommended at 5 years for a single large ($\geq$ 10-mm) lesion, or three or more small (< 10-mm) lesions.

3. For patients diagnosed as having HPS, colonoscopy is recommended every 1 to 2 years with resection of all lesions larger than 5 mm if possible. This resection is best performed at a tertiary center with a special interest in the condition. First-degree relatives of an index case should be offered colonoscopic screening with pancolonic dye-spray.

4. After piecemeal resection of an SSA, patients should undergo repeat colonoscopy at 2 to 6 months to review the polypectomy site for recurrence, per adenoma guidelines.

5. After diagnosis of an SSA, a large hyperplastic polyp, or HPS, strong consideration should be given to optimizing surveillance detection through pancolonic chromoendoscopy.

6. Extending surveillance beyond the age of 75 years should be considered because of the potential for rapid neoplastic transformation and the occurrence in older patients of cancers from these precursor lesions, but this strategy should be weighed carefully against the risk of further colonoscopy.

7. Surveillance intervals may require modification in the presence of other risk factors such as age, family or personal history of colorectal cancer, comorbidity, and the accuracy and completeness of the colonoscopic examination. It is subject to modification by new data.

8. Pathologists should acquire diagnostic expertise to diagnose SSA.

These recommendations based on grade D, level V evidence (Oxford Center for Evidence-based Medicine) should be considered a starting point for research to promulgate definitive recommendations.

these lesions are not detected well by any screening strategy except colonoscopy, and even detection by colonoscopy is challenging.

Case-control studies provide evidence that the same lifestyle factors associated with adenomas and colorectal cancer also are associated with hyperplastic polyps. Smoking, alcohol, consumption of red meat, and increased body mass index all increase the risk of hyperplastic polyps. High consumption of dietary calcium or dietary fiber; the use of aspirin, nonsteroidal anti-inflammatory drugs, and possibly hormone replacement therapy; and physical exercise all decrease the risk. Most hyperplastic polyps in these studies were detected in the distal colorectum, however, and the relevance to proximal hyperplastic polyps, which are more likely to be SSAs, is unclear [89–93].

SUMMARY

This article describes evidence underlying an alternative pathway to colorectal cancer implicating hyperplastic polyps and allied lesions. The genetic, molecular, and morphologic features of hyperplastic polyps and two types of serrated adenomas (traditional and sessile) are presented. The importance of *BRAF* mutations is discussed. Pathologists are incorporating these evolving concepts clinically. There is a need for improved diagnostic criteria and an internationally agreed classification for these polyps. The risks associated with sporadic serrated polyps and syndromic serrated polyps in the hyperplastic polyposis syndrome are outlined. Problems associated with the colonoscopic detection and treatment of sessile serrated polyps are highlighted, as are the benefits of chromoendoscopy to enhance lesion detection and the pros and cons of resecting large, proximal SSAs. Prevention though lifestyle measures is outlined. Guidelines for management and surveillance of sporadic sessile serrated adenomas and the hyperplastic polyposis syndrome based on current knowledge are suggested.

References

[1] Kinzler KW, Nilbert MC, Su LK, et al. Identification of FAP locus genes from chromosome 5q21. Science 1991;253:661–5.

[2] Fodde R, Smits R, Clevers H. APC, signal transduction and genetic instability in colorectal cancer. Nat Rev Cancer 2001;1:55–67.

[3] Kinzler KW, Vogelstein B. Lessons from hereditary colorectal cancer. Cell 1996;87:159–70.

[4] Ionov Y, Peinado MA, Malkhosyan S, et al. Ubiquitous somatic mutations in simple repeated sequences reveal a new mechanism for colonic carcinogenesis. Nature 1993;363:558–61.

[5] Thibodeau SN, Bren G, Schaid D. Microsatellite instability in cancer of the proximal colon. Science 1993;260:816–9.

[6] Loukola A, Eklin K, Laiho P, et al. Microsatellite marker analysis in screening for hereditary nonpolyposis colorectal cancer (HNPCC). Cancer Res 2001;61:4545–9.

[7] Grady WM, Rajput A, Myeroff L, et al. Mutation of the type ii transforming growth factor-beta receptor is coincident with the transformation of human colon adenomas to malignant carcinomas. Cancer Res 1998;58:3101–4.

[8] Huang J, Papadopoulos N, McKinley AJ, et al. APC mutations in colorectal tumors with mismatch repair deficiency. Proc Natl Acad Sci U S A 1996;93:9049–54.

[9] Olschwang S, Hamelin R, Laurent-Puig P, et al. Alternative genetic pathways in colorectal carcinogenesis. Proc Natl Acad Sci U S A 1997;94:12122–7.

[10] Salahshor S, Kressner U, Pahlman L, et al. Colorectal cancer with and without microsatellite instability involves different genes. Genes Chromosomes Cancer 1999;26:247–52.

[11] Kambara T, Simms LA, Whitehall VLJ, et al. BRAF mutation is associated with DNA methylation in serrated polyps and cancers of the colorectum. Gut 2004;53:1137–44.

[12] Weisenberger DJ, Siegmund KD, Campan M, et al. CpG island methylator phenotype underlies sporadic microsatellite instability and is tightly associated with BRAF mutation in colorectal cancer. Nat Genet 2006;38:787–93.

[13] Kane MF, Loda M, Gaida GM, et al. Methylation of the hMLH1 promoter correlates with lack of expression of hMLH1 in sporadic colon tumors and mismatch repair-defective human tumor cell lines. Cancer Res 1997;57:808–11.

[14] Longacre TA, Fenoglio-Preiser CM. Mixed hyperplastic adenomatous polyps/serrated adenomas: a distinct form of colorectal neoplasia. Am J Surg Pathol 1990;14:524–37.

[15] Iino H, Jass JR, Simms LA, et al. DNA microsatellite instability in hyperplastic polyps, serrated adenomas, and mixed polyps: a mild mutator pathway for colorectal cancer? J Clin Pathol 1999;52:5–9.

[16] Williams GT, Arthur JF, Bussey HJ, et al. Metaplastic polyps and polyposis of the colorectum. Histopathology 1980;4:155–70.

[17] Cooper HS, Patchefsky AS, Marks G. Adenomatous and carcinomatous changes within hyperplastic colonic epithelium. Dis Colon Rectum 1979;22:152–6.

[18] Jass JR, Iino H, Ruszkiewicz A, et al. Neoplastic progression occurs through mutator pathways in hyperplastic polyposis of the colorectum. Gut 2000;47:43–9.

[19] Torlakovic E, Snover DC. Serrated adenomatous polyposis in humans. Gastroenterology 1996;110:748–55.

[20] Torlakovic E, Skovlund E, Snover DC, et al. Morphologic reappraisal of serrated colorectal polyps. Am J Surg Pathol 2003;27:65–81.

[21] Miwa S, Mitomi H, Igarashi M, et al. Clinicopathologic differences among subtypes of serrated adenomas of the colorectum. Hepatogastroenterology 2005;52.437–40.

[22] Matsumoto T, Mizuno M, Shimizu M, et al. Serrated adenoma of the colorectum: colonoscopic and histologic features. Gastrointest Endosc 1999;49:736–42.

[23] Yang S, Farraye FA, Mack C, et al. BRAF and KRAS Mutations in hyperplastic polyps and serrated adenomas of the colorectum: relationship to histology and CpG island methylation status. Am J Surg Pathol 2004;28:1452–9.

[24] Jass JR, Young J, Leggett BA. Hyperplastic polyps and DNA microsatellite unstable cancers of the colorectum. Histopathology 2000;37:295–301.

[25] Jass JR, Baker K, Zlobec I, et al. Advanced colorectal polyps with the molecular and morphological features of serrated polyps and adenomas: concept of a 'fusion' pathway to colorectal cancer. Histopathology 2006;49:121–31.

[26] Lee EJ, Choi C, Park CK, et al. Tracing origin of serrated adenomas with BRAF and KRAS mutations. Virchows Arch 2005;447:597–602.

[27] O'brien MJ, Yang S, Mack C, et al. Comparison of microsatellite instability, CpG island methylation phenotype, BRAF and KRAS status in serrated polyps and traditional adenomas indicates separate pathways to distinct colorectal carcinoma end points. Am J Surg Pathol 2006;30:1491–501.

[28] Ajioka Y, Watanabe H, Jass JR, et al. Infrequent K-ras codon 12 mutation in serrated adenomas of human colorectum. Gut 1998;42:680–4.

[29] Sawyer EJ, Cerar A, Hanby AM, et al. Molecular characteristics of serrated adenomas of the colorectum. Gut 2002;51:200–6.

[30] Uchida H, Ando H, Maruyama K, et al. Genetic alterations of mixed hyperplastic adenomatous polyps in the colon and rectum. Jpn J Cancer Res 1998;89:299–306.

[31] Yamamoto T, Konishi K, Yamochi T, et al. No major tumorigenic role for beta-catenin in serrated as opposed to conventional colorectal adenomas. Br J Cancer 2003;89: 152–7.

[32] Burt RW, Jass JR. Hyperplastic polyposis. In: Hamilton SR, Aaltonen LA, editors. WHO classification of tumours. Pathology and genetics. Tumours of the digestive system. Berlin: Springer-Verlag; 2000.

[33] Beach R, Chan AO, Wu TT, et al. BRAF mutations in aberrant crypt foci and hyperplastic polyposis. Am J Pathol 2005;166:1069–75.

[34] Rashid A, Houlihan PS, Booker S, et al. Phenotypic and molecular characteristics of hyperplastic polyposis. Gastroenterology 2000;119:323–32.

[35] Makinen MJ. Colorectal serrated adenocarcinoma. Histopathology 2007;50:131–50.

[36] Jass JR, Whitehall VLJ, Young J, et al. Emerging concepts in colorectal neoplasia. Gastroenterology 2002;123:862–76.

[37] Ogino S, Kawasaki T, Kirkner GJ, et al. Molecular correlates with MGMT promoter methylation and silencing support CpG island methylator phenotype-low (CIMP-low) in colorectal cancer. Gut 2007;56:1564–71.

[38] Goldstein NS, Bhanot P, Odish E, et al. Hyperplastic-like colon polyps that preceded micro-satellite-unstable adenocarcinomas. Am J Clin Pathol 2003;119:778–96.

[39] Robertson DJ, Greenberg ER, Beach M, et al. Colorectal cancer in patients under close colonoscopic surveillance. Gastroenterology 2005;129:34–41.

[40] Farrar WD, Sawhney MS, Nelson DB, et al. Colorectal cancers found after a complete colonoscopy. Clin Gastroenterol Hepatol 2006;4:1259–64.

[41] Sawhney MS, Farrar WD, Gudiseva S, et al. Microsatellite instability in interval colon cancers. Gastroenterology 2006;131:1700–5.

[42] Jass JR. Hyperplastic-like polyps as precursors of microsatellite-unstable colorectal cancer. Am J Clin Pathol 2003;119:773–5.

[43] O'brien MJ, Yang S, Clebanoff JL, et al. Hyperplastic (serrated) polyps of the colorectum: relationship of CpG island methylator phenotype and K-ras mutation to location and histologic subtype. Am J Surg Pathol 2004;28:423–34.

[44] Snover DC, Jass JR, Fenoglio-Preiser C, et al. Serrated polyps of the large intestine: a morphologic and molecular review of an evolving concept. Am J Clin Pathol 2005;124:380–91.

[45] Ansher AF, Lewis JH, Fleischer DE, et al. Hyperplastic colonic polyps as a marker for adeno-matous colonic polyps. Am J Gastroenterol 1989;84:113–7.

[46] Provenzale D, Garrett JW, Condon SE, et al. Risk for colon adenomas in patients with rectosigmoid hyperplastic polyps. Ann Intern Med 1990;113:760–3.

[47] Rex DK, Smith JJ, Ulbright TM, et al. Distal colonic hyperplastic polyps do not predict proximal adenomas in asymptomatic average-risk subjects. Gastroenterology 1992;102:317–9.

[48] Jass JR, Young PJ, Robinson EM. Predictors of presence, multiplicity, size and dysplasia of colorectal adenomas. A necropsy study in New Zealand. Gut 1992;33:1508–14.

[49] Goldstein NS. Small colonic microsatellite unstable adenocarcinomas and high-grade epithelial dysplasias in sessile serrated adenoma polypectomy specimens: a study of eight cases. Am J Clin Pathol 2006;125:132–45.

[50] Oh K, Redston M, Odze RD. Support for hMLH1 and MGMT silencing as a mechanism of tumorigenesis in the hyperplastic-adenoma-carcinoma (serrated) carcinogenic pathway in the colon. Hum Pathol 2005;36:101–11.

[51] Lynch HT, Smyrk T, Jass JR. Hereditary nonpolyposis colorectal cancer and colonic adeno-mas: aggressive adenomas? Semin Surg Oncol 1995;11:406–10.

[52] Sheridan TB, Fenton H, Lewin MR, et al. Sessile serrated adenomas with low- and high-grade dysplasia and early carcinomas: an immunohistochemical study of serrated lesions ''caught in the act''. Am J Clin Pathol 2006;126:564–71.

[53] Imperiale TF, Wagner DR, Lin CY, et al. Risk of advanced proximal neoplasms in asymp-tomatic adults according to the distal colorectal findings. N Engl J Med 2000;343:169–74.

[54] Lieberman DA, Weiss DG, Bond JH, et al. Use of colonoscopy to screen asymptomatic adults for colorectal cancer. N Engl J Med 2000;343:162–8.

[55] Imperiale TF, Ransohoff DF, Itzkowitz SH, et al. Fecal DNA versus fecal occult blood for colorectal-cancer screening in an average-risk population. N Engl J Med 2004;351:2704–14.

[56] Spring KJ, Zhao ZZ, Karamatic R, et al. High prevalence of sessile serrated adenomas with BRAF mutations: a prospective study of patients undergoing colonoscopy. Gastroenterology 2006;131:1400–7.

[57] Waldock A, Ellis IO, Armitage NC, et al. Histopathological assessment of bleeding from polyps of the colon and rectum. J Clin Pathol 1989;42:378–82.

[58] Sobin LH. The histopathology of bleeding from polyps and carcinomas of the large intestine. Cancer 1985;55:577–81.

[59] Jin YM, Li BJ, Qu B, et al. BRAF, K-ras and BAT26 mutations in colorectal polyps and stool. World J Gastroenterol 2006;12:5148–52.

[60] Taylor SA, Laghi A, Lefere P, et al. European Society of Gastrointestinal and Abdominal Radiology (ESGAR): consensus statement on CT colonography. Eur Radiol 2007;17: 575–9.

[61] Park SH, Ha HK, Kim AY, et al. Flat polyps of the colon: detection with 16-MDCT colonography: preliminary results. Am J Roentgenol 2006;186:1611–7.

[62] Park SH, Ha HK, Kim MJ, et al. False-negative results at multi-detector row CT colonography: Multivariate analysis of causes for missed lesions. Radiology 2005;235:495–502.

[63] Pickhardt PJ, Nugent PA, Choi JR, et al. Flat colorectal lesions in asymptomatic adults: implications for screening with CT virtual colonoscopy. Am J Roentgenol 2004;183:1343–7.

[64] Fidler JL, Johnson CD, MacCarty RL, et al. Detection of flat lesions in the colon with CT colonography. Abdom Imaging 2002;27:292–300.

[65] Mang TG, Schaefer-Prokop C, Maier A, et al. Detectability of small and flat polyps in MDCT colonography using 2D and 3D imaging tools: results from a phantom study. Am J Roentgenol 2005;185:1582–9.

[66] Rembacken BJ, Fujii T, Cairns A, et al. Flat and depressed colonic neoplasms: a prospective study of 1000 colonoscopies in the UK. Lancet 2000;355:1211–4.

[67] Harrison M, Singh N, Rex DK. Impact of proximal colon retroflexion on adenoma miss rates. Am J Gastroenterol 2004;99:519–22.

[68] Barclay RL, Vicari JJ, Doughty AS, et al. Colonoscopic withdrawal times and adenoma detection during screening colonoscopy. N Engl J Med 2006;355:2533–41.

[69] East JE, Suzuki N, Arebi N, et al. Position changes improve visibility during colonoscope withdrawal: a randomized, blinded, crossover trial. Gastrointest Endosc 2007;65:263–9.

[70] Froehlich F, Wietlisbach V, Gonvers JJ, et al. Impact of colonic cleansing on quality and diagnostic yield of colonoscopy: the European Panel of Appropriateness of Gastrointestinal Endoscopy European multicenter study. Gastrointest Endosc 2005;61:378–84.

[71] Yano T, Sano Y, Iwasaki J, et al. Distribution and prevalence of colorectal hyperplastic polyps using magnifying pan-mucosal chromoendoscopy and its relationship with synchronous colorectal cancer: Prospective study. J Gastroenterol Hepatol 2005;20:1572–7.

[72] Brooker JC, Saunders BP, Shah SG, et al. Total colonic dye-spray increases the detection of diminutive adenomas during routine colonoscopy: a randomized controlled trial. Gastrointest Endosc 2002;56:333–8.

[73] Hurlstone DP, Cross SS, Slater R, et al. Detecting diminutive colorectal lesions at colonoscopy: a randomised controlled trial of pan-colonic versus targeted chromoscopy. Gut 2004;53:376–80.

[74] Lapalus MG, Helbert T, Napoleon B, et al. Does chromoendoscopy with structure enhancement improve the colonoscopic adenoma detection rate? Endoscopy 2006;38:444–8.

[75] Le Rhun M, Coron E, Parlier D, et al. High resolution colonoscopy with chromoscopy versus standard colonoscopy for the detection of colonic neoplasia: a randomized study. Clin Gastroenterol Hepatol 2006;4:349–54.

[76] Lee YS. Adenomas, metaplastic polyps and other lesions of the large bowel: an autopsy survey. Ann Acad Med Singap 1987;16:412–20.

[77] Togashi K, Radford-Smith G, Hewett D, et al. The use of indigocarmine spray increases the colonoscopic detection rate of flat adenomas and large sessile hyperplastic polyps [abstract]. Gastrointest Endosc 2004;59:P96.

[78] Rex DK. Maximizing detection of adenomas and cancers during colonoscopy. Am J Gastroenterol 2006;101:2866–77.

[79] East JE, Suzuki N, Stavrinidis M, et al. Narrow band imaging for colonoscopic surveillance in hereditary non-polyposis colorectal cancer. Gut 2008;57:65–70.

[80] Kudo S, Tamura S, Nakajima T, et al. Diagnosis of colorectal tumorous lesions by magnifying endoscopy. Gastrointest Endosc 1996;44:8–14.

[81] Brooker JC, Saunders BP, Shah SG, et al. Treatment with argon plasma coagulation reduces recurrence after piecemeal resection of large sessile colonic polyps: a randomized trial and recommendations. Gastrointest Endosc 2002;55:371–5.

[82] Dunlop MG. Guidance on gastrointestinal surveillance for hereditary non-polyposis colorectal cancer, familial adenomatous polyposis, juvenile polyposis, and Peutz-Jeghers syndrome. Gut 2002;51(Suppl 5):V21–7.

[83] Carvajal-Carmona L, Howarth K, Lockett M, et al. Molecular classification and genetic pathways in hyperplastic polyposis syndrome. J Pathol 2007;212:378–85.

[84] Winawer SJ, Zauber AG, Fletcher RH, et al. Guidelines for colonoscopy surveillance after polypectomy: a consensus update by the US Multi-Society Task Force on Colorectal Cancer and the American Cancer Society. Gastroenterology 2006;130:1872–85.

[85] Atkin WS, Saunders BP. Surveillance guidelines after removal of colorectal adenomatous polyps. Gut 2002;51(Suppl 5):V6–9.

[86] Rex DK, Cutler CS, Lemmel GT, et al. Colonoscopic miss rates of adenomas determined by back-to-back colonoscopies. Gastroenterology 1997;112:24–8.

[87] Kiesslich R, Neurath MF. Surveillance colonoscopy in ulcerative colitis: magnifying chromoendoscopy in the spotlight. Gut 2004;53:165–7.

[88] Wallace MH, Frayling IM, Clark SK, et al. Attenuated adenomatous polyposis coli: the role of ascertainment bias through failure to dye-spray at colonoscopy. Dis Colon Rectum 1999;42:1078–80.

[89] Martinez ME, McPherson RS, Levin B, et al. A case-control study of dietary intake and other lifestyle risk factors for hyperplastic polyps. Gastroenterology 1997;113:423–9.

[90] Shin A, Shrubsole MJ, Ness RM, et al. Meat and meat-mutagen intake, doneness preference and the risk of colorectal polyps: the Tennessee Colorectal Polyp Study. Int J Cancer 2007;121:136–42.

[91] Wallace K, Baron JA, Karagas MR, et al. The association of physical activity and body mass index with the risk of large bowel polyps. Cancer Epidemiol Biomarkers Prev 2005;14:2082–6.

[92] Morimoto LM, Newcomb PA, Ulrich CM, et al. Risk factors for hyperplastic and adenomatous polyps: Evidence for malignant potential? Cancer Epidemiol Biomarkers Prev 2002;11:1012–8.

[93] Lieberman DA, Prindiville S, Weiss DG, et al. Risk factors for advanced colonic neoplasia and hyperplastic polyps in asymptomatic individuals. J Am Med Assoc 2003;290:2959–67.

Gastroenterol Clin N Am 37 (2008) 47–72

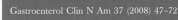

GASTROENTEROLOGY CLINICS
OF NORTH AMERICA

SEVIER
UNDERS

Syndromic Colon Cancer: Lynch Syndrome and Familial Adenomatous Polyposis

Tusar K. Desai, MD[a,b,*], Donald Barkel, MD[a,b]

[a]Division of Gastroenterology, Department of Medicine, William Beaumont Hospital, 3601 West Thirteen Mile Road, Royal Oak, MI 48073, USA
[b]Department of Surgery, William Beaumont Hospital, 3601 West Thirteen Mile Road, Royal Oak, MI 48073, USA

Colon cancer, the third leading cause of mortality from cancer in the United States, afflicts about 150,000 patients annually. More than 10% of these patients exhibit familial clustering [1]. The most common and well characterized of these familial colon cancer syndromes is hereditary nonpolyposis colon cancer syndrome (HNPCC or Lynch syndrome), which accounts for about 2% to 3% of all cases of colon cancer in the United States [1].

Lynch syndrome, an autosomal dominant condition with incomplete penetrance, was initially defined by clinical and family history criteria, known as the Amsterdam criteria (Box 1). Subsequently, genetic mutations in six distinct DNA mismatch repair genes have been identified, and testing for three of these genes (MLH1, MSH2, MSH6) has become widely available to clinicians. Lynch syndrome now refers to patients who have mutations in one of four DNA mismatch repair (MMR) genes–MLH1, MSH2, MSH6, and PMS2–regardless of whether the Amsterdam criteria for family history are met [2,3]. About 1 in 1000 to 1 in 3000 Americans are carriers for MMR gene mutations [4,5], and 100,000 to 300,000 Americans have Lynch syndrome. Genetic testing for these mutations is now used for the diagnosis, although genetic testing is limited by its cost of more than $2000 and concerns regarding privacy. Patients may be reluctant to be identified as a carrier of a cancer-causing genetic mutation that may limit their ability to obtain insurance, home mortgage loans, or employment. This aversion to being identified, potentially publicly, as a cancer gene carrier, has impeded the diagnosis of Lynch syndrome even in European countries where nationalized health care renders concerns about insurability irrelevant [6].

*Corresponding author. Department of Medicine, William Beaumont Hospital, 3601 West Thirteen Mile Road, Royal Oak, MI 48073. E-mail address: tusardesai@aol.com (T.K. Desai).

0889-8553/08/$ – see front matter
doi:10.1016/j.gtc.2007.12.006

Box 1: Amsterdam criteria: family risk for hereditary nonpolyposis colorectal cancer[a]

At least three relatives have a cancer associated with hereditary nonpolyposis colorectal cancer[b]

One should be first-degree relative of the other two relatives.

At least two successive generations should be affected.

At least one relative should be diagnosed before age 50 years.

Familial adenomatous polyposis should be excluded.

Tumors should be verified by pathologic examination.

[a]About half of the families meeting Amsterdam I criteria have Lynch syndrome (hereditary DNA mismatch repair gene mutation); conversely, many families that have Lynch syndrome do not meet these criteria.
[b]Colorectal cancer, cancer of the endometrium, small bowel, or renal pelvis. Amsterdam I criteria included only colorectal cancer. Amsterdam II criteria included all cancers listed.

We review the current knowledge of familial cancer syndromes, with an emphasis on Lynch syndrome and familial adenomatous polyposis (FAP).

MISMATCH MUTATION REPAIR GENE FUNCTION

Six MMR genes have been identified (Box 2). The two major genes are MLH1 and MSH2. The four minor MMR genes are MSH6, MSH3, PMS2, and MLH3. Mutations in MLH3 and MSH3 are not believed to cause malignancy [3]. MMR genes work as dimers or in pairs: MLH1 can pair with PMS2 or MLH3, whereas MSH2 can pair with MSH3 or MSH6. A mutation in MSH3 can therefore be overcome as MSH2 pairs with MSH6, and MSH6 mutations can be overcome by MSH2 pairing with MSH3 [3]. Similarly, a mutation in PMS2 can be overcome as MLH1 pairs with MLH3. A mutation in MLH1, however, leads to loss of MLH1 function and also PMS2 and MLH3 function because these two latter genes cannot function without MLH1. A mutation in MSH2 leads to loss of function for MSH3 and MSH6 because the protein products of these genes require the MSH2 protein for stabilization [3]. Mutations in MSH6 and PMS2 therefore lead to an attenuated form of familial cancer and Lynch syndrome, although there is one case report of a family with individuals who had colon cancer, uterine cancer, and three other cancers all occurring before age 25 associated with homozygous PMS2 mutations [7]. Gene sequencing for PMS2 is not commercially available.

Mutations in these genes can be truncating, leading to highly abbreviated mRNA transcription and complete lack of normal protein function, resulting in complete absence of immunohistochemical staining. MMR gene mutations often are missense mutations, however, which lead to single amino acid substitutions in MMR proteins. Such mutations may or may not express the cancer phenotype [3]. Missense mutations in MSH2 are almost always pathogenic [8],

> **Box 2: DNA mismatch repair genes**
>
> MLH1: Mutations lead to classic form of Lynch syndrome; 30% of mutations are missense mutations
>
> PMS2: Usually leads to attenuated form of Lynch syndrome
> > MSI-H cancers
> >
> > Onset cancer 7 to 8 years later than classic Lynch
>
> MLH3: Not pathogenic
>
> MSH2: Classic form of Lynch syndrome
>
> MSH6: Usually leads to attenuated form of Lynch syndrome
> > Onset cancer 7 to 8 years later
> >
> > Cancers often MSI-L or stable
>
> MSH3: Not pathogenic

whereas nontruncating missense mutations in MSH6 are usually not associated with MMR dysfunction and a high cancer risk [9]. MLH1 mutations are the most common MMR gene mutation found; 30% of these mutations are missense mutations. Some pathologic missense MLH1 gene mutations result in a minimally functional protein, which leads to falsely positive immunohistochemical staining [3].

LYNCH SYNDROME: CLINICAL PRESENTATION AND DIAGNOSIS

Insofar as every patient who has colon cancer should undergo a detailed family history, the Amsterdam criteria, listed in Box 1, represents the starting point for evaluating the genetic basis of colon cancer. Genetic testing, however, reveals MMR gene mutations in only half of patients who meet the Amsterdam criteria [10]. Conversely, at least half of patients who have genetic mutations that define Lynch syndrome do not meet the Amsterdam criteria [11–14]. The Amsterdam criteria are, therefore, obsolete. They are clinically useful only when a patient and family meet the Amsterdam criteria; in this case one may proceed directly to genetic testing for MMR mutations (Fig. 1). In the dominant familial colon cancer pedigree, a family meets the Amsterdam criteria in number of colon cancers, but all family members developed the cancer after age 50. If, however, a patient does not meet the Amsterdam criteria, then the Bethesda guidelines should be followed. The revised Bethesda guidelines (Box 3) were established to identify patients who had colon cancer who should undergo testing for either microsatellite instability or immunohistochemistry for MMR proteins as a prelude to genetic testing [15]. Testing for microsatellite instability is beyond the capability of most community hospitals, but immunohistochemical testing for MMR proteins is technically easier and can be

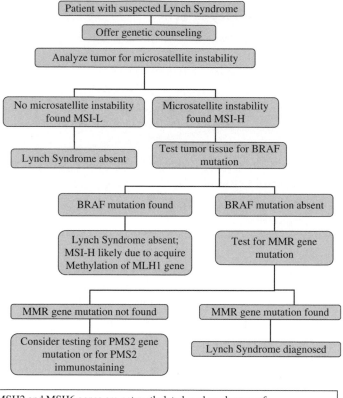

Fig. 1. Diagnostic algorithm for Lynch syndrome using microsatellite instability.

performed in most pathology laboratories [4]. Missense mutations, however, can lead to weakly false-positive immunostaining for the MMR protein.

Each of the above genes except MLH1 has in its coding sequence a nucleotide repeat of seven or more elements, so they are particularly susceptible to mutation in the event of MMR gene dysfunction.

The finding of microsatellite instability should lead to genetic testing because it is found in more than 90% of patients who have Lynch syndrome, but in only 15% to 20% of patients who have sporadic colon cancer. Sporadic colon cancer that has high microsatellite instability (MSI-H) is believed to arise from serrated adenomas due to hypermethylation of the MLH1 gene promoter [4,16]. MLH1 gene hypermethylation is an age-related process [17]. Sporadic colon cancer that is MSI-H thus usually occurs after age 60.

Box 3: Revised Bethesda guidelines[a]

Tumors should be tested for microsatellite instability when one or more of the
  following exist:
Colorectal cancer diagnosed in a patient who is younger than 50 years

Presence of colorectal cancers that are synchronous (simultaneous) or metachronous (diagnosed at different times) or other tumors associated with hereditary
  nonpolyposis colorectal cancer,[b] regardless of age

Colorectal cancer with a high amount of microsatellite instability[c] or histology[d]
  diagnosed in a patient who is younger than 60 years[e]

Colorectal cancer or tumor associated with hereditary nonpolyposis colorectal
  cancer[b] diagnosed before age 50 years in at least one first-degree relative[f]

Colorectal cancer or tumor associated with hereditary nonpolyposis colorectal
  cancer[b] diagnosed at any age in two first- or second-degree relatives[f]

[a]These guidelines are intended for colorectal cancer patients to identify those who may benefit from tumor microsatellite instability testing. The guidelines are not diagnostic criteria for
hereditary nonpolyposis colorectal cancer or Lynch syndrome. When a tumor is not available for testing, germline DNA testing can be offered if clinical presentation is strongly suggestive of Lynch syndrome.
[b]Includes colorectal, endometrial, stomach, ovarian, pancreas, ureter and renal pelvis, biliary tract, and brain (usually glioblastoma as seen in Turcot syndrome) tumors, sebaceous
gland adenomas, and keratoacanthomas in Muir-Torre syndrome, and carcinoma of the
small bowel.

[c]Refers to changes in two or more of the five panels of microsatellite markers recommended
by the National Cancer Institute.

[d]Presence of tumor infiltrating lymphocytes, Chrohn disease–like lymphocytic reaction,
mucinous or signet-ring differentiation, or medullary growth pattern.

[e]There was no consensus among the Bethesda workshop participants on whether to include
the age criteria in guideline 3 above; participants voted to keep age younger than 60 years
in the guidelines.

[f]Criteria 4 and 5 have been reworded to clarify the revised Bethesda guidelines.

Up to 50% of MSI-H colon cancers diagnosed before age 60 are related to
Lynch syndrome [17,18]. Only 20% to 25% of patients who have MSI-H colon cancer have an MMR gene mutation and Lynch syndrome [11,13]. Patients who have microsatellite instability and do not have MMR gene
mutation are believed to have hypermethylation and inactivation of the
MLH1 gene [4,16]. This situation frequently correlates with BRAF proto-oncogene mutations and may represent the pathway from serrated adenomas to
sporadic colon cancer [19,20].

Microsatellites refer to long segments of nontranscribed DNA that are composed of a repeating mononucleotide (eg, AAAAAAAAAAAAAAAA) or dinu-
cleotide sequences (eg, GTGTGTGTGTGTGT). These long DNA sequences
provide a simple indicator of genetic mutation rate and risk because mutations
are readily apparent in these long repeating sequences. For example, in the

sequence AAAAAAAAAAAAAAACAAAAAA, the C is an obvious mutation. Microsatellite instability is tested at five loci, the best known of which are BAT 26 and BAT 25, which consist of 25 and 26 adenine nucleotides in a row, respectively. BAT 25 or 26 is short for Big A Nucleotide Tract 25 or 26, respectively. Short nucleotide repeats of 7 to 8 elements are commonly present in the expressed portion of various genes. These genes are susceptible to mutation when MMR dysfunction exists.

The test sites for MSI are not involved in the carcinogenic process. Thirty-two genes in the human genome have mononucleotide repeats of more than 7 elements [21]. These long repetitive sequences are believed to be more prone to mutation than nonrepetitive sequences. Common target genes for mutation attributable to mismatch repair deficiency are the TGFB1R2 gene, the neurofibroma 1 gene, and the four minor mismatch repair genes themselves (MSH6, MSH3, MLH3, PMS2) [22]. Each of these six genes has a repetitive sequence of eight or more nucleotides in its coding sequence, whereas MSH2, a major MMR gene, has an A7 repeat sequence in its coding region. The presence of microsatellites within the coding region of MSH2, MSH6, and MSH3 and their susceptibility to MMR deficiency leads to a vicious cycle whereby a mutation in one MMR gene leads to mutations in other MMR genes. This phenomenon may account for the rapid development of adenomas and their rapid transition to cancer in Lynch syndrome [23].

TGFBR2 mutations are found in more than 90% of Lynch colorectal cancers, but are not found in nonmalignant tissues of Lynch patients, nor are they found in sporadic colorectal cancer without MMR deficiency [24,25].

Once microsatellite instability is found in a resected cancer, genetic testing may be offered to the patient or family members. Some 70% to 75% of patients whose cancer demonstrates microsatellite instability do not demonstrate mutations in the MMR genes. The high cost of genetic testing, coupled with the observation that genetic testing is negative in more than 70% of patients who have MSI, has led to a search for other cancer markers. Mutations in the BRAF proto-oncogene are nearly always absent in patients who have Lynch syndrome [19,20]. Testing for BRAF gene mutations in the cancer tissue may be performed for approximately $200.

Some authorities have suggested the protocol outlined in Fig. 1. Candidates for MSI testing are identified according to the Bethesda guidelines. If MSI is detected, then BRAF gene mutation should be tested. If the BRAF gene has a mutation, genetic testing is unnecessary because the presence of this mutation suggests hypermethylation. If the BRAF gene does not have a mutation, genetic testing should be performed. If a patient who has MSI-H lacks all of the above (ie, has no mutations in MMR genes, BRAF genes, or abnormal methylation) then it is currently speculated that this patient has an undetectable MMR gene mutation. One possibility is mutation of the PMS2 gene, as discussed below. The cost of genetic testing to identify mutations in the MMR genes is approximately $2200. If a proband is diagnosed with a specific MMR gene mutation, however, family members can be checked for mutations within this specific gene at a cost of approximately $300 per patient. The cost effectiveness of these various approaches has not been evaluated. It seems that for families, screening the proband for MMR gene mutations is cost effective. Genetic diagnosis is important because of the high lifetime risk of 70% for cancer in these patients [26]. Moreover, the average age of the initial cancer diagnosis is only 44 years of age. Once an index patient is identified, therefore, the $300 per person cost to identify family members who need intensive screening is cost effective. The lifetime risk for cancers associated with Lynch syndrome is provided in Box 4.

Immunohistochemistry to stain a resected cancer specimen for functional MLH1 and its heterodimer partner PMS2, MSH2, or MSH6 protein has been used to screen for Lynch syndrome (Fig. 2). Staining for MLH1 or PMS2 is often absent in sporadic colon cancer because of hypermethylation of these genes. If immunohistochemistry shows the absence of either of these two proteins, testing for hypermethylation or the BRAF mutation should be performed, and if hypermethylation or the BRAF mutation are found, genetic testing is not indicated. If hypermethylation or the BRAF mutation are not found, genetic testing is indicated. If immunohistochemistry reveals an absence of MSH2 or MSH6, one may proceed directly to genetic testing without testing for hypermethylation [12]. Missense mutations in MLH1 or MSH6 may lead to defective function with a weakly staining protein on immunohistochemistry.

Immunohistochemistry for PMS2 is usually not performed for PMS2 but should be included in any investigation of familial cancer or MSI-H cancer. Among 12 patients who had MSI-H cancer and staining for MLH1, MSH2, and MSH6, 8 patients showed a loss of PMS2 staining. Five of these patients had an MMR gene mutation in either MLH1 or PMS2 [27]. Of 775 patients who had familial colon cancer undergoing immunohistochemical stains for MLH1, MSH2, MSH6, and PMS2, 8 patients had loss of only PMS2, of whom 7 had PMS2 gene mutations associated with MSI-H [28]. Finally, a kindred with PMS2 mutations has recently been reported that

Box 4: Lifetime risk for cancer in Lynch syndrome

Colon cancer 70%

Endometrial cancer 60% to 70%

Ovarian cancer 7% to 10%

Gastric cancer 13% (higher in East Asia)

Small bowel cancer 4% (age at onset 40; 50% within range of upper endoscope)

Brain cancer 3.5%

Pancreas cancer

Renal ureteral

Sebaceous adenoma

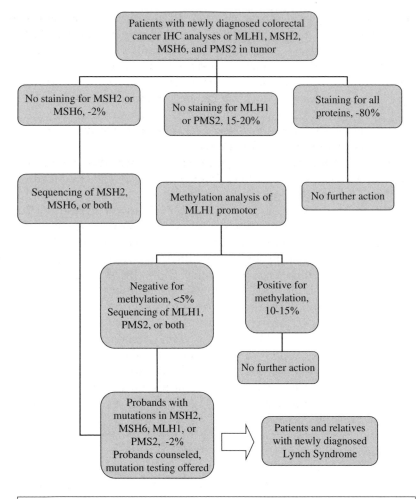

MSH2 and MSH6 genes are not methylated, and so absence of immunostaining for these genes does not lead to studies for methylation. One may proceed directly to testing for gene mutations. One advantage of IHC is that microsatellite stable tumors related to MSH6 mutations can be detected.

Fig. 2. Diagnostic algorithm for Lynch syndrome using immunohistochemistry.

met the Amsterdam criteria; all the children had homozygous biallelic mutations for PMS2 [7].

Colon cancer related to Lynch syndrome tends to be proximal and have a specific histologic appearance characterized by a heavy infiltration of lymphocytes, medullary growth pattern, and a mucinous or signet ring differentiation [2]. Colon cancers with these histologic characteristics in a patient who is less than 60 years of age, or has had other HNPCC-related cancers, should undergo testing for MSI. The clinicopathologic features most predictive of MSI-H cancers are lymphocytic infiltration and proximal cancer location [29]. There is considerable heterogeneity in the pathologic appearance of colon cancers from family members who have the same MMR gene mutation, and even among metachronous colorectal cancers from the same individual, suggesting that factors other than MMR gene mutations influence carcinogenesis [30]. Distal cancers are less likely than proximal cancers to demonstrate the characteristic pathologic features of Lynch colon cancer [30].

The initial Bethesda guidelines suggested that patients who have adenomas diagnosed before age 40 undergo evaluation for HNPCC. A small study of such patients, however, found that none of the adenomas demonstrated MSI or lacked immunohistochemical markers for MSH1 or MLH2 [31]. Microsatellite instability occurs in 40% to 80% of benign adenomas from patients who have documented colon cancer and MMR gene mutations [32,33]. The revised Bethesda guidelines no longer suggest detailed evaluation of patients who have adenoma before age 40 unless the adenoma demonstrates high-grade dysplasia or multiple adenomas are found.

Cancers associated with HNPCC are listed in Box 4. Gynecologic cancers may be more common than colon cancer in patients who have HNPCC, and some gynecologists have proposed changing the name to not refer to colon cancers or to also mention endometrial cancer [34]. These gynecologists argue that it is difficult to raise awareness of this syndrome when the name of the syndrome includes colon cancer but not the frequently associated gynecologic malignancies [34]. It has been proposed that all patients younger than age 50 years who have endometrial cancer be tested for Lynch syndrome mutations. In one study, 34% of women who had endometrial cancer younger than age 50 had HNPCC mutations [35].

The phenotypic expression of Lynch syndrome varies according to ethnicity. In Korea and China, gastric cancer is far more common among patients who have Lynch syndrome than in Holland [36,37]. The high risk for endometrial cancer seems to affect all ethnic groups, however. A study of 385 Japanese women who had endometrial cancer reported that 0.5% satisfied the Amsterdam criteria for family history, 30% demonstrated MSI-H in the cancer tissue, and 8.3% demonstrated MMR gene mutations [38].

Other cancers associated with Lynch syndrome include stomach, pancreas, biliary tract, small bowel, renal pelvis and ureter, and brain (see Box 3) [2]. The cumulative lifetime risk for gastric cancer in patients who have Lynch syndrome is estimated at 13% [39]. It is much higher in East Asia and lower in the West [36,37]. In China and Korea, the risk for gastric cancer exceeds the risk for endometrial cancer among MMR gene mutation carriers [36,37]. The relative risk for brain tumors among patients who have MMR gene mutations is six times the baseline in the general population [40]. Despite this high relative risk, the lifetime risk for brain tumor among patients who have Lynch syndrome is only 3.5%, so screening for this tumor is not recommended [40].

The lifetime risk for small bowel cancer among MMR gene mutation carriers is estimated at 4%, which is too low to justify screening [41]. Up to 50% of small bowel cancers are located in the duodenum or proximal jejunum within reach of the upper endoscope [42]. The average age of onset of small bowel cancer is 39 years. In about 50% of patients who have small bowel cancer, this cancer was the first indicator of Lynch syndrome [42]. This cancer exhibits intense lymphocytic infiltration similar to that for colon cancer [42]. There have been reports of cancer of the prostate and thyroid in association with HNPCC, with microsatellite instability in these cancers [43].

Confounding Features of Microsatellite Instability Testing

Cancers from about 6% of patients who have Lynch syndrome do not manifest microsatellite instability; these patients usually have MSH6 mutation [44,45]. MSH6 mutations account for approximately 8% of all Lynch syndrome cancers.

There are data suggesting that cigarette smoking increases the risk for colonic adenomas [46,47], but the link to colon cancer has been harder to establish. It has been recently found, however, that cigarette smoking selectively increases the risk for colon cancer that is MSI-H [48,49]. Similarly, the incidence of colon cancer is 1.2–fold higher in African Americans than Caucasians. In two small series from Washington DC a high level of microsatellite instability was found in more than 40% of cancers in African Americans, representing a doubling of the rate found in cancers in Caucasians [50]. The colon cancers found with MSI-H were proximal, well differentiated, and mucinous, a pattern suggestive of colon cancer in Lynch syndrome [50]. The proportion of patients who have MSI who have defective expression of MMR gene function is similar in African Americans and in Caucasians. In African Americans, females accounted for 68% of the cancers with MSI-H, whereas in Caucasians, most patients who had MSI-H colon cancer were male [11,12]. Alpha-1-antitrypsin deficiency is also associated with MSI-H colon cancer [51].

Management of Patients Who Have Amsterdam Criteria

Approximately half of the families who meet the Amsterdam criteria do not demonstrate microsatellite instability or MMR gene mutation. They are classified as familial colon cancer X. They seem to have a colon cancer risk intermediate between that of Lynch syndrome and the general population [10]. The standardized incidence ratio of colon cancer in familial colon cancer X is 2.3, compared with 6 for Lynch syndrome. These patients do not seem to be at risk for other cancers. Patients who have familial colon cancer X syndrome develop colon cancer at an older age, with a mean age of about 60 years [10].

Colon cancer screening of these families should probably be more aggressive than the recommendations of the American Cancer Society for patients who have one family member who has colon cancer or polyps before age 60 of undergoing colonoscopy every 5 to 10 years starting at age 40 or 10 years before the age of the youngest immediate family member who developed cancer. It therefore seems reasonable to advise these patients to undergo colonoscopy every 5 years beginning 5 years earlier than the age of the youngest family member to develop cancer. Colon cancer in these patients tends to be proximal and associated with multiple adenomas, whereas more than three adenomas is rare in Lynch syndrome [52].

Mutational Heterogeneity

Among patients who have documented MMR gene mutations, 90% have mutations in MLH1 and MSH2. The risk for cancer presumably varies according to the specific mutation, but guidelines are presented for mutations in aggregate. The risk for various cancers in patients who have Lynch mutations is presented in Box 3. It varies according to ethnicity. A study from the German HNPCC registry reported that families that have the MSH6 mutation have a lower risk for colon cancer and a later age of cancer onset [53]. A large series from the Dutch HNPCC database reported that the risk for cancer in MSH6 carriers is related to sex and the type of cancer. Among women who have the MSH6 mutation the risk for colon cancer was significantly less than the risk for colon cancer among women who have MLH1 or MSH2 mutations, whereas the risk for endometrial cancer in women who have MSH6 mutation was significantly higher than that for women who have MLH1 or MSH2 mutation [54]. About 70% of women who have MSH6 mutation develop endometrial cancer by age 70 [54]. Among men who have MSH6 mutations, the risk for colon cancer was less, but the difference was not statistically significant. MSH6-related cancers are usually microsatellite stable [44,45]. Missense mutations of MSH6 lead to weakly (false) positive immunostaining for the MSH6 protein, but deficient MMR function [3].

Mutations of the PMS2 gene lead to an attenuated form of Lynch syndrome with onset of cancer at a later age, like mutations in the MSH6 gene. Cancers in patients who have PMS2 mutations are MSI-H, however [27,28]. Interestingly, families who have mutations in either PMS2 or MSH6 tend to be small and not meet the Amsterdam criteria [28]. The largest series of families that had PMS2 mutations reported breast cancer to be the second most common cancer after colon cancer [28].

Screening for Patients/Families Who Have Lynch Syndrome

A proband identified as having Lynch syndrome should undergo subtotal colectomy for colon cancer and screening for the other associated cancers. The evaluation of immediate family members depends on their willingness to undergo genetic testing. If family members who have a documented MMR gene mutation refuse genetic testing, colonoscopy should be offered every 1 to 2 years starting at age 20 to 25 years. If genetic testing is negative, screening colonoscopy should still be offered in a program similar to that for the family colon cancer X syndrome, at every 5 years starting at age 10 years before the youngest family member to develop cancer. If genetic testing is positive, screening is intensive and prophylactic surgery may be considered. The adenoma-to-carcinoma progression in Lynch syndrome is believed to occur more rapidly than in sporadic colon cancer, and may occur in flat adenomas that are easily missed by colonoscopy. Colonoscopic screening was shown to be effective in reducing the rate of colon cancer and overall mortality among 133 patients who had Lynch syndrome, as compared with 119 patients who had Lynch syndrome who refused screening colonoscopy [55]. Colon cancer was found in 8 screened subjects and in all cases it was local and potentially curable, with no deaths of colon cancer. Colon cancer occurred in 19 controls who refused screening, of whom 9 died of colon cancer [55]. Despite intensive counseling and education, almost 50% of patients told that they had a 70% lifetime risk for colon cancer from Lynch syndrome refused screening [55]. This finding has been confirmed. The Netherlands launched a large-scale surveillance program in the late 1980s, and a retrospective analysis of the national cancer registry revealed that mortality from colon cancer decreased among patients who had Lynch syndrome after the introduction of this surveillance program [56]. In this study, there was no absolute excess mortality for any of Lynch syndrome–related cancers, except for colon and brain cancers [56].

Among 394 primary relatives of patients who had Lynch syndrome undergoing surveillance colonoscopy, 5 patients developed an interval colon cancer within 3.5 years of a reportedly normal colonoscopy [57]. This presumed high miss rate has led to the performance of frequent colonoscopies on these patients, and the use of chromoendoscopy to increase mucosal contrast and improve detection of flat adenomas. Back-to-back colonoscopy using indigo carmine dye during the second colonoscopy was performed in 25 patients who met the Amsterdam criteria, of whom 84% had MSH2 or MLH1 germline mutations. The initial colonoscopy revealed 24 lesions in 10 patients, but the segmental pancolonic chromogen dye contrast colonoscopy revealed 52 lesions in 15 patients. One cancer in this series was detected by conventional colonoscopy, but 7 conventional adenomas with high-grade dysplasia and 4 serrated adenomas were found by chromogen dye colonoscopy that were missed on conventional colonoscopy [58]. This intriguing study should stimulate further study of chromocolonoscopy in this high-risk population.

Lecomte and colleagues [59], after performing a conventional colonoscopy, sprayed indigocarmine dye into only the proximal colon and then re-evaluated the proximal colon with chromocolonoscopy in 36 patients from HNPCC families. Conventional colonoscopy revealed 25 lesions, whereas chromocolonoscopy of the proximal colon revealed an additional 45 lesions. Most missed lesions detected by chromocolonoscopy were less than 5 mm, flat, and hyperplastic [59]. East and colleagues [60] compared use versus nonuse of narrow band imaging (NBI) with high-definition colonoscopes in 62 patients from HNPCC families who already underwent a prior clearing colonoscopy. Conventional colonoscopy detected 25 adenomas in 17 patients, whereas NBI colonoscopy detected an additional 21 adenomas. Because the progression from adenoma to cancer can occur within 2 years in patients who have Lynch syndrome, the enhanced detection rate of these newer colonoscopic techniques seems to be clinically significant. The above data suggest that chromocolonoscopy or high-definition colonoscopy with NBI may be highly useful in this high-risk population.

Virtual CT colonography has been proposed for screening of sporadic colon cancers, but this would likely be inappropriate for patients who have proven or suspected Lynch syndrome who are at high risk for flat adenomas. In a study from Finland both CT colonography and optical colonoscopy were performed in 78 patients who had proven MMR gene mutations [61]. Two colon cancers were detected by both modalities. A total of 26 polyps were found (13 adenomatous and 13 hyperplastic). The sensitivity of CT colonography for detecting polyps was only 27%, and for polyps greater than 1 cm the sensitivity was only 80% [61]. Given the rapid progression of adenomas to carcinomas in Lynch syndrome, CT colonography seems inadequate for screening these patients. Among patients who have documented Lynch syndrome who have not had colon cancer, colonoscopy should be performed every 2 years starting at age 25 to 30, depending on the age of onset of the colon cancer in the family.

Natural History of Lynch Syndrome Colon Cancer

Large population-based studies have reported that survival of patients who have colon cancer related to MMR gene mutations is similar to survival of patients who have sporadic colon cancer [11,62,63]. Patients who have Lynch syndrome who have distal colon cancer may develop metachronous colon cancer more quickly than those who have proximal colon cancer.

MSI-H cancers, considered as a group, including Lynch syndrome and acquired methylation of MLH1, have different clinical characteristics. Patients who have MSI-H colon cancer exhibit improved survival for all cancer stages, so that the improved survival is not because of earlier detection [64]. Patients who have stage I or II colorectal cancer have 5-year survivals of 90% or more [64]. Among patients who have stage II and III colon cancer, microsatellite stability may affect the response to chemotherapy. Patients who have MSI-H cancers are less likely to respond to alkylating agents or 5-FU [65,66] but are more likely to respond to irinotecan than patients who have MSI-L colon cancers [67]. In vitro studies of MSI-H cell lines suggest that demethylating agents can restore sensitivity to alkylating agents and 5-FU [68].

Postoperative Surveillance for Rectal Cancer

Patients who have colon cancer related to Lynch syndrome should undergo subtotal colectomy and then undergo aggressive endoscopic surveillance of the rectum. A retrospective study estimated the risk for rectal cancer to be 12% during 12 years after abdominal colectomy [69].

Gynecologic Management

Gynecologic malignancies may be as common in Lynch syndrome as colon cancer. The lifetime risk in Lynch syndrome for colon cancer is 70%, for endometrial cancer is 50%, and for ovarian cancer is 10% to 20%. These risks may be overestimated because of ascertainment bias and may actually be lower [70].

Among 543 unselected patients who had endometrial cancer, 22% were MSI-H or had abnormal immunohistochemistry. Ten patients demonstrated MMR gene mutations. Remarkably, 7 of these 10 patients would not have met any published criteria for HNPCC, and 6 of these patients were more than 50 years old [35].

About 2% to 4% of women who have ovarian cancer carry MMR gene mutations, compared with 11% of women who carry BRCA gene mutations [71]. If the BRCA mutation has been excluded in patients who have familial ovarian cancer, genetic testing for Lynch syndrome should be considered [71]. The lifetime risk for endometrial cancer may be underestimated because so many women have a hysterectomy for benign causes. Prophylactic hysterectomy and bilateral salpingo-oophorectomy have been proposed as an alternative to intensive annual screening. Prophylactic surgery is generally accepted as a cost-effective measure for women between 30 and 35 years old [72]. A retrospective study comparing 245 women who had an MMR gene mutation who did not undergo hysterectomy and salpingo-oophorectomy to 61 women who did undergo surgery, for either prophylaxis or a benign indication, reported that endometrial cancer occurred in 33% of women who did not have surgery, whereas no woman undergoing preventive surgery developed gynecologic cancers [72]. Patients who have ovarian cancer related to Lynch syndrome have a survival similar to that of patients who have sporadic ovarian cancer [73].

Homozygous Mutations

Lynch III syndrome refers to patients who are either homozygous or compound heterozygotes for MMR gene mutations, rather than simple heterozygotes. These patients develop malignancies of the colon, endometrium, brain, and hematopoietic system at a very young age in the first through third decades of life (Box 5) [74]. Café-au-lait spots and neurofibromas frequently occur [7]. The neurofibroma gene may undergo mutation because of MMR gene mutation [75]. MLH1 deficiency accelerates the development of leukemia in mice heterozygous for the neurofibromatosis gene [76]. Among children who have neurofibromatosis, MLH1 mutations lead to a higher likelihood of hematologic malignancy [77] and an earlier onset of cancer [78].

A literature review revealed 59 individuals among 24 families with members who had café-au-lait spots and biallelic gene mutations [7]. Among these 59

Box 5: Lynch syndrome homozygotes or compound heterozygotes

Cancer onset in first 3 decades of life

Pediatric malignancies

Leukemia lymphoma

Brain cancer

Café-au-lait spots

If suspected check normal tissue for microsatellite instability. If normal tissue MSI-H suspect biallelic mutations.

individuals 42 (71%) developed colon cancer at a mean age of 32, and 28 individuals developed a brain tumor at a mean age of 16. Remarkably, 2 of these families had only PMS2 mutation, but in 1 of these families it was a homozygous PMS2 mutation [7]. In a study of consecutive children who developed cancer before age 15 years, 6% to 10% of children were homozygous for MMR gene mutations [79]. Among children who had 6 or more café-au-lait spots, 80% had a serious disease [80].

Patients who have complete absence of MMR function present with hematologic and brain malignancies in the first 2 decades of life, whereas those who have biallelic mutations and minimal residual MMR function present with gastrointestinal and endometrial cancer in the third and fourth decades of life [74]. In carriers of biallelic mutations, MSI-H can be found in normal tissue [81]. When a Lynch syndrome–associated cancer is found in a very young patient (<30 years old), normal tissue should be checked for microsatellite instability, and if detected, biallelic mutations should be searched for.

Muir-Torre Syndrome

Muir-Torre syndrome refers to the occurrence of sebaceous adenomas on the skin of patients who have cancers related to Lynch syndrome [82]. These adenomas demonstrate microsatellite instability and MMR gene mutations. The presence of sebaceous adenomas should trigger screening for colonic and gynecologic malignancy and testing for MSI.

Colon Cancer Prevention

Observational studies have shown that aspirin reduces the risk for sporadic colon cancer, but prospective randomized controlled trials have shown no benefit [83], possibly because of the low dose of aspirin used in prospective trials [83]. There are no data among patients who have Lynch syndrome. Nonsteroidal anti-inflammatory drugs, particularly sulindac, have been studied to prevent colon cancer in high-risk groups, such as FAP, but a recent study of sulindac in patients who had Lynch syndrome was disappointing [84]. The investigators analyzed epithelial proliferation as a surrogate marker for carcinogenesis before and after a 1-month course of orally administered sulindac. Such studies have shown reduced colonic epithelial cell proliferation in patients who had sporadic adenomas and familial adenomatous polyposis [85]. In patients who had Lynch syndrome, however, sulindac did not suppress colonic epithelial proliferation, and it stimulated epithelial cell proliferation in the proximal colon [84].

Folic acid has been suggested to reduce the risk for sporadic colon cancer [86] and for colon cancer among patients who have ulcerative colitis [87], but there are no data among patients who have Lynch syndrome. Calcium supplementation has been shown to reduce the risk for benign adenomas and the rate of epithelial proliferation in patients who have adenomas [88], but calcium supplementation did not reduce the rate of epithelial proliferation among patients who had Lynch syndrome [89].

Cigarette smoking was shown to increase the risk for cancer in patients who had Lynch syndrome, whereas alcohol use did not alter the colon cancer risk

[90]. This study reported that a mean cigarette consumption of 24 pack-years increased the hazard ratio for colon cancer to 1.43. This study was limited by the lack of a dose–response relationship and lack of a tobacco history in 236 of the 596 study patients [90]. Patients who have familial colon cancer should be advised to follow a healthy lifestyle that incorporates exercise and a diet low in fat and red meat and high in whole grains, legumes, fruits, and vegetables.

Barriers to Screening

Few physicians follow a systematic protocol to evaluate for Lynch syndrome, even among patients who present with colon or uterine cancer before age 50. Clinicians typically do not obtain a family history for the Amsterdam criteria. Screening for gynecologic cancer is particularly inadequate because of provider- and patient-related factors. In a highly educated population in Northern California, only 69% of women who had HNPCC had undergone screening for endometrial and ovarian cancer, and only 12% underwent this screening as a result of the advice of their gynecologist [91]. In a survey of 2845 women in California's Silicon Valley, 313 were identified as being at risk for familial cancer syndromes, and yet when contacted, less than 25% were interested in follow-up, cancer screening, or genetic testing [92].

A survey in 2002 reported that only 51% of 815 gastroenterologists who were members of the American Gastroenterological Association referred patients for genetic counseling before cancer predisposition testing. When presented with a family history consistent with Lynch syndrome, only 26% advised genetic testing and only 16% advised appropriate screening [93]. Pathologists may not screen for microsatellite instability or immunohistochemistry even when pathologic criteria are present in a patient who is younger than 50 years of age. The pathologist has the additional burden of the cost of the MSI or immunohistochemical testing, which may not be reimbursed by insurance. Even if insurance paid for these tests, the insurance company might inquire about the test results or infer positive results from a subsequent request for genetic testing. Once MMR mutations have been identified, the insurance company might decline further coverage for the patient or primary relatives. In the Netherlands, where there is universal health coverage, 40% of healthy carriers of MMR gene mutations experienced problems obtaining disability or life insurance or a home mortgage [6].

Patient-Related Lapses in Screening

After an index patient is diagnosed with Lynch syndrome, there remain barriers to identify family members who are carriers and to ensure proper screening of affected relatives. Patients may not inform their primary relatives, partly because of their natural reluctance to reveal that they have a life-threatening genetic disorder. If the health care providers take the initiative by contacting family members, this poses a time burden on a busy physician, infringes on patient privacy, and potentially violates doctor–patient confidentiality. Both studies that proposed direct physician communication with relatives of Lynch probands were conducted outside the United States [94,95]. Canadian patients felt that a physician did not have the right to inform relatives without the patient's permission [94]. There may be legal risks to not informing the relatives of a Lynch proband, however. Three lawsuits have been filed in the United States against physicians who failed to warn family members about the risk for a hereditary disease [96]. Even after relatives have been informed of the risk for carrying an MMR gene and the potential of a 70% lifetime risk for cancer, 28% to 40% of at-risk relatives decline genetic testing [97,98].

Among those who accept genetic testing and are proved to be carriers, only about 75% comply with colonoscopy; most of these studies have been performed in Australia or Europe where cost is not an issue because of universal health care coverage [55,99,100]. Finally, less than 65% of female carriers of the MMR gene comply with gynecologic screening in Australia and the United States [99,100]. Relatives may decline genetic testing or subsequent screening because of a lack of interest in prevention or a fatalistic attitude toward the disease.

The current cost of genetic testing for MMR gene mutations is estimated at about $2700, but this cost will certainly decline as technological advances in gene sequencing revolutionize medicine. Complete human genome sequencing currently costs $100,000 but should decline to $10,000 within 5 years.

CLASSICAL FAMILIAL ADENOMATOUS POLYPOSIS

FAP is a dominantly inherited syndrome in which affected people develop hundreds, if not thousands, of colonic polyps that inevitably lead to colon cancer at a relatively young age. It is caused by mutations of the APC gene, a tumor-suppressor gene located on chromosome 5q21-q22 [101]. The APC gene normally blocks DNA transcription that would otherwise lead to uncontrolled cellular growth, helps control cell adhesion, and helps regulate migration of enterocytes [102]. APC gene mutation and protein inactivation trigger the growth of the numerous polyps found in this syndrome. The specific location of the mutation on the APC gene predicts the specific phenotype.

Classical FAP occurs in about 1 in 20,000 live births. It affects both sexes equally. It represents less than 1% of the total colon cancer risk in the United States. It is caused by mutations in exon 15 of the APC gene [103]. Variants of FAP include Turcot syndrome (FAP associated with brain tumors), Gardner syndrome (FAP associated with extraintestinal manifestations), and attenuated FAP (aFAP). Genetic evaluation has shown that 10% to 30% of patients who have classical FAP do not have an APC mutation and up to 90% who have aFAP do not have a detectable APC mutation. One third of patients who have FAP have no family history of the syndrome and represent de novo germline APC mutations [104].

Up to 10% of patients who have FAP eventually develop periampullary cancer. Other neoplasms triggered by FAP include gastric polyps, small intestinal adenomas, osteomas, and adrenal, liver, and thyroid tumors. These associations historically led to the use of eponyms, such as Turcot syndrome and Gardner syndrome, but these associations represent variant presentations of FAP. Other features occurring in FAP include abdominal desmoid tumors and congenital hypertrophic retinal pigment epithelium.

Attenuated Familial Adenomatous Polyposis

Attenuated FAP is caused by mutations in the 5′ or 3′ end of the APC gene. Attenuated expression occurs because these mutations can be bypassed by an internal translation initiation site in the APC gene [105]. Patients who have attenuated FAP have fewer polyps, a later age of diagnosis, and more frequent involvement of the proximal colon [106]. These patients can develop the extracolonic features of classical FAP.

MUTYH-Associated Polyposis

MUTYH-associated polyposis is an autosomal recessive form of FAP. The MUTYH gene is located on the p-arm of chromosome 1. This gene results in the production of an enzyme involved in DNA repair. Mutations allow for an accumulation of mutations in the APC gene that can lead to a form of FAP. MUTYH mutation most frequently results in the development of numerous polyps, typically fewer than 100 polyps, but up to 1000 polyps, and can result in cancer even without polyps [107]. These patients can also manifest the extracolonic features of FAP. Most cancers in MUTHY-associated polyposis are right-sided.

I1307K

This APC mutation, which affects 6% of the Ashkenazi Jewish population, leads to an increased risk for colon polyps and cancer. Ashkenazi Jews are descended from Jewish communities from middle or eastern Europe. Ashkenazi Jews constitute approximately 80% of Jews worldwide [108]. The I1307K mutation is so named because it involves codon 1,307 in exon 15 of the APC gene. This mutation is autosomal dominant, is of low penetrance, and has no detectable effect on APC function, but seems to render the gene more susceptible to additional mutations that can then lead to the development of colon cancer. An individual who has the I1307K mutation has a 10% to 20% lifetime risk for colorectal cancer.

Screening

Recognition of these and other inherited colorectal cancer syndromes is essential to reduce colorectal cancer risks and to advise at-risk family members regarding screening. The diagnosis of FAP is straightforward in a patient presenting with hundreds to thousands of colonic polyps. Suspicion should also be raised when patients present with colon cancer when they are younger than age 45, adenomatous polyps younger than age 40, or multiple colonic malignancies; when patients develop more than 10 polyps in their lifetime together with a positive family history; or when a family has multiple generations with colon cancer and clustering of extracolonic cancers [109].

Screening: familial adenomatous polyposis
Patients affected with FAP and their first-degree relatives should be offered genetic counseling. An affected patient should undergo APC gene testing and if positive, at-risk family members should be tested. If no APC mutation is found in the affected member, additional gene testing is not indicated. If the family mutation is known, genetic testing of at-risk family members can determine if they have FAP. If the family mutation is unknown or the affected family member is unavailable, at-risk family members can still be tested but a negative result in this setting is inconclusive. It is inadvisable to genetically test children before the age of 10 years because it does not change treatment strategy and can lead to emotional and family conflicts [110]. Gene carriers or at-risk family members who have inconclusive results should begin annual endoscopic surveillance starting at age 10 to 12.

Screening: attenuated familial adenomatous polyposis
Genetic screening of patients and families that have suspected aFAP is similar to that for classical FAP. Fewer of these individuals have a detectable mutation, however. As right-sided tumors predominate in aFAP, it is mandatory to use colonoscopy as the screening tool in at-risk individuals.

Screening: MUTYH-associated polyposis
Patients who have FAP or aFAP phenotypes who have negative genetic tests for APC mutations should undergo MUTYH genetic testing. About 10% to 20% of such patients test positive for MYH-associated polyposis (MAP) [106]. Siblings of patients who have MAP should be considered for this genetic test. Children of MAP patients are carriers (MAP is autosomal recessive), and therefore screening of their partners to determine risk for MAP in any future children should be considered.

Screening: duodenal adenomas
Patients should undergo screening esophagogastroduodenoscopy beginning at age 20 because of their high risk for developing duodenal adenomas [111]. The rate of conversion of a duodenal adenoma to invasive cancer is low and therefore the aim of esophagogastroduodenoscopy in these patients is to detect severe dysplasia rather than to eradicate all neoplasia. Adenomas greater than 1 cm or with known dysplasia should be removed [112]. Endoscopic removal of these lesions is often incomplete and duodenectomy must be considered for lesions with high-grade dysplasia.

Screening: I1307K
A person of Ashkenazi heritage who has a personal or family history of colonic neoplasia may consider gene testing. Because these patients are already considered at increased risk, however, knowledge of their I1307 status is unlikely to change the screening guidelines, which call for colonoscopic surveillance at 3- to 5-year intervals [113].

Treatment

Treatment of FAP is surgical removal of the colon and rectum. The timing and type of surgery depend on the severity of the polyposis phenotype and to a lesser extent on the genotype, age, and clinical and social circumstances of the patient. Cancer is rare under the age of 20 [114]. If the syndrome is severe or symptomatic, surgery is done as soon as convenient. If the disease is mild, surgery can be delayed to the mid-teen years.

The three main surgical options are: colectomy and ileorectal anastomosis (IRA), total proctocolectomy and ileostomy (TPC), and proctocolectomy with ileal pouch–anal anastomosis (IPAA). TPC is almost never done as the first operation, except when IPAA is contraindicated. Contraindications include mesenteric desmoids, advanced low rectal cancer, or poor anal sphincter function. IRA has the advantage of better functional outcome, but has the disadvantage of a continuing risk for rectal cancer. Because this cancer risk is related to the severity of polyposis, IRA is a reasonable option in patients who have mild disease (<20 rectal adenomas, <1000 colonic adenomas) [115]. Proponents of IPAA for FAP cite rectal cancer risk after IPA and studies showing equivalent quality of life after the two operations [116]. Technical factors, including the type of pouch constructed and whether it is hand-sewn, stapled, or with or without mucosectomy, have little functional impact [117].

Follow-up After Surgery

Patients must undergo yearly endoscopic surveillance after IRA or IPAA surgery for FAP. Rectal polyps occurring after IRA should be removed if greater than 5 mm in diameter. Random mucosal biopsies should be performed to exclude severe dysplasia even in patients who do not have polyps. Sulindac and celecoxib reduce the polyp load, but do not completely prevent cancers. Long-term chemoprevention for rectal polyposis is therefore of doubtful benefit [118]. Annual endoscopic evaluation of the pouch is necessary after IPAA because polyposis can occur in ileal pouches. The impact of pouch polyposis will not be known until a large number of FAP patients who have IPAA reach 20 years of follow-up, because 20 years is the time for development of most ileostomy cancers. It is disturbing that cancer in patients who have IPAA is beginning to be reported [119].

References

[1] Lynch HT, de la Chapelle A. Hereditary colorectal cancer. N Engl J Med 2003;348:
919–32.

[2] Lindor NM, Petersen GM, Hadley DW, et al. Recommendations for the care of individuals
with an inherited predisposition to Lynch syndrome. JAMA 2006;296:1507–17.

[3] Boland CR, Koi M, Chang D, et al. The biochemical basis of microsatellite instability and
abnormal immunohistochemistry and clinical behavior in Lynch syndrome: from bench to
bedside. Fam Cancer 2007 July.

[4] Boland CR. Decoding hereditary colorectal cancer. N Engl J Med 2006;354:2815–7.

[5] Dunlop MG, Farrington SM, Nicholl I, et al. Population carrier frequency of hMSH2 and
hMLH1 mutations. Br J Cancer 2000;83:1643–5.

[6] Wagner A, Van Kessel I, Kriege MG, et al. Long term follow-up of HNPCC gene mutation carriers: compliance and satisfaction with counseling and screening procedures. Fam Cancer 2005;4(4):295–300.

[7] Trimbath JD, Petersen GM, Erdman SH, et al. Café-au-lait spots and early onset colorectal neoplasia: a variant of HNPCC? Fam Cancer 2001;1(2):1010–5.

[8] Ollila S, Sarantaus L, Kariola R, et al. Pathogenicity of MSH2 missense mutations is typically associated with impaired repair capability of the mutated protein. Gastroenterology 2006;131:1408–17.

[9] Kariola R, Hamel H, Frankel WL, et al. MSH6 missense mutations are often associated with no or low cancer susceptibility. Br J Cancer 2004;91:1287–92.

[10] Lindor NM, Rabe K, Petersen GM, et al. Lower cancer incidence in Amsterdam-I criteria families without mismatch repair deficiency. Familial colorectal cancer type X. JAMA 2005;293:1979–85.

[11] Barnetson RA, Tenesa A, Farrington SM, et al. Identification and survival of carriers of mutations in DNA mismatch-repair genes in colon cancer. N Engl J Med 2006;356(26): 2751–63.

[12] Hampel H, Frankel WL, Martin E, et al. Screening for the Lynch syndrome (hereditary non-polyposis colorectal cancer). N Engl J Med 2005;352:1851–60.

[13] Aaltonen LA, Saloraara R, Kristp P, et al. Incidence of hereditary non-polyposis colorectal cancer and the feasibility of molecular screening for the disease. N Engl J Med 1998;338: 1481–7.

[14] Casey G, Lindor NM, Papadopoulos N, et al. Conversion analysis for mutation detection in MLH1 and MLH2 patients with colorectal cancer. JAMA 2005;293:799–809.

[15] Umar A, Boland CR, Syngal S, et al. Revised Bethesda guidelines for hereditary non-polyposis colorectal cancer (Lynch Syndrome) and microsatellite instability. J Natl Cancer Inst 2004;96:261–8.

[16] Herman JG, Umar A, Plyak K, et al. Incidence and functional consequences of hMLH1 promoter hypermethylation in colorectal carcinoma. Proc Natl Acad Sci 1998;95: 6870–5.

[17] Kakar S, Burgart LJ, Thibodeau SN, et al. Frequency of loss of MLH1 expression in colorectal cancer increases with advancing age. Cancer 2003;97(6):1421–7.

[18] Farrington SM, Lin-Goerke J, Ling J, et al. Systematic analysis of MSH2 and MLH1 in young colon cancer patients and controls. Am J Hum Genet 1998;63:749–59.

[19] Deng G, Bell J, Crawley S, et al. BRAF mutation is frequently present in sporadic colorectal cancer with methylated hMLH1 but not in hereditary non-polyposis colorectal cancer. Clin Cancer Res 2004;10:191–5.

[20] Kambara T, Simms LA, Whitehall VLJ, et al. BRAF mutation is associated with DNA methylation in serrated polyps and cancers of the colorectum. Gut 2004;53:1137–44.

[21] Duval A, Hamelin R. Mutations at coding repeat sequences in mismatch repair-deficient human cancers: toward a new concept of target genes for instability. Cancer Res 2002;62(9):2447–54.

[22] Chang DK, Metzgar D, Wills C, et al. Microsatellites in the eukaryotic DNA mismatch repair genes as modulators of evolutionary mutation rate. Genome Res 2001;11(7): 1145–6.

[23] Perucho M. Microsatellite instability: the mutator that mutates the other mutator. Nat Med 1996;2(6):630–1.

[24] Markowitz S, Wang J, Myeroff L, et al. Inactivation of the type II TGF-beta receptor in colon cancer cells with microsatellite instability. Science 1995;268(5215):1336–8.

[25] Parsons R, Myeroff LL, Liu B, et al. Microsatellite instability and mutations of the transforming growth factor beta type II receptor gene in colorectal cancer. Cancer Res 1995; 55(23):5548–50.

[26] Dunlop MG, Farrington SM, Carothers AD, et al. Cancer risk associated with germline DNA-mismatch-repair gene mutation. Hum Mol Genet 1997;6:105–10.

[27] Halvarsson B, Lindblom A, Rambech E, et al. The added value of PMS2 immunostaining in the diagnosis of hereditary non-polyposis colorectal cancer. Fam Cancer 2006;5(4): 353–8, Epub 2006 July 12.

[28] Hendriks Y, Jagmohan-Changur S, Van Der Klift H, et al. Heterozygous mutations in PMS2 cause hereditary non-polyposis colorectal carcinoma (Lynch syndrome). Gastroenterology 2006;130:312–22.

[29] Jenkins MA, Hayashi S, O'Shea M, et al. Pathology features in Bethesda guidelines predict colorectal cancer microsatellite instability; a population-based study. Gastroenterology 2007;133:48–56.

[30] Halvarsson B, Muller W, Planck M, et al. Phenotypic heterogeneity in hereditary non-polyposis colorectal cancer: identical germline mutations associated with variable tumor morphology and immunohistochemical expression. J Clin Pathol 2007;60:781–6.

[31] Velayos FS, Allen BA, Conrad PG, et al. Low rate of microsatellite instability in young patients with adenomas: reassessing the Bethesda guidelines. Am J Gastroenterol 2005;10:1143–9.

[32] DeJong AE, Morreau H, Van Puijenbroek M, et al. The role of mismatch repair gene defects in the development of adenomas in patients with HNPCC. Gastroenterology 2004;126: 42–8.

[33] German HNPCC Consortium, Muller A, Beckman C, et al. Prevalence of mismatch-repair-deficient phenotype in colonic adenomas arising in HNPCC patients: results of a 5-year follow-up study. Int J Colorectal Dis 2006;21(7):642–4.

[34] Lu HK, Broaddus RR. Gynecologic cancers in Lynch syndrome. Fam Cancer 2005;4(3): 249–54.

[35] Hampel H, Frankel W, Panescu J, et al. Screening for Lynch syndrome among endometrial cancer patients. Cancer Res 2006;66(15):7810–7.

[36] Cai SJ, Xu Y, Cai GX, et al. Clinical characteristics and diagnosis of patients with hereditary non-polyposis colorectal cancer. World J Gastroenterol 2003;9:284–7.

[37] Park YJ, Shin KH, Park JG. Risk of gastric cancer in hereditary non-polyposis colorectal cancer in Korea. Clin Cancer Res 2000;6:2994–8.

[38] Banno K, Susumu N, Yanokura M, et al. Association of HNPCC and endometrial cancers. Int J Clin Oncol 2004;9(4):262–9.

[39] Aarnio M, Sankila R, Pukkala E, et al. Cancer risk in mutation carriers of DNA-mismatch repair genes. Int J Cancer 1999;81:214–8.

[40] Vasen HF, Sanders EA, Taal BG, et al. The risk of brain tumors in hereditary non-polyposis colorectal cancer. Int J Cancer 1996;65(4):422–5.

[41] Ten Kate GL, Kleibeuker JR, Nagengast FM, et al. Is surveillance of the small bowel indicated for Lynch syndrome families? Gut 2007;56:1198–201.

[42] Schulmann K, Brasch FE, Kunstanann E, et al. HNPCC associated small bowel cancer: clinical and molecular characteristics. Gastroenterology 2005;128(3):590–9.

[43] Maul JS, Warner NR, Kuwanda SK, et al. Extra-colonic cancers associated with hereditary non-polyposis colorectal cancer in the Utah population database. Am J Gastroenterology 2006;101(7):1591–6.

[44] Wu Y, Berends MJ, Mensink RG, et al. Association of hereditary non-polyposis colorectal cancer-related tumors displaying low microsatellite instability with MSH6 germline mutations. Am J Hum Genet 1999;65:1291–8.

[45] Wijnen J, de Leeuw W, Vasen H, et al. Familial endometrial cancer in female carriers of MSH6 germline mutations. Nat Genet 1999;23:142–4.

[46] Martinez ME, McPherson RS, Annegers JF, et al. Cigarette smoking and alcohol consumption as risk factors for colorectal adenomatous polyps. J Natl Cancer Inst 1995;87:274–9.

[47] Kikendall JW, Bowen PE, Burgess MB, et al. Cigarettes and alcohol as independent risk factors for colonic adenomas. Gastroenterology 1989;97:660–4.

[48] Neugut AI, Terry MB. Cigarette smoking and microsatellite instability: casual pathway or marker-defined subset of colon tumors? J Natl Cancer Inst 2000;92:1791–3.

[49] Samovitz WS, Albertsen H, Sweeney C, et al. Association of smoking CpG Island methylator phenotype, and V600E BRAF mutations in colon cancer. J Natl Cancer Institute 2006;98:1731–8.

[50] Ashktorab H, Smoot DT, Carethers JM, et al. High incidence of microsatellite instability in colorectal cancer from African-Americans. Clin Cancer Res 2003;9(3):1112–7.

[51] Yang P, Cunningham JM, Halling KC, et al. Higher risk of mismatch-repair deficient colorectal cancer in alpha-antitrypsin deficiency carriers and cigarette smokers. Mol Genet Metab 2000;71:639–45.

[52] Dove-Edwin J, Dejong AE, Adams T, et al. Prospective results of surveillance colonoscopy in dominant familial colorectal cancer with and without Lynch syndrome. Gastroenterology 2006;130:1995–2000.

[53] Plaschke J, Engel C, Kruger S, et al. Lower incidence of colorectal cancer and later age of disease onset in 27 families with pathogenic MSH6 germline mutations compared with families with MLH1 or MSH2 mutations; the German HNPCC consortium. J Clin Oncol 2004;22(22):4486–94.

[54] Hendriks YM, Wagner A, Morreau H, et al. Cancer risk in hereditary nonpolyposis colorectal cancer due to MSH6 mutations: impact on counseling and surveillance. Gastroenterology 2004;127(1):17–25.

[55] Jarvinen HJ, Aarnio M, Mustonen H, et al. Controlled 15-year trial on screening for colorectal cancer in families with hereditary non-polyposis colorectal cancer. Gastroenterology 2000;118:829–34.

[56] DeJong AE, Hendriks YM, Kleibeuker JF, et al. Decrease in mortality in Lynch syndrome families because of surveillance. Gastroenterology 2006;130(3):655–71.

[57] Vasen H, Nagenast F, Meera Khan P. Interval cancer in hereditary non-polyposis colorectal cancer (Lynch syndrome). Lancet 1995;345:1183–4.

[58] Hurlstone DP, Karajeh M, Cross SC, et al. The role of high-magnification chromoscopic colonoscopy in hereditary non-polyposis colorectal cancer screening: a prospective "back to back" endoscopic study. Am J Gastroenterol 2005;100:2167–73.

[59] Lecomte T, Cellier C, Meatchi T, et al. Chromoendoscopic colonoscopy for detecting preneoplastic lesions in hereditary nonpolyposis colorectal cancer. Clin Gastroenterol Hepatol 2005;3:897–902.

[60] East JE, Suzuki N, Starrinidis M, et al. Narrrow band imaging for colonoscopic surveillance in hereditary nonpolyposis colorectal cancer. Gut 2008;57:65–70.

[61] Renkonen-Sinisablo L, Kivisaari A, Kivisaari L, et al. Utility of computed tomographic colonography in surveillance for hereditary nonpolyposis colorectal cancer syndrome. Fam Cancer; 2007 [Epub ahead of print].

[62] Bertario L, Russo A, Sala P, et al. Survival of patients with hereditary colorectal cancer in comparison to sporadic colorectal cancer. Int J Cancer 1999;80:183–7.

[63] Goecke T, Schulmann K, Engel C, et al. Genotype-phenotype comparison of German MLH1 and MSH2 mutation carriers clinically affected with Lynch syndrome. J Clin Oncol 2006;24(26):4285–92.

[64] Gryfe R, Kim H, Hsieh ETK, et al. Tumor microsatellite instability and clinical outcome in young patients with colorectal cancer. N Engl J Med 2000;342:69–77.

[65] Ribic CM, Sargent DJ, Moore MJ, et al. Tumor microsatellite-instability as a predictor of benefit from fluorouracil-based adjuvant chemotherapy for colon cancer. N Engl J Med 2003;349(3):247–57.

[66] Jover R, Zapater P, Castells A, et al. Mismatch repair status in the prediction of benefit from adjuvant fluorouracil chemotherapy in colorectal cancer. Gut 2006;55(6):848–55.

[67] Fallik D, Borrini F, Boige V, et al. Microsatellite instability is a predictive factor of the tumor response to irinotecan in patients with advanced colorectal cancer. Cancer Res 2003;63(18):5738–44.

[68] Arnold CN, Goel A, Castells CR. Role of hMLH1 promoter hypermethylation in drug resistance to 5-fluorouracil in colorectal cancer cell lines. Int J Cancer 2003;106(1):66–73.

[69] Rodriguez-Bigas MA, Vasen HF, Pekka-Mecklin J, et al. Rectal cancer risk in hereditary non-polyposis colorectal cancer after abdominal colectomy. Ann Surg 1997;225:202–7.

[70] Risk of colorectal and endometrial cancers for carriers of mutations of hMLH1 and hMSH2 gene: correction for ascertainment. J Med Genetics 2005;42(6):491–6.

[71] Farrell C, Lyman M, Freitag k, et al. The role of hereditary non-polyposis colorectal cancer in the management of familial ovarian cancer. Genet Med 2006;8(10):653–7.

[72] Scmeler KM, Lynch HT, Chen LM, et al. Prophylactic surgery to reduce the risk of gynecologic cancers in the Lynch syndrome. N Engl J Med 2006;354:261–9.

[73] Crijnen TE, Janssen-Heijnen ML, Gelderblom H, et al. Survival of patients with ovarian cancer due to mismatch repair defect. Fam Cancer 2005;4(4):301–5.

[74] Bandipalliam P. Syndrome of early onset colon cancers, hematologic malignancies and features of neurofibromatosis in HNPCC families with homozygous mismatch repair gene mutations. Fam Cancer 2005;4(4):323–33.

[75] Wang Q, Montmain G, Ruano E, et al. Neurofibromatosis type 1 gene as a mutational target in a mismatch repair-deficient cell type. Hum Genet 2003;112(2):117–23.

[76] Kort BR. Diagnostic outcome in children with multiple café-au-lait spots. Pediatrics 1992; 90:924–7.

[77] Gutmann DH, Winkeler E, Kabbarah O, et al. M1H1 deficiency accelerates myeloid leukemogensis in neurofibromatosis 1 (Nf1) heterozygous mice. Oncogene 2003;22(29): 4581–5.

[78] Wang Q, Lasset C, Desseigne F, et al. Neurofibromatosis and early onset of cancers in hMLH1-deficient children. Cancer Res 1999;59:294–7.

[79] Ricciardone MD, Ozcelik T, Cevher B, et al. Human MLH1 deficiency predisposes to hematological malignancy and neuro-fibromatosis type 1. Cancer Res 1999;59:290–3.

[80] Poley JW, Wagner A, Hoogmans MM, et al. Biallelic germline mutations of mismatch-repair genes: a possible cause for multiple pediatric malignancies. Cancer 2007;109: 2349–56.

[81] DeRosa M, Fasano C, Panariello L, et al. Evidence for recessive inheritance of Turcot's syndrome caused by a compound heterozygous mutations in the PMS2 gene. Oncogene 2000;19:1719–23.

[82] Jones B, Oh C, Mangold E, et al. Muir Torre syndrome: diagnostic and screening guidelines. Australas J Dermatol 2006;47(4):266–9.

[83] Dubé C, Rostom A, Lewin G, et al. The use of aspirin for primary prevention of colorectal cancer; a systematic review prepared for the U.S. Preventive service task force. Ann Intern Med 2007;146:365–75.

[84] Rijcken FE, Hollema H, van der Zee AG, et al. Sulindac treatment in hereditary non-polyposis colorectal cancer. Eur J Cancer 2007;43:1251–6.

[85] Giardello FM, Yang VW, Hylind LM, et al. Primary chemoprevention of familial adenomatous polyposis with sulindac. N Engl J Med 2002;346:1054–9.

[86] Pufulete M, Al-Ghnaniem R, Leather AJ, et al. Folate status, genomic DNA hypomethylation, and the risk of colorectal adenoma and cancer: a case control study. Gastroenterology 2003;124:1240–8.

[87] Chan EP, Lichtenstein GR. Chemoprevention: risk reduction with medical therapy of inflammatory bowel disease. Gastroenterol Clin North Am 2006;35:675–712.

[88] Baron JA, Beach M, Mandel JS, et al. Calcium supplement for the prevention of colorectal adenomas. Calcium polyp prevention study group. N Engl J Med 1999;340(2):101–7.

[89] Cats A, Kleibeuker JH, van der Meer R, et al. Randomized double blinded, placebo-controlled intervention study with supplemental calcium in families with hereditary non-polyposis colorectal cancer. J Natl Cancer Inst 1995;87(8):598–603.

[90] Watson P, Ashwathnarayan R, Lynch HT, et al. Tobacco use and increased colorectal cancer risk in patients with hereditary non-polyposis colorectal cancer. Arch Intern Med 2004;164:2429–31.

[91] Yang K, Allen B, Conrad P, et al. Awareness of gynecologic surveillance in women from hereditary non-polyposis colorectal cancer families. Fam Cancer 2006;5(4):405–9, Epub 2006 Aug 26.

[92] Manuel MR, Lilja J, Kieran S, et al. Cancer risk assessment in a community setting: prevalence of patients with high risk family histories (abstract). Gynecol Oncol 2007;104(535):15.

[93] Batra S, Valdimarsdottir H, McGovern M, et al. Awareness of genetic testing for colorectal cancer predisposition among specialists in gastroenterology. Am J Gastroenterol 2002;97(3):729–33.

[94] Kohut K, Manno M, Gallinger S, et al. Should healthcare providers have a duty to warn family members of individual with an HNPCC-causing mutation? A survey of patients from the Ontario Familial Colon Cancer Registry. J Med Genet 2007;44(6): 404–7.

[95] Aktan-Collan K, Haukkala A, Pylvänäinen K, et al. Direct contact in inviting high-risk members of hereditary colon cancer families to genetic counseling and DNA-testing. J Med Genet 2007;44:732–8.

[96] Offit K, Groeger E, Turner S, et al. The "duty to warn" a patient's family members about hereditary disease risks. JAMA 2004;292(12):1469–73.

[97] Halbert CH, Lynch H, Lynch J, et al. Colon cancer screening practices following genetic testing for hereditary non-polyposis colon cancer (HNPCC) mutations. Arch Intern Med 2004;164(17):1881–7.

[98] Ponz de Leon M, Benatti P, Di Gregorio C, et al. Genetic testing among high-risk individuals in families with hereditary non-polyposis colorectal cancer. Br J Cancer 2004;90(4): 882–7.

[99] Collins V, Meiser B, Gaff C, et al. Screening and preventive behaviors one year after predictive genetic testing for hereditary non-polyposis colorectal carcinoma. Cancer 2005;104(2):273–81.

[100] Hadley DW, Jenkins JF, Dimond E, et al. Colon cancer screening practices after genetic counseling and testing for hereditary non-polyposis colorectal cancer. J Clin Oncol 2004;22(1):39–44.

[101] Burt RW, DiSario JA, Cannon-Albright L. Genetics of colon cancer: impact of inheritance on colon cancer risk. Annu Rev 1995;46:371–9.

[102] Grady WM, Markowitz SD. Genetic and epigenetic alterations in colon cancer. Annu Rev Genomics Hum Genet 2002;3:101–28.

[103] Russell AM, Zhang J, Luz J, et al. Prevalence of MYH germline mutations in Swiss APC mutation-negative polyposis patients. Int J Cancer 2006;118:1937–40.

[104] Hernegger GS, Moore HG, Guillem JG. Attenuated familial polyposis: an evolving and poorly understood entity. Dis Colon Rectum 2002;45:827–34.

[105] Heppner GK, Trzepacz C, Tuohy TM, et al. Attenuated APC alleles produce functional protein from internal translation initition. Proc Natl Acad Sci U S A 2002;99:8161–6.

[106] Galiatsatos P, Foulkes WD. Familial adenomatous polyposis. Am J Gastroenterol 2006;101:385–98.

[107] Wang L, Baudhuin I, Boardman L, et al. MYH mutations in patients with attenuated and classic polyposis and with young-onset colorectal cancer without polyps. Gastroenerology 2004;127:9–16.

[108] Elazar DJ. Can Sephardic Judaism be reconstructed? Jerusalem center for public affairs. Available at: (www.jcpa.org/dje/articles3/sephardic.htm). Accessed August 31, 2007.

[109] Kaz AM, Brentnall TA. Genetic testing for colon cancer. Nat Clin Pract Gastroenterol Hepatol 2006;3:670–9.

[110] American Society of Clinical Oncology Policy Statement Update: genetic testing for cancer susceptibility. J Clin Oncol 2003;21:2397.

[111] Wallace MH, Phillips RK. Upper gastrointestinal disease in patients with familial adenomatous polyposis. Br J Surg 1998;85:742–50.

[112] Church J, Simmang C. Practice parameters for the treatment of patients with dominantly inherited colorectal cancer (familial adenomatous polyposis and hereditary nonpolyposis colorectal cancer). Dis Colon Rectum 2003;46:1001–12.

[113] Strul H, Barenboim E, Lehno M, et al. The I1307K adenomatous polyposis coli gene variant does not contribute in the assessment of the risk for colorectal cancer in Ashkenazi Jews. Cancer Epidemilo Biomarkers Prev 2003;12:1012–5.

[114] Church JM, McGannon E, Burke C, et al. Teenagers with familial adenomatous polyposis: what is their risk for colorectal cancer? Dis Colon Rectum 2002;45:887–9.

[115] Church J, Burke C, McGannon E, et al. Predicting polyposis severity by proctoscopy: how reliable is it? Dis Colon Rectum 2001;44:1249–54.

[116] Ambroze WL Jr, Dozois RR, Pemberton JH, et al. Familial adenomatous polyposis: results following ileal pouch-anal anastomosis and ileorectostomy. Dis Colon Rectum 1992;35: 12–5.

[117] von Roon AC, Tekkis PP, Clark SK, et al. The impact of technical factors on outcome of restorative proctocolectomy for familial adenomatous polyposis. Dis Colon Rectum 2007;50:952–61.

[118] Lynch HT, Thorson AG, Smyrk T. Rectal cancer after prolonged sulindac chemoprevention. A case report. Cancer 1995;75:936–8.

[119] Church J. Ileoanal pouch neoplasia in familial adenomatous polyposis: an underestimated threat. Dis Colon Rectum 2005;48:1708–13.

Gastroenterol Clin N Am 37 (2008) 73–82

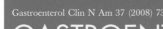

GASTROENTEROLOGY CLINICS
OF NORTH AMERICA

Prevention of Colorectal Cancer: Diet, Chemoprevention, and Lifestyle

James R. Marshall, PhD

Roswell Park Cancer Institute, Elm and Carlton, Buffalo, NY 14263, USA

This article describes primary prevention of colon cancer (ie, interventions that do not involve the removal of diseased tissue or chemotherapy for known colon cancer). Although screening with ablation of adenomas has a significant impact on colon cancer [1], the logistics of screening are complicated [2–4]. These issues are addressed in accompanying articles. This article focuses on preventing the initiation and promotion of neoplastic growth, particularly with dietary measures. A goal of dietary epidemiology is to identify chemopreventive agents and strategies. The effects of diet are analyzed by observational approaches and experimental dietary, nutritional, or chemopreventive interventions.

The adenomatous polyp or adenoma is an important surrogate endpoint for colon cancer [5–7]. The adenoma often remains indolent for years, so prevalence can be analyzed. The adenoma is common among older individuals, especially those more than 50 years old. As many as 30% to 50% of individuals older than 50 years of age harbor one or more adenomatous polyps [8].

The adenoma is usually asymptomatic and is generally discovered only during routine screening. The adenoma is the key premalignant lesion that leads to colon cancer [5,6]. Many, if not most, adenomas never progress to colon cancer, but most colon cancers emerge from adenomas (adenoma-to-carcinoma sequence). As the adenoma is more common than colon cancer and new adenomas develop in individuals who have had previous adenomas that were ablated, studies of interventions designed to prevent colon cancer usually analyze the adenoma as a surrogate marker. This strategy is based on preventing colon cancer by preventing adenomas. The weakness of this strategy is that the formation of adenomas does not guarantee that an individual is at increased colon cancer risk, but this weakness has not deterred investigators from studying the adenoma as a surrogate marker for human colon cancer.

The proportion of colon cancer attributable to genetic syndromes—familial adenomatous polyposis and hereditary nonpolyposis colon cancer—seems to be small, so that screening for these two syndromes is unlikely to substantially reduce the incidence of colon cancer. Although these syndromes are powerful

E-mail address: james.marshall@roswellpark.org

0889-8553/08/$ – see front matter
doi:10.1016/j.gtc.2007.12.008

predictors of colon cancer, they are uncommon and contribute a relatively small proportion to the total colon cancer burden.

OBSERVATIONAL EPIDEMIOLOGY

The epidemiologic literature is replete with studies that claim that various dietary factors affect colon cancer risk, either by reducing or increasing the risk. This epidemiologic literature must be read critically. The possibility of small-sample variation and of outright bias in studies is great. In addition, the study design—the means by which data were collected—may affect the nature and quality of the findings. A historically important study design has been the ecologic method. In this design, political entities, rather than individuals, are the unit of analysis. The cancer risk or mortality of several countries is analyzed together with the typical exposure level within each country; the analytic task is to then correlate each country's cancer risk or mortality with the country's mean exposure level [9].

A better and more common study design is the case-control method, in which a sample of cases diagnosed with the disease is enrolled along with a sample of controls. The prior exposure of cases versus controls is then analyzed. If a given exposure increases the risk for disease, those who have the disease should have experienced greater exposure than the controls [10]. Case-control studies are efficient and are relatively inexpensive to perform.

The cohort method is regarded as the scientifically most valid observational epidemiologic study design. The exposure of each member of an assembled cohort is assessed using a standardized measure, such as a questionnaire [11]. Occasionally, the exposure data are obtained from a biologic sample, such as blood. After exposure data are procured, the cohort is followed over time, and the analysis considers whether those who have greater exposure to a putative risk factor experience a greater incidence of the disease. Because the risk for a particular cancer within a brief period is small, cohort studies must be large, and the cohorts must be followed for several years.

CLINICAL TRIALS

Several dietary hypotheses have emerged from observational studies, such as case-control and prospective cohort studies; in almost every case, however, attempts to experimentally validate these findings have failed.

Because of the ambiguities of observational studies, researchers have increasingly instituted prevention trials to identify means of preventing colon cancer. A key element in these trials is random assignment to one intervention or another, or nonintervention, so that intervention is independent of any other characteristic of trial participants. Experimental and control subjects tend to be alike in baseline height, weight, smoking, social class, physical activity, and other characteristics.

Prevention trials directly test an intervention; they evaluate whether dietary, nutritional, or chemopreventive intervention alters the risk for an individual. Observational studies merely focus on the association between dietary practice or nutrient exposure and risk for disease (ie, whether variance in practice or exposure predicts elevated or diminished disease risk). Analyses based on cross-sectional variance in practice assume that changing an individual's exposure can alter individual risk. If, for example, greater red meat consumption predicts elevated risk for colon cancer, individuals who have above-average intake should decrease their colon cancer risk by decreasing their red meat consumption. This assumption, although reasonable, is largely unproved. Furthermore, the length of time required for the risk to change is generally unknown and would be daunting to accurately specify empirically.

A complication of prevention trials involving altered behavior or environmental exposure is that they often cannot be administered under conditions of blinding: subjects know whether they are assigned to an intervention. In addition, behavioral change is difficult to implement and to maintain long term. The Polyp Prevention Trial required subjects to adopt and maintain a dietary change for 4 years [12]. Recidivism among experimental subjects diminishes the differences between them and control subjects. Behavioral changes rarely happen in isolation. The goal of experiments is often to identify the impact of a single change, such as smoking cessation, increased physical activity, or a dietary change.

DIET AND COLON CANCER PREVENTION

The analysis of dietary data is highly complex. Hundreds of food items are commonly consumed in Western societies, and the number of dietary elements—macronutrients, micronutrients, and minerals—extracted from foods, is in the thousands. Analysis of these items is therefore complex.

The Western Diet: Fat and Fiber

Dr. Burkitt [13] observed in 1971 that the diets and stools of the native peoples of South Africa were much different from those of Westerners and they had a different incidence of colon cancer. He proposed that the high fiber content of these peoples could protect against colon cancer. Formal analyses of ecologic data revealed strong positive associations of dietary fat, and strong negative associations of dietary fiber, with colon cancer risk [9]. An early case-control study indicated that a history of elevated dietary fat intake increased risk [14]. Although a study based on a large, hospital-based sample of cases and controls provided no evidence that dietary fat was associated with increased risk [15], an equally large and well-executed case-control analysis revealed a strong association of dietary fat with colon cancer risk [16]. One of the best studies of diet and colon cancer, the prospective Nurses Health Study, indicated that dietary fiber does not affect the risk for subsequent colon cancer [17]. Although some fruits and vegetables, which contribute fiber to the diet, may be protective, dietary fiber alone seems to have no impact on colon cancer risk [17].

Alberts and colleagues [18] directly tested Burkitt's provocative hypothesis in a double-blind, placebo-controlled clinical prevention trial. They randomized 1429 patients who had adenoma to a high-fiber versus a low-fiber cereal supplement. Compliance with the study protocol was high. Recurrence rates among experimental and placebo subjects were virtually identical. Although experimental subjects were slightly less likely than placebo patients to take their supplement, adjustment for imperfect compliance made no difference; assignment to the high-fiber supplement did not affect the risk for recurrence.

Although interest in the role of dietary fat and fiber in the genesis of colon cancer has persisted, the accumulated evidence has been unconvincing. The strongest of the cohort studies indicates that dietary fat, per se, does not increase the risk for colon cancer [17,19], but that some foods that contribute fat to the diet, especially red meat, may increase the risk [19].

Fruit and Vegetable Consumption

The analysis by Graham and colleagues [15] indicated that intake of cruciferous vegetables, such as broccoli, cabbage, and cauliflower, decreased the cancer risk. A subsequent report by Graham and colleagues [20], with a more detailed dietary assessment, showed cases consumed fewer fruits and vegetables than controls. Nonetheless, no association between cruciferous vegetable consumption and risk was observed. A recently published compendium of case-control studies indicated that cruciferous vegetable consumption was associated with a modest (15%) decrease in colon cancer risk [21]. Cohort and prospective studies provide stronger evidence that dietary cruciferous vegetable intake decreases the colon cancer risk by approximately 25% [21]. The evidence regarding colon cancer protection is stronger for cruciferous than for other vegetables. A meta-analysis of case-control studies suggests that fruit and vegetable consumption in general is associated with a slight decrease in the risk for colon cancer [22]. For example, fruit consumption is associated with a 13% decrease in colon cancer risk, and vegetable consumption is associated with a 40% decrease. The strength of the association is, however, variable. Furthermore, the cohort evidence is less compelling [22,23].

The Polyp Prevention Trial constitutes an important attempt to analyze the effect of dietary intervention among patients who have adenomatous polyps in preventing polyp recurrence [12,24]. The intervention achieved statistically significant changes in dietary practice, whereas the diets of the control subjects did not change, as confirmed by analysis of blood tests [12]. Nevertheless, dietary intervention had no impact on the recurrence of adenomatous polyps compared with control subjects, including the total number of adenomas, the number of adenomas by site, or the number of high-risk or advanced adenomas [12]. A 17-year follow-up revealed no impact of this 4-year dietary intervention on the total adenoma rate or colon cancer risk [25]. The Women's Health Initiative dietary intervention trial reported similarly disappointing results [26]. In this randomized trial of dietary intervention of some 48,000 women followed for an average of more than 8 years, the subsequent risk for colon cancer for experimental and control patients was virtually identical [26].

Antioxidants

There is excellent evidence that oxidative stress contributes to the risks for chronic diseases, including cancers [27]. Whether this mechanism is important in colorectal cancer is not completely clear. It was hoped that antioxidant dietary constituents, including vitamins C and E and carotenoids, might protect against oxidative stress and thereby decrease cancer risk [28]. An important interventional trial reported no evidence of reduction of the risk for adenoma recurrence from administration of beta carotene and vitamins C and E, however [29]. Compliance with study medications, as reflected by blood nutrient levels, was extremely high.

NONSTEROIDAL ANTI-INFLAMMATORY DRUGS

Interest in the use of nonsteroidal anti-inflammatory drugs stemmed from the observation that individuals who chronically used large amounts of aspirin had decreased mortality from colorectal cancer [30]. This finding was supported by other studies [31–33]. Subsequent reports based on clinical trials have generally supported this observation. In a study of 635 patients randomized to receive either 325 mg/d of aspirin or placebo after colorectal cancer surgery, the relative risk for adenoma among those randomized to aspirin was approximately 0.65 [32]. In a study of 1121 patients who had a history of adenoma randomized to receive placebo, 81 mg aspirin, or 325 mg aspirin daily, the relative risk for adenoma recurrence was 0.81 in the 81 mg group and 0.96 in the 325 mg group [34]. Why 81 mg/d of aspirin significantly decreased adenoma recurrence, while 325 mg/d did not, is puzzling [34]. Although these results are encouraging, the use of aspirin as a chemopreventive agent entails risks: as an anticoagulant it can lead to excessive bleeding, and as an inhibitor of cyclooxygenase 1 activity it can lead to intestinal bleeding. Other anti-inflammatory drugs were therefore studied [35,36]. These agents unfortunately have cardiovascular toxicity that renders them unsuitable for chemoprevention [37].

SELENIUM

The trial by Clark and colleagues [38] of selenium supplementation among patients who had nonmelanoma skin cancer was partly motivated by ecologic data indicating that regions of the United States where ambient soil selenium levels were low had elevated risks for several cancers. This intervention resulted in a nearly 50% decrease in colon cancer risk among patients receiving selenium supplementation; unfortunately, the statistical significance of the decrease in risk was marginal because of the small number of patients in the study who developed colon cancer. Extended follow-up analysis of the data reveals that assignment to selenium supplementation was also associated with a decreased risk for developing adenomatous polyps [39]. Numerous animal studies have shown that selenium has antineoplastic properties [40]. In addition observational studies have revealed decreases in colon cancer risk among those who have elevated selenium intake [41].

CALCIUM

Observational epidemiologic evidence suggests that calcium protects against colon cancer [42]. The [34] randomized, controlled trial reported by Baron and colleagues [34] provided even stronger evidence. The relative risk for adenoma recurrence among those assigned to receive calcium was 0.85, and the ratio of adenomatous polyps among experimental versus control patients was 0.76. Both effects were statistically significant. The decline in adenoma risk associated with calcium supplementation was only 15%, however. Whether this small decrease would justify widespread calcium supplementation is debatable. No subgroup of subjects was affected enough to alter the standard colon cancer screening schedule.

FOLATE

Evidence derived from in vitro and in vivo models strongly suggests that folate should protect against colon cancer [43,44]. Baron and colleagues [45] in a cohort study conducted within a randomized clinical trial found that folate intake at baseline was associated with a statistically significant reduced risk for adenoma recurrence. Adjustment for likely confounders, for total energy, and for dietary fiber intake, however, obliterated this effect. On the other hand, alcohol intake, which diminishes folate levels, was associated with a greater than twofold increase in adenoma recurrence [46]. The reduction in risk with folate may be as high as 40%. In a study of male health professionals, a high dietary folate intake was weakly associated with a decreased risk for colon cancer [47]. A more recent study found that folate intake for more than 15 years was associated with a sizeable, statistically significant decrease in colon cancer. In these studies, alcohol intake was again associated with increased colon cancer risk, and this association was stronger than that for folate.

LIFESTYLE

Several aspects of lifestyle, including body mass, physical activity, and smoking, have been analyzed as possible colon cancer risk factors.

Body Mass

Elevated body mass, or obesity, partly represents energy balance, or the juxtaposition of energy intake and expenditure. On an ecologic level, Western industrialized countries have increased obesity and an increased colon cancer risk. The epidemiologic literature is relatively consistent: case-control and prospective studies show obesity is associated with increased risk [42]. The mechanisms of the association are not well understood; hormonal factors for women or insulin metabolism have been proposed [42]. Alteration of inflammatory processes is possible; Martinez and colleagues [48] reported a strongly positive association between body mass index and prostaglandin E2, a marker of inflammation and inflammatory responses. There have been no experimental evaluations of this association or whether weight loss can decrease colon cancer risk.

Physical Activity

Physical activity, a component of energy expenditure and energy balance, may by itself be associated with decreased colon cancer risk [42]. Much of the recent literature has emphasized recreational physical activity [48,49]. The mechanisms of this effect are poorly understood. Martinez and colleagues [48] showed a statistically significant, positive association between rectal mucosal prostaglandin E2 levels and body mass, and a negative association between rectal mucosal prostaglandin E2 levels and physical activity.

Smoking

The pathogenicity of tobacco smoking for pulmonary and urologic cancers and for heart and lung disease is well established and understood. Early studies of colon cancer did not show smoking to be associated with increased risk [50]. It now appears that the effects of smoking on colon cancer require decades of exposure. Only individuals who have long periods of smoking have increased risk for adenomatous polyps [41,42]; this risk may be increased as much as threefold. The increased risk for colon cancer may take even longer to manifest; competing causes of death may diminish the impact of smoking.

The association between smoking and colon cancer is not as strong as those between smoking and pulmonary cancers. Nonetheless, the effect is significant, and attempts to prevent colon cancer should include control of smoking. The risk for colon cancer among long-term smokers is approximately doubled [51,52]. Smoking thus increases the risk for colon cancer more than any known chemopreventive agent decreases the risk. The mechanisms of this association are poorly understood; carcinogenic smoking byproducts are carried in the blood and could infuse the colon, whereas smoke entering through the mouth could be ingested with food and transported to the colonic lumen.

CHALLENGES FOR FUTURE PROGRESS IN COLON CANCER PREVENTION

Major questions concerning the etiology of colon cancer remain to be resolved. Two major exposure routes are possible: the fecal stream within the colonic lumen and transmission by way of the blood circulation to the colon. For example, the concentration of deoxycholate and related compounds in stool has received much attention [53]. Blood is the major, if not only, means by which compounds initiating and promoting neoplastic growth could be transmitted to many other tissues—breast, prostate, liver, brain. Factors transmitted by the circulatory system could be related to the cause, and hence to the prevention, of colon cancer. Clearly, further understanding of the etiology of colon cancer is needed.

Several options are available to prevent colon cancer. The most important is screening [1,2,4]. The costs of screening are considerable [4], however, and there are at present not enough trained medical personnel to screen the entire eligible population of the United States.

Diet may play a moderate role in colon cancer risk, but the effect of diet may be underestimated because of imprecise dietary measurements attributable to the complexity of the diet [54,55]. Short-term trials that alter intermediate biomarkers that are more sensitive than the adenoma to interventions may be necessary. The same logic needs to be applied to chemoprevention. Nonsteroidal anti-inflammatory drugs, calcium, and selenium have some individual effects that could be potentiated if added together. The current evidence is that the combined effect of all three agents is modest, compared with the effects of screening, or even those of smoking cessation.

References

[1] Mandel JS, Church TR, Bond JH, et al. The effect of fecal occult-blood screening on the incidence of colorectal cancer. N Engl J Med 2000;343(22):1603–7.

[2] Byers T, Levin B, Rothenberger D, et al. For the American Cancer Society Detection and Treatment Advisory Group on Colorectal Cancer. American cancer society guidelines for screening and surveillance for early detection of colorectal polyps and cancer: update 1997. CA Cancer J Clin 1997;47(3):154–60.

[3] Lance P, Grossman S, Marshall JR. Screening for colorectal cancer. Semin Gastrointest Dis 1992;3:22–33.

[4] Marshall JR, Fay D, Lance P. Potential costs of flexible sigmoidoscopy-based colorectal cancer screening. Gastroenterology 1996;111(6):1411–7.

[5] Schatzkin A, Freedman LS, Schiffman MH, et al. Validation of intermediate end points in cancer research. J Natl Cancer Inst 1990;82(22):1746–52.

[6] Schatzkin A, Freedman LS, Dorgan J, et al. Surrogate end points in cancer research: a critique. Cancer Epidemiol Biomarkers Prev 1996;5(12):947–53.

[7] Vogelstein B, Fearon ER, Hamilton SR, et al. Genetic alterations during colorectal-tumor development. N Engl J Med 1988;319(9):525–32.

[8] Schatzkin A, Freedman LS, Dawsey S, et al. Interpreting precursor studies: what polyp trials tell us about large bowel cancer. J Natl Cancer Inst 1994;86:1053–7.

[9] Winder EL, Reddy BS. Metabolic epidemiology of colorectal cancer. Cancer 1974;34:801–6.

[10] Cornfield J. A statistical problem arising from retrospective studies. In: Neyman JE, editor. Proceedings of the third Berkeley symposium. Berkeley (CA): University of California Press; 1956. p. 135–48.

[11] Willett WC, Stampfer MJ, Colditz GA, et al. Dietary fat and the risk of breast cancer. N Engl J Med 1987;316(1):22–8.

[12] Schatzkin A, Lanza E, Corle D, et al. Lack of effect of a low-fat, high-fiber diet on the recurrence of colorectal adenomas: the polyp prevention trial study group. N Engl J Med 2000;342(16):1149–55.

[13] Burkitt DP. Epidemiology of cancer of the colon and rectum. Cancer 1971;28:3–13.

[14] Wynder EL. Amount and type of fat/fiber in nutritional carcinogenesis. Prev Med 1987;16:451–9.

[15] Graham S, Dayal H, Swanson M, et al. Diet in the epidemiology of cancer of the colon and rectum 79. J Natl Cancer Inst 1978;61:709–14.

[16] Howe GR, Miller AB, Jain M, et al. Dietary factors in relation to the etiology of colorectal cancer. Cancer Detect Prev 1982;5:331–4.

[17] Fuchs CS, Giovannucci EL, Colditz GA, et al. Dietary fiber and the risk of colorectal cancer and adenoma in women. N Engl J Med 1999;340(3):169–76.

[18] Alberts DS, Martinez ME, Roe DJ, et al. Lack of effect of a high-fiber cereal supplement on the recurrence of colorectal adenomas. N Engl J Med 2000;342(16):1156–62.

[19] Willett WC, Stampfer MJ, Colditz GA, et al. Relation of meat, fat, and fiber intake to the risk of colon cancer in a prospective study among women. N Engl J Med 1990;323(24): 1664–72.

[20] Graham S, Marshall J, Haughey B, et al. Dietary epidemiology of cancer of the colon in western New York. Am J Epidemiol 1988;128(3):490–503.

[21] International Agency for Research on Cancer. Cruciferous vegetables, isothiocyanates and indoles. Lyon (France): IARC Press; 2004.

[22] International Agency for Research on Cancer. Fruit and vegetables. Lyon (France): IARC Press; 2003.

[23] Michels KB, Giovannucci E, Joshipura KJ, et al. Prospective study of fruit and vegetable consumption and incidence of colon and rectal cancers. J Natl Cancer Inst 2000;92(21): 1740–52.

[24] Schatzkin A, Lanza E, Freedman LS, et al. The polyp prevention trial I: rationale, design, recruitment, and baseline participant characteristics. Cancer Epidemiol Biomarkers Prev 1996;5:375–83.

[25] Schatzkin A, Mouw T, Park Y, et al. Dietary fiber and whole-grain consumption in relation to colorectal cancer in the NIH-AARP diet and health study. Am J Clin Nutr 2007;85(5): 1353–60.

[26] Beresford SAA, Johnson KC, Ritenbaugh C, et al. Low-fat dietary pattern and risk of colorectal cancer the Women's Health Initiative Randomized Controlled Dietary Modification Trial. JAMA 2006;295(6):643–54.

[27] Institute of Medicine (IOM). Dietary reference intakes for vitamin C, vitamin E, selenium, and carotenoids. Washington (DC): National Academy Press; 2000.

[28] Block G, Subar AF. Estimates of nutrient intake from a food frequency questionnaire: the 1987 National Health Interview Survey. J Am Diet Assoc 1992;92(8):969–77.

[29] Greenberg ER, Baron JA, Tosteson TD, et al. A clinical trial of antioxidant vitamins to prevent colorectal adenoma. N Engl J Med 1994;331(3):141–7.

[30] Thun MJ, Calle EE, Namboodiri MM, et al. Risk factors for fatal colon cancer in a large prospective study. J Natl Cancer Inst 1992;84(19):1491–500.

[31] Neugut AI, Jacobson JS, De Vivo I. Epidemiology of colorectal adenomatous polyps. Cancer Epidemiol Biomarkers Prev 1993;2:159–76.

[32] Peipins LA, Sandler RS. Epidemiology of colorectal adenomas. Epidemiol Rev 1994;16: 273–97.

[33] Arber N. Do NSAIDs prevent colorectal cancer? Can J Gastroenterol 2000;14:299–307.

[34] Baron JA, Cole BF, Sandler RS, et al. A randomized trial of aspirin to prevent colorectal adenomas. N Engl J Med 2003;348(10):891–9.

[35] Steinbach G, Lynch PM, Phillips RKS, et al. The effect of celecoxib, a cyclooxygenase-2 inhibitor, in familial adenomatous polyposis. N Engl J Med 2000;342:1946–52.

[36] Gupta RA, Dubois RN. Colorectal cancer prevention and treatment by inhibition of cyclooxygenase-2. Nat Rev Cancer 2001;1:11–21.

[37] Bertagnolli MM, Eagle CJ, Zauber AG, et al. Celecoxib for the prevention of sporadic colorectal adenomas. N Engl J Med 2006;355(9):873–84.

[38] Clark LC, Combs GF, Turnbull BW, et al. Effects of selenium supplementation for cancer prevention in patients with carcinoma of the skin. A randomized controlled trial. JAMA 1996;276(24):1957–63.

[39] Reid ME, Duffield-Lillico AJ, Sunga A, et al. Selenium supplementation and colorectal adenomas: Analysis of the nutritional prevention of cancer trial. International Journal of Cancer 2006;118:1777–81.

[40] Combs GF, Combs SB. The role of selenium in nutrition. New York: Academic Press; 1986.

[41] Martinez ME, Marshall JR, et al. Environmental and life style issues in colorectal cancer. In: Levin B, Kelsen DP, Daly JM, editors. Gastrointestinal oncology: principles and practices. Philadelphia: Lippincott Williams and Wilkins; 2002. p. 665–83.

[42] Giovannucci E, Wu K. Cancers of the colon and rectum. In: Schottenfeld D, Fraumeni JF, editors. Cancer epidemiology and prevention. 3rd edition. New York: Oxford; 2006. p. 809–29.

[43] Kim YI, Christman JK, Fleet JC, et al. Moderate folate deficiency does not cause global hypomethylation of hepatic and colonic DNA of c-myc-specific hypomethylation of colonic DNA in rats. Am J Clin Nutr 1995;61(5):1083–90.

[44] Choi SW, Mason JB. Folate and carcinogenesis: an integrated scheme. J Nutr 2000;130: 129–32.

[45] Baron JA, Sandler RS, Haile RW, et al. Folate intake, alcohol consumption, cigarette smoking, and risk of colorectal adenomas 371. J Natl Cancer Inst 1998;90(1):57–62.

[46] Giovannucci E, Stampfer MJ, Colditz GA, et al. Folate, methionine, and alcohol intake and risk of colorectal adenoma 75. J Natl Cancer Inst 1993;85:875–84.

[47] Giovannucci E, Rimm EB, Ascherio A, et al. Alcohol, low-methionine–low-folate diets, and risk of colon cancer in men. J Natl Cancer Inst 1995;87(4):265–73.

[48] Martinez EM, Heddens D, Earnest DL, et al. Physical activity, body mass index, and prostaglandin E2 levels in rectal mucosa. J Natl Cancer Inst 1999;91(11):950–3.

[49] Martinez EM, Giovannucci E, Spiegelman D, et al. Leisure-time physical activity, body size, and colon cancer in women. J Natl Cancer Inst 1997;89(13):948–55.

[50] Doll R, Peto R. Mortality in relation to smoking: 20 years' observations on male British doctors. Br Med J 1976;273(ii):1525–36.

[51] Giovannucci E, Colditz GA, Stampfer MJ, et al. A prospective study of cigarette smoking and risk of colorectal adenoma and colorectal cancer in U.S. women [see comments]. J Natl Cancer Inst 1994;86(3):192–9.

[52] Giovannucci E, Rimm EB, Stampfer MJ, et al. A prospective study of cigarette smoking and risk of colorectal adenoma and colorectal cancer in U.S. men [see comments]. J Natl Cancer Inst 1994;86(3):183–91.

[53] Marshall JR, Alberts DS. Future strategies for the medical prevention of colorectal cancer. In: Schmiegel W, Scholmerich J, editors. Colorectal cancer molecular mechanisms, premalignant state and its prevention. Hingham (MA): Kluwer Academic Publishers BV; 1999. p. 267–76.

[54] Marshall JR, Hastrup JL. Mismeasurement and the resonance of strong confounders: uncorrelated errors. Am J Epidemiol 1996;143(10):1069–78.

[55] Marshall J, Hastrup JL, Ross JS. Mismeasurement and the resonance of strong confounders: correlated errors. Am J Epidemiol 1999;150(1):88–96.

Gastroenterol Clin N Am 37 (2008) 83–95

GASTROENTEROLOGY CLINICS
OF NORTH AMERICA

Implementation of Colon Cancer Screening: Techniques, Costs, and Barriers

Anthony B. Miller, MD

Department of Public Health Sciences, University of Toronto, 392 Lakeshore Road East, Oakville, Ontario, L6J 1J8, Canada

Colorectal cancer and breast cancer are the only cancer sites for which evidence on the efficacy of screening is available from randomized trials. The trials on colon cancer screening in the United States and Europe used the fecal occult blood test (FOBT) as the primary screen, but randomized trial data are not yet available on endoscopy (flexible sigmoidoscopy to 60 cm), and no randomized, controlled trials of colonoscopy as a screening test are in progress. In an accompanying article in this issue the currently available guidelines for screening for colorectal cancer in the United States are described. In this article colorectal cancer screening is reviewed from an epidemiologist's perspective to provide the theoretic evidence-based underpinning for the role of the gastroenterologist in colorectal screening.

THE THEORY OF A SCREENING TEST

Screening, sometimes termed "secondary prevention," is a major component of disease control, the others comprising primary prevention, diagnosis, treatment, rehabilitation after treatment or disability, and palliative care. Ideally, the control of a disease should be achievable either by preventing the disease from occurring or, if it does occur, by curing those who develop it by appropriate treatment. Completely successful prevention would render treatment obsolete. Completely successful treatment would not make prevention obsolete, however, because there are costs and undesirable sequelae of the disease itself (especially diseases such as cancer, diabetes and hypertension) and of the treatment that patients and society would like to avoid if possible. At present, neither prevention nor treatment is completely successful for most diseases; they will continue to complement each other for many diseases, and screening can be regarded as complementary to either of these approaches.

E-mail address: ab.miller@sympatico.ca

0889-8553/08/$ – see front matter
doi:10.1016/j.gtc.2007.12.015

Because of a strong belief among physicians that "early diagnosis" of disease is beneficial, many regard screening as necessarily effective. This belief, however, is not necessarily true, as explained later. This article describes important epidemiologic considerations relevant to screening for colon cancer.

DEFINITION OF SCREENING

Screening, as defined by the Commission on Chronic Illness, is "the presumptive identification of unrecognized disease or defect by the application of tests, examinations or other procedures that can be applied rapidly" [1]. A screening test is not intended to be diagnostic. Rather, a positive finding is confirmed by special diagnostic procedures. Screening, by definition, is offered to those who do not suspect that they have a disease. This lack of suspicion is subtly different from being asymptomatic. Symptoms may be revealed by careful questioning related to the organ of interest, not regarded by the individual attending for screening as being related to a possible disease.

An ideal screening test is simple, inexpensive, accurate in terms of being positive if disease is present (sensitivity) or negative if disease is absent (specificity), relatively safe, and acceptable to the patient. Some of these desirable features of an ideal screening test are lacking in the currently available screening tests for colon cancer. Two of these features, sensitivity and specificity, measure a screening test's validity. Clinicians, however, also are interested in another feature, the predictive value of the screening test, as a practical measure of test utility. The positive predictive value, the proportion of those who test positive who actually have the disease, is of great interest. False positives, persons who test positive but who are found on further investigation not to have the disease, suffer anxiety and the costs and risks of investigation. The negative predictive value indicates the extent to which a negative test truly indicates the absence of disease rather than being a false-negative test. These attributes of a screening test are interrelated, as illustrated in Table 1.

There is a reciprocal interrelationship between sensitivity and specificity if the test limits for positive and negative can be changed, when a semiquantitative test is used. Maneuvers that increase sensitivity tend to reduce specificity, and vice versa. This phenomenon occurred when rehydration of the FOBT was

Table 1
Relationship between true state and screening test results with derived validity (sensitivity and specificity) and process (predictive) measures*

Test result	True state		
	Disease	No disease	Total
Positive	True positive (TP)	False positive (FP)	TP + FP
Negative	False negative (FN)	True negative (TN)	FN + TN
Total	TP + FN	FP + TN	

*Sensitivity: TP/TP + FN; specificity: TN/FP + TN; positive predictive value: TP/TP + FP; negative predictive value: FN/FP + TN.

introduced in the Minnesota screening trial. Rehydration substantially increased sensitivity but substantially reduced specificity, resulting in an enormous increase in the load on the diagnostic services [2]. Consequently, the European trials of FOBT used nonrehydrated slides, and nearly all organizations that have made recommendations for population-based FOBT screening have followed suit. This example illustrates that in population-based screening specificity should be optimized, even at the cost of some small reduction in sensitivity to reduce costs from screening tests with low specificity [3]. A solution to this dilemma would be to develop a better test with higher sensitivity without poorer specificity—hence the interest in immunologically based FOBTs as successors to guaiac-based tests.

THE CONDITIONS SOUGHT BY SCREENING

For appropriate screening, the disease should be an important health problem. Colorectal cancer fulfills this prerequisite. It is the third most important cancer site, with a lifetime incidence of about 5% in both men and women [4]. The goal of screening, however, is not merely early detection; the main goal is reduced mortality. In epidemiologic parlance, this goal is a reduction in disease-specific mortality, that is, a reduction in the numbers of deaths from the disease in a defined population. This reduction is not equivalent to improving the survival of screen-detected cases: the diagnosis is made earlier by screening, resulting in lead-time bias introduced by screening that automatically will increase survival. In length bias, rapidly progressive cancers tend to present clinically in the intervals between screens when screening is applied intermittently, so that cancers detected by screening will have a better prognosis than those that are not. In selection bias, those who volunteer for screening tend to be more health conscious than those who do not and therefore would have a better prognosis even without screening. Thus even if detection improves observed survival, it is not necessarily beneficial in terms of reduced disease mortality.

In addition, some cancers detected by screening will be fatal despite earlier detection. Some cancers detected by screening would have been cured even if they had presented clinically later in the normal way. Some cancers identified by screening never would have presented in the subject's lifetime, because the subject was destined to die earlier from another cause of death. The latter phenomenon, called "overdiagnosis," has been demonstrated for breast, lung, and prostate screening but not yet definitively shown for colorectal screening.

Colorectal cancer is, however, different from breast, lung, and prostate cancer in that screening, with the appropriate test, can detect cancer precursors, that is, adenomatous polyps. Detection of cancer precursors reduces the incidence of the relevant cancer, as has been well demonstrated for cervical cancer screening and for colorectal cancer screening using the FOBT [5]. Endoscopic screening also is expected to reduce the incidence of colorectal cancer, but this reduction has not yet been demonstrated in randomized screening trials. The disadvantage of screening for cancer precursors is that most detected lesions will not develop into cancer during the subject's lifetime (eg, about 75% in the case of colorectal cancer). Persons found to have nonprogressive polyps therefore will be subjected to unnecessary diagnostic tests and treatment. Furthermore, colorectal cancers may arise from "flat" adenomas that are not detectable by currently available screening tests. As yet it is not known whether or how often this phenomenon occurs. Much of this information will come from ongoing randomized trials of flexible sigmoidoscopy in the United States and Europe for cancers within reach of the sigmoidoscope.

THE ETHICS OF SCREENING

The interaction between a patient and a physician is governed by ethical principles. Patients generally consult physicians for symptoms or for reassurance that all is well. Because screening is promoted by professional and sometimes by lay organizations, patients increasingly initiate the screening in the expectation of personal benefit. This places the onus on ensuring that patients benefit from the screening on the organizations that promote screening and on the physicians who administer the screening tests. It is unethical to promote screening unless patients benefit from these tests. Benefit is demonstrated unequivocally only by randomized screening trials [6]. A major problem is that only a small proportion of those screened will benefit from the screening. In North America, the average man or woman has a lifetime risk of dying from colorectal cancer of 2% to 3% [4]. The randomized trials of FOBT screening on average showed only a 20% reduction in mortality, or less than 1 in 100 deaths. The same computation related to incidence indicates a benefit of 1 to 2 per 100; that is, 98% of those screened by FOBT derive no benefit, and many of them incur risks of harm from diagnostic interventions and inconvenience and expense of the screening and the diagnosis that follows. The physician recommending the screening therefore must ensure that the potential benefits and harms are described accurately. Further, the physician should ensure that those patients in whom an abnormal screening result is reported do attend for diagnosis—and treatment if necessary—and are negotiated through the difficulties in reaching the correct conclusion with the accepted treatment.

IMPLEMENTATION OF COLORECTAL SCREENING

In Europe and Canada, organizations concerned with cancer control established mechanisms to implement screening, and many now are applying these mechanisms to colorectal cancer. They generally follow the principles established many years ago for organized screening programs for cervical cancer [7]:

- The target population is identifiable.
- Measures are available to guarantee insurance coverage and patient attendance.
- Enough facilities are available that perform high-quality screening tests.
- The referral system for diagnosis and treatment of abnormalities is effective.
- There are adequate facilities for diagnosis and treatment.

Although the Centers for Disease Control has established some organized programs for disadvantaged groups, especially for breast and cervical cancer screening, screening in the United States generally is not implemented in an organized way. This lack of a unified strategy results in part from the absence of the health care organizations that are active in other countries, which often are pejoratively called "socialized medicine" in the United States.

Expecting all subjects in the target group to volunteer for screening, labeled "opportunistic screening," has been shown in cervical cancer to be largely ineffective on a population and disease-control basis and to lead to major overexpenditures from unnecessarily frequent screening and investigations [8]. Despite this experience, gastroenterologists in the United States probably will continue to have the implicit responsibility of ensuring screening of referred patients. Clearly, gastroenterologists cannot be expected to recruit people who do not consult them. It is, however, reasonable for gastroenterologists to promulgate screening actively to the public in their catchment area, if opportunities arise (either through the local division of the American Cancer Society, or through the media), and to promote screening actively to family physicians or internists in their area. Gastroenterologists should promote the accepted guidelines and contribute to revisions of these guidelines as new data emerge.

For patients who fall into the target age group for screening, including those referred for other reasons, it is appropriate for gastroenterologists to ensure that their computer system is set up to remind patients automatically of their next screening test date. Some physicians have expressed doubt as to whether mailing screening reminders to healthy people is in accordance with established principles of medical practice. In Canada medical and legal authorities have confirmed that such reminders are appropriate, ethical, and legal. The author doubts that different opinions would be rendered in the United States.

EVALUATION OF SCREENING EFFECTIVENESS

The evaluation of screening effectiveness involves research and operational phases. The research phase depends on randomized screening trials demonstrating whether, under ideal or nearly ideal situations, the screening test is efficacious in reducing disease mortality in those screened and, if a precursor is removed, in reducing the disease incidence [6]. Designs that are less efficient than randomized trials have been used. For example, screening for cervical cancer is believed to be effective, even though no randomized screening trial has ever been performed to demonstrate its effectiveness. It took many decades of effort and controversy to demonstrate its efficacy, however, and therefore randomized trials now are regarded as essential for other cancer sites.

The operational phase begins when clinicians accept that screening is effective and begin to apply the tests. Determining whether screening is effective in practice is complicated. For example, even though trials have demonstrated the efficacy of breast screening in women over the age of 50 years, the reduction in breast cancer mortality now seen in many countries may not result exclusively from screening. Improvements in treatment seem to have had at least an equal impact [9]. The recently noted declines in the incidence of colon cancer may result partly from changes in diet, and the reduction in mortality may result partly from improved therapy.

DETERMINING THE EFFICACY OF NEW SCREENING TESTS

New screening tests may not have had their efficacy demonstrated by randomized screening trials because of insufficient research funding and clinicians' unwillingness to wait for a trial to implement a promising new test. Clinicians, however, should understand the pitfalls in blythely assuming a new test is superior, even if a small-scale study has demonstrated superior test sensitivity and/or specificity compared with an established test that had its efficacy demonstrated in a randomized screening trial. This situation is arising for new immunologically based tests compared with guaiac tests for occult blood and for colonoscopy compared with flexible sigmoidoscopy.

Screening tests tend to identify a spectrum of abnormalities associated with colon cancer. A new, apparently more sensitive test will identify an additional spectrum of abnormalities not detected by the older test. It cannot be assumed that this newly identified spectrum of abnormalities will have the same propensity to progress to cancer as those identified by the older test. Indeed, cervical dysplasia and carcinoma in situ often regress rather than progress to cervical cancer. This situation probably also occurs for colorectal cancer. Forty percent or more of the elderly have adenomas demonstrated at autopsy. A test with improved sensitivity for preclinical cancer or cancer precursors therefore may not have as great an increase in efficacy as might be expected by the degree of improved sensitivity. Indeed, at the extreme, this increased sensitivity might result in an increase in overdiagnosis of cancer and an increase in the number of nonprogressive polyps identified and treated. The only way to determine the extent to which a new test is superior to an older one is a randomized, comparative screening trial using the appropriate end points of mortality for detected cancers and of cancer incidence for detected cancer precursors. Unfortunately, such trials are performed rarely and have not been proposed to compare the new immunologic occult blood tests with guaiac-based tests or colonoscopy with flexible sigmoidoscopy.

Instead, in comparative studies, there is a tendency to compare the new test simultaneously with the currently used test in the same subjects in a single-arm study. Such a design has several disadvantages. If the test currently used as the reference standard has the disadvantage of detecting nonprogressive lesions, a test that failed to detect these lesions might be inappropriately judged adversely. Further, it could be regarded as ethically indefensible to fail to act on positive findings with either test. Although the two tests could be compared in terms of counts of detected cases and their characteristics, one of the fundamental means to assess sensitivity—the rate of interval cancers in comparison with the expected incidence [10]—could not be measured for the two tests independently. The only way to assess each test independently is to randomize sufficient individuals to each test to determine the detection rate at the initial and repeat screens and the interval cancer rate between those screens. This trial design was not used in comparing digital mammography with film-screen mammography in screening for breast cancer [11]. The conclusion that digital mammography is preferable in screening younger women therefore may be false, but without a proper study design the results are not conclusive. This design flaw should be avoided. The same principle can be adapted to compare the sensitivity of conventional versus virtual colonoscopy in detecting cancer precursors. The two tests are administered to comparable randomized groups, and, following established prospectively criteria, appropriately sized lesions are removed. After an interval (eg, 2 years), during which interval cancers are counted and the rates compared, the test that is thought to be more sensitive (eg, conventional colonoscopy) is administered to the two groups. The number of lesions detected larger than the previously established size in the subjects in the two groups is counted. The group having the smallest number of newly detected lesions was administered the more sensitive initial test. It is important to ensure that the administrators for both tests are trained to the same standard; otherwise, what is being assessed would be the sensitivity of the examiners rather than the sensitivity of the test.

Breast cancer screening provides another lesson concerning assessment of sensitivity. A series of breast cancer screening trials beginning in the 1960s has continued, until recently, to suggest a benefit of screening mammography in women aged 50 to 69 years. The sensitivity of mammography undoubtedly has improved during these 40 years, but the reduction in breast cancer mortality has remained fixed at about 20% to 30% [12]. At the same time, the specificity has improved, but not to the degree that would be anticipated if the improvement in sensitivity had indeed been accompanied by an improvement in disease mortality.

WHO ADMINISTERS THE SCREENING TEST?

When a screening test is simple, it is likely to be self-administered (eg, breast self-examination) or administered by a primary care practitioner. For FOBT, a combination of the two methods is used: the primary care practitioner advises the test should be done, and instructs the screenee in the use of the test, and the screenee performs the test. Because of the shortage of gastroenterologists, many screening programs in countries other than the United States will continue to use tests that can be simply administered, such as the FOBT, unless more sophisticated test are proven to be markedly superior.

For endoscopy, a specialist must be involved. Even if an ancillary health care worker (eg, a nurse) actually inserts the endoscope, a professional, the gastroenterologist, must interpret the findings. The use of nurse-endoscopists for flexible sigmoidoscopy was evaluated in the Prostate, Lung, Colorectal, and Ovarian (PLCO) screening trial conducted at 10 centers in the United States [13,14]. In several centers, video cameras were used to monitor the examinations for quality-control purposes. Such an approach is compatible with the theory of screening: a screening test is not intended to be diagnostic but is expected to identify people who probably have the disease. When such a process is introduced, sensitivity rather than specificity is emphasized, so large numbers of false-positive examinations occur. With increased experience, however, the examiner finds it easier to separate the abnormal from the normal, so that specificity improves without loss of sensitivity. This phenomenon occurred with nurse examiners performing screening clinical breast examinations in the Canadian National Breast Screening Study [15]. Although their breast examinations proved as effective as mammography [16], the lure of technology and the pressure from specialist groups resulted in the Canadian Breast Screening programs concentrating on mammography. A similar process may be happening with regard to colonoscopy in North America, as discussed later in this article.

DIAGNOSIS AND FOLLOW-UP

If a subject has an abnormal screening test (eg, a positive FOBT), should this test be repeated for confirmation, or should the diagnostic test be administered? Given that most FOBTs are falsely positive, there is merit in considering a repeat test (ie, a more sensitive FOBT), especially if there is a suspicion that the dietary guidelines were not followed at the time of the original test. If the repeat test also is positive, further investigations are indicated, but if the repeat test is negative, and the subject is asymptomatic, a repeat test in 3 and then 6 months would be in order. The patient may have to be reminded to have these follow-up tests.

Following an abnormal screening test, the current reference standard for diagnosis is colonoscopy, although in the past a combination of rectal examination, sigmoidoscopy, and barium enema would have been usual. Colonoscopy has the advantage of being diagnostic and therapeutic, allowing simultaneous polypectomy for identified polyps. If the lesion is extensive, or if an invasive cancer is found, surgery may be required.

In the flexible sigmoidoscopy component of the PLCO screening trial, 18% of women and 28% of men had an abnormal initial sigmoidoscopy, and another 15% and 7%, respectively, had an inadequate examination [14]. The diagnostic protocol was not specified in this trial; the screening centers reported the results to the participating physician, who then, if deemed necessary, made the referral for diagnosis, which was made in 74% of those with abnormal screens. Subjects who had only small polyps detected by screening were less likely than subjects who had at least one large polyp to have diagnostic follow-up, 69% of women and 65% of men versus 86% and 81%, respectively. Only 6% underwent repeat sigmoidoscopy, without colonoscopy. Of the subjects who had diagnostic follow-up, 1.6% had colorectal cancer, 19% had advanced adenomas, and 31% had non-advanced adenomas.

COST EFFECTIVENESS

The costs of screening include

- Costs to the subjects from attendance for screening, including potentially lost income

- Costs of the screening test
- Costs of diagnostic tests needed
- Costs of unnecessary treatment, if the cancer is overdiagnosed

Additionally, screening involves opportunity costs; that is, the funds invested in screening might have been better used for another health- or non-health–related purpose.

Screening also has a psychologic toll:

- Patients may be embarrassed by the test.
- Patients may experience anxiety about what may be found.
- Health-related quality of life will be reduced, if cancer is diagnosed, and this reduced quality of life is potentially prolonged, because the lead time from screening will ensure that the patient knows about having cancer for a longer time than if the cancer had been detected when symptomatic.

Physical costs to the subject include

- Test hazards
- False-positive results
- True-positive results with no benefit

Offsetting these harms are the potential benefits from screening:

- Reassurance from a negative test
- Extension of life from true-positive detection, providing treatment is effective
- Simpler therapy, if the disease is detected at an earlier stage
- Fewer complications of therapy if the disease is detected at an earlier stage
- Reduced costs of therapy if the disease is detected at an earlier stage

Various techniques can be used to compare the costs of screening with the potential benefits. A cost–benefit analysis has been defined as "an analysis in which the costs of medical care and the benefits of reduced loss of net earnings due to preventing premature death or disability are considered" [17], or "an analysis in which the costs and effectiveness of similar activities are compared with determine the degree they will obtain the desired outcome" [17]. This latter analysis could be used to compare the costs of detecting cancers by two different screening tests. A cost–utility analysis is "an analysis in which the outcomes of alternative procedures are compared in terms of a single 'utility-based' unit, such as 'Quality-adjusted life years'" [17].

The US Preventive Services Task Force [18] noted that among six high-quality cost-effectiveness analyses examining only direct costs, the average cost-effectiveness ratio for screening adults older than 50 years for colorectal cancer with each of the recommended major strategies was less than $30,000 per life-year saved (in year-2000 dollars) [19]. Studies varied as to which strategy was most cost effective, however. The Canadian National Committee for Colorectal Screening estimated that the overall cost per life-year gained from a 25-year screening program using FOBT every 2 years with lifetime follow-up, assuming 67% participation of subjects aged 50 to 74 years, and with a rescreen rate of 93% was $Cad11,907 (ie, approximately $US10,000 in year-2000 dollars). When the assumptions were changed in a sensitivity analysis (ie, increased costs for some procedures), however, the cost increased to $Cad18,074 with 5% discounting (approximately $US16,600) [20]. The committee pointed out that costs increased substantially if screening commenced at age 40 years rather than 50 years. Even though more life years were gained with screening at younger ages, the cost of such screening was greater than $100,000 per life-year saved. Extending screening beyond the age of 80 years did not increase life expectancy significantly.

The differences between these two analyses relate partly to differences in health care in the United States and Canada. In both analyses, the estimated costs were comparable with the costs of other life-saving procedures that are generally accepted. Note, however, that screening entails a net cost, even though some savings accrue from screening (eg, reduced costs of diagnosis and treatment), because of the substantial costs associated with administering screening tests to large numbers of people who do not benefit from screening.

SCREENING OF AFRICAN AMERICANS

The incidence of colon cancer is higher at all ages up to age 75 years in African American men than non-Hispanic white men in the United States, although the rates in African American and white women are similar [4]. The differences, however, are not sufficiently large to justify initiating screening at a lower age in African Americans. In all races, the probability of developing colon cancer in the next 5 years is less than 1% before the age of 60 years and is much lower at ages below 50 years. Therefore, for all races, initiating screening before the age of 50 years is not cost effective.

African Americans, however, probably require targeted education, so that they recognize that they have an important risk of developing colorectal cancer and should participate in screening. This situation is no different from the educational needs for the whole community, although specially designed materials providing culturally relevant examples are desirable.

BARRIERS IN IMPLEMENTATION OF COLON CANCER SCREENING

It takes many years to establish a culture of screening. Papanicolaou smears for screening for cervical cancer became part of standard medical care in North America after many years of public and professional education led by the American and Canadian Cancer Societies. A similar process has been largely successful for mammography screening. Even though educational efforts for colorectal screening began 1 decade ago, they have not been very successful, partly because of the public distaste for manipulation of feces and the discomfort and costs associated with endoscopic screening. In a cluster randomized Italian trial, based on general (family) medical practices, higher compliance was obtained from invitations for FOBT than for flexible sigmoidoscopy

(17% and 7%, respectively) [21]. Compliance with FOBT was higher among the upper socioeconomic group. It would be interesting to perform a similar study in the United States where there might be higher compliance for a specialist-conducted procedure. In the Italian study the compliance levels were very low for both tests, however, and were much below the program's targeted participation level of 70% or more in the at-risk group. These barriers are overcome only if persons eligible for screening perceive it is advantageous to surmount them. Further research is needed on means to overcome barriers.

Several Canadian provinces are attempting to introduce organized population-based FOBT screening programs. From the experience in breast and cervical cancer screening in Canada, these programs probably will be successful only if the full spectrum of requirements for organized programs is instituted, especially mechanisms to identify and recruit at-risk groups for screening. In planning these programs, however, another barrier has been appreciated: the shortage of gastroenterologists to perform the vast numbers of required diagnostic colonoscopies. Special projects now are being planned, including innovative ways of providing incentives for participation, to ensure that the programs reach their theoretic participation and success rates.

THE ROLE OF COLONOSCOPY IN SCREENING

Colonoscopy does not comply with many of the criteria for a screening test. It is not simple, it often is unacceptable to the client (largely because of the extensive bowel preparation required), it is expensive, and it requires highly trained physicians for its application. Colonoscopy, however, is gradually replacing other screening tests in North America because it avoids most of the disadvantages of other colorectal screening tests: colonoscopy is more sensitive and can often be used to administer definitive treatment, especially for adenomatous polyps. There is not, however, unequivocal evidence of its efficacy in reducing the incidence and mortality of colorectal cancer, and no randomized screening trials have been established to determine its efficacy.

Colonoscopy may not be as effective for screening as expected. First, more rapidly progressive and highly lethal colorectal cancers may not pass through a prolonged preclinical (adenomatous polyp) stage and therefore may be missed by colonoscopy performed at the recommended frequency (length bias). Second, colonoscopy may miss flat adenomas, which may have a greater tendency to metastasize than cancers arising from adenomatous polyps. Third, the routine nature of screening, and its lack of interest for many specialists, may result in either less careful examination or in less qualified individuals administering the test, producing a decline in performance quality. Unfortunately, the absence of randomized trial data on the efficacy of colonoscopy for screening will limit the evidence base that specialty organizations, such as the US Preventive Services Task Force, require for promulgating guidelines. In the absence of such data, those in charge of cancer control programs will have to establish mechanisms to monitor and evaluate the impact of the changes in practice currently occurring. The new Canadian Partnership Against Cancer (a federally funded initiative) is attempting to establish such mechanisms.

Virtual colonoscopy, a CT visualization of the interior of the colon, is an alternative to standard colonoscopy. Some initial studies were encouraging [22], but virtual colonoscopy does not seem to be replacing standard colonoscopy, except for scattered enthusiastic radiologists, perhaps because bowel preparation still is required, and a standard colonoscopy is still required for more accurate visualization and for treatment when an abnormality is detected.

The boundaries that will restrict further improvements in imaging technology have not been reached; it is possible that in several years technical improvements in virtual colonoscopy will render screening by conventional colonoscopy obsolete. This development currently seems unlikely to occur in the near future.

SUMMARY

This article has reviewed difficulties in implementing screening for colorectal cancer. For successful implementation, it is necessary to pay attention to the details, especially in program organization. High compliance with recommended guidelines does not guarantee a major impact on the disease. It will be necessary to assess trends in incidence and mortality from colorectal cancer carefully during the next decade to determine whether current initiatives in screening are successful.

References

[1] Commission on Chronic Illness. Chronic illness in the United States: prevention of chronic illness. Cambridge (MA): Harvard University Press; 1957.

[2] Mandel JS, Bond JH, Church TR, et al. Reducing mortality from colorectal cancer by screening for fecal occult blood. Minnesota Colon Cancer Control study. N Engl J Med 1993;328: 1365–71 [published erratum appears in N Engl J Med 1993;329:672].

[3] Cole P, Morrison AS. Basic issues in population screening for cancer. J Natl Cancer Inst 1980;64:1263–72.

[4] Ries LAG, Melbert D, Krapcho M, et al, editors. SEER cancer statistics review, 1975–2004. Bethesda (MD): National Cancer Institute; 2007. Based on November 2006 SEER data submission, posted to the SEER Website. Available at: http://seer.cancer.gov/csr/ 1975_2004/. Accessed June 2007.

[5] Mandel JS, Church TR, Bond JH, et al. The effect of fecal occult-blood screening on the incidence of colorectal cancer. N Engl J Med 2000;343:1603–7.

[6] Miller AB. Design of cancer screening trials/randomized trials for evaluation of cancer screening. World J Surg 2006;30:1152–62.

[7] Hakama M, Chamberlain J, Day NE, et al. Evaluation of screening programmes for gynecological cancer. Br J Cancer 1985;52:669–73.

[8] Nieminen P, Kallio M, Antilla A, et al. Organised vs. spontaneous Pap-smear screening for cervical cancer: a case-control study. Int J Cancer 1999;83:55–8.

[9] Berry DA, Cronin KA, Plevritis SK, et al. Effect of screening and adjuvant therapy on mortality from breast cancer. N Engl J Med 2005;353:1784–92.

[10] Day NE. Evaluating the sensitivity of a screening test. J Epidemiol Community Health 1985;39:364–6.

[11] Pisano ED, Gatsonis C, Hendrick E, et al. Diagnostic performance of digital versus film mammography for breast-cancer screening. N Engl J Med 2005;353:1773–83.

[12] Vainio H, Bianchini F, editors. IARC handbooks on cancer prevention, Vol 7, breast cancer screening. Lyon (France): IARC Press; 2002.

[13] Gohagen JK, Levin DL, Prorok PC, et al, editors. The prostate, lung, colorectal and ovarian (PLCO) cancer screening trial. Control Clin Trials 2000;21(6 Suppl):249S–406S.

[14] Weissfeld JL, Schoen RE, Pimsky PF, et al. Flexible Sigmoidoscopy in the PLCO Cancer Screening Trial: Results From the Baseline Screening Examination of a Randomized Trial. J Natl Cancer Inst 2005;97:989–97.

[15] Miller AB, Baines CJ, Turnbull C. The role of the nurse-examiner in the National Breast Screening Study. Can J Public Health 1991;82:162–7.

[16] Miller AB, To T, Baines CJ, et al. Canadian National Breast Screening Study-2: 13-year results of a randomized trial in women age 50–59 years. J Natl Cancer Inst 2000;92: 1490–9.

[17] Last JM. A dictionary of epidemiology. 3rd edition. New York: Oxford University Press; 1995.

[18] Pignone M, Rich M, Teutsch SM, et al. Screening for colorectal cancer in adults at average risk: summary of the evidence for the U.S. Preventive Services Task Force. Ann Intern Med 2002;137:132–41.

[19] Pignone M, Rich M, Teutsch SM, et al. Screening for colorectal cancer in adults. Systematic Evidence Review No. 7 (Prepared by the Research Triangle Institute-University of North Carolina Evidence-based Practice Center under Contract No. 290-97-0011). AHRQ Publication No. 02-S003. Rockville (MD): Agency for Healthcare Research and Quality; 2002. Available at: www.ahrq.gov/clinic/serfiles.htm.

[20] National Committee for Colorectal Screening: technical report. 2002. Available at: http:// www.phac-aspc.gc.ca/publicat/nccs-cndcc/techrep_e.html.

[21] Federici A, Marinacci C, Mangia M, et al. Is the type of test used for mass colorectal cancer screening a determinant of compliance? A cluster-randomized controlled trial comparing fecal occult blood testing with flexible sigmoidoscopy. Cancer Detect Prev 2006;30: 347–53.

[22] Fenlon HM, Nunes DP, Schroy PC, et al. A comparison of virtual and conventional colonoscopy for the detection of colorectal polyps. N Engl J Med 1999;341:1496–503.

Gastroenterol Clin N Am 37 (2008) 97–115

GASTROENTEROLOGY CLINICS
OF NORTH AMERICA

Screening for Colorectal Cancer

Jack S. Mandel, PhD, MPH

Department of Epidemiology, Rollins School of Public Health, Emory University,
1518 Clifton Road NE, Room 430, Atlanta, GA 30322, USA

I n 1993 Winawer [1] declared that colorectal cancer screening had come of age. Fifteen years later we have not yet achieved the goal of screening most of the eligible population despite the availability of multiple screening tests. Current screening rates in the United States are inadequate, with particularly poor rates in some segments of the population [2,3]. The Behavioral Risk Factor Surveillance System has reported that among people aged 50 years or older only 18.7% had a fecal occult blood test (FOBT) within the prior year, 50.6% had either flexible sigmoidoscopy or colonoscopy within the past 10 years, and 57.3% had one or both of these tests within these time periods [2]. In a national household survey using in-person interviews conducted by the National Health Interview Survey, about 50% of adults older than 50 years of age never had colorectal cancer screening and only 37.1% were current in their screening [3]. This study reported small variability in screening rates according to age and between men and women but reported large variability based on educational level, insurance availability, family history of colorectal cancer, and race, with black women less likely to be screened than white women. Somewhat surprising was the relatively low rate of colorectal cancer screening in the Medicare population despite the insurance coverage available for this screening and governmental efforts to increase screening in this population [4]. Results from randomized controlled clinical trials (RCT) have shown that with current technology, screening can greatly reduce colorectal cancer mortality and incidence [5–8]. The development and implementation of population-based screening programs has so far not successfully achieved what was envisioned in 1993.

In the United States, colorectal cancers represent 10% of incident cancers and cancer deaths [9]. About 6% of the population will develop colorectal cancer in their lifetime. In 2007, there will be an estimated 153,760 new cases and 52,180 deaths from colorectal cancer [9]. Globally, there are about 1 million new cases and about 500,000 deaths per year [10].

E-mail address: jsmande@sph.emory.edu

0889-8553/08/$ – see front matter
doi:10.1016/j.gtc.2007.12.007

In the United States, colorectal cancer is the third leading cause of cancer death among white, black, Asian/Pacific Islander, and Indian/Alaska Native men, but second among Hispanic men [11]. It is the second leading cause of cancer death among American women. In the United States, the colorectal cancer incidence rates are 60.4 and 44.2 per 100,000 population and the death rates are 23 and 16.1 per 100,000 population for men and women, respectively. Rates are generally higher in the Midwest and the Northeast.

The incidence has declined from about 60 per 100,000 in 1975 to about 50 per 100,000 in 2004. The decrease in colorectal cancer mortality in the United States has recently accelerated [11]. The rate decreased from about 29 per 100,000 population in 1970 to about 18 per 100,000 in 2004. The decline has been similar for men and women, although the decline for men began several years after that for women. Overall, the mortality among white men and women has declined by about 40%, but the mortality has changed little for black men and women. Since 1990, the mortality in blacks has decreased from about 30 to 25 per 100,000 population. The mortality has been consistently higher in men than women and since about 1980 the mortality has been higher in blacks than whites.

To further emphasize the importance of early detection, 5-year survival rates are strikingly different by stage, ranging from 90% for localized disease to 10% for distant disease, clearly arguing for early detection [11]. Five-year survival rates are similar for men and women, but are notably higher for whites than blacks; this difference may reflect in part the larger percentage of distant cancers in blacks compared with whites (24% versus 18%). For both sexes and all races, 5-year survival rates have increased from about 50% between 1975 and 1979 to 65% between 1996 and 2003, with a somewhat greater increase for white men and women than black men and women.

METHODS FOR COLORECTAL CANCER SCREENING

The American Cancer Society recommends several screening methods, ranging from stool blood tests to semi-invasive procedures, such as colonoscopy (Box 1) [12]. The recommendation to begin screening at age 50 for people at average risk is based on the age distribution of colorectal cancer rates, which shows a significant increase in the sixth decade of life. There is no specific evidence to suggest that the optimal effect of screening is achieved by starting at age 50 and continuing indefinitely, however. Recently, in the United Kingdom, colorectal cancer screening has been recommended for average-risk people aged 60 to 69 [13].

The guaiac-based fecal occult blood test (Hemoccult) is the only screening test proved to be effective by RCTs [5–8,14–18]. Other screening tests, such as immunochemical-based fecal occult blood tests, although never tested in an RCT, have been evaluated against guaiac-based tests and have performed at least as well, with higher compliance rates [19–23]. Colorectal cancer is the only cancer for which the diagnostic test, colonoscopy, is recommended as a screening test.

Box 1: Recommendations from the American Cancer Society

Beginning at age 50, men and women should follow one of these five testing schedules:

Yearly fecal occult blood test (FOBT)[a] or fecal immunochemical test (FIT)

Flexible sigmoidoscopy every 5 years

Yearly FOBT[a] or FIT, plus flexible sigmoidoscopy every 5 years[b]

Double-contrast barium enema every 5 years

Colonoscopy every 10 years

All positive tests should be followed up with colonoscopy

People should talk to their doctors about starting colorectal cancer screening earlier or undergoing screening more often if they have any of the following colorectal cancer risk factors:

A personal history of colorectal cancer or adenomatous polyps

A strong family history of colorectal cancer or polyps (cancer or polyps In a first-degree relative [parent, sibling, or child] younger than 60 or in two first-degree relatives of any age)

A personal history of chronic inflammatory bowel disease

A family history of a hereditary colorectal cancer syndrome (familial adenomatous polyposis or hereditary nonpolyposis colon cancer)

[a]For FOBT, the take-home multiple sample method should be used.
[b]The combination of yearly FOBT or FIT and flexible sigmoidoscopy every 5 years is preferred over either of these options alone.

FECAL OCCULT BLOOD TESTS
Guaiac-Based Tests

The only screening test for colorectal cancer that has been proved to be effective is the guaiac-based Hemoccult test, which detects the pseudoperoxidase activity of heme. Fecal excretion of heme as a screening test is based on the propensity of colon cancers and adenomas to bleed microscopically. The test must be performed multiple times on multiple occasions to be sensitive, however, because of the intermittent nature of this bleeding. Three RCTs conducted in the United States, England, and Denmark have demonstrated that multiple testing with Hemoccult applied annually and biennially significantly reduces colorectal cancer mortality [5–7]. One of the trials further demonstrated that such screening reduces the cancer incidence [8]. A recent Cochrane Review concluded from a review of the three RCTs and unpublished data from a Swedish trial that biennial screening with the Hemoccult test reduced mortality by 16% overall, or by 25% when adjusted for missed screening appointments [24].

These three RCTs used Hemoccult as the screening test, generally screened men and women between the ages of 45 and 80 years, incorporated some form of dietary restriction, used colorectal cancer mortality as the primary endpoint, and included a biennial test group. The results from all three trials were consistent and statistically significant. In a fourth, unpublished RCT, the Hemoccult test performed on men and women aged 60 to 64 years living in Sweden revealed a similar 16% reduction in mortality, as reported by Hewitson and colleagues [24,25]. A study in which geographic areas rather than individuals were randomized to evaluate the Hemoccult test on men and women aged 45 to 74 years also reported a 16% colorectal cancer mortality reduction from biennial screening [26]. The mortality reduction was 33% for compliers, who completed at least one screen.

Despite the deficiencies that guaiac-based tests are not specific for human blood and that not all cancers or adenomas bleed, the Hemoccult test has consistently been shown to reduce mortality when applied repeatedly over time, either annually or biennially, in an average-risk asymptomatic population between the ages of 45 through 80 years. Several observational studies showed similar results. Immunochemical tests seem to be superior to guaiac-based tests to detect fecal occult blood and would therefore be expected to also demonstrate a beneficial effect.

Immunochemical Tests

Immunochemical tests use monoclonal or polyclonal antibodies to detect the globin protein in human hemoglobin [27]. These tests do not react with non-human hemoglobin or with foods that contain peroxidase activity and are therefore more specific than guaiac tests. They detect only human hemoglobin from the lower, not the upper, gastrointestinal tract [28]. There has been no RCT of a fecal immunochemical test (FIT), but there have been numerous observational studies, including studies comparing an immunochemical test to Hemoccult.

In a paired comparison of Hemoccult and Insure, a fecal immunochemical test, FIT was more sensitive for cancers and significant adenomas [21]. For the FIT, the subject sampled the stool surface by swishing the brush over the stool and then wiping the brush onto the test card, as opposed to collecting a direct stool sample for the Hemoccult test. In a comparison of Insure with Hemoccult Sensa and FlexSure OBT, the participation rate was highest for Insure, which was likely because of the simplified sampling technique and lack of dietary restrictions [19]. Another study of Insure showed that the sensitivity and specificity could be adjusted to increase sensitivity but at the cost of reduced specificity [29]. Quantitative FITs have the advantage of calibration of positivity to adjust the population-based screening program according to the funding level. Applying FIT to patients scheduled for colonoscopy, Levi and colleagues [30] showed the advantages of a quantitative test to determine the cutoff for positivity. The investigators varied the hemoglobin level for a positive test from 50 to 150 ng/mL using three fecal samples and computed sensitivity and specificity for different levels. The average fecal hemoglobin levels increased from normal mucosa through non-advanced adenoma and advanced adenoma to cancer. The fecal hemoglobin level in the most non-advanced adenomas was less than 75 ng/mL.

Screening with a 1-day immunochemical hemagglutination test (Immudia-Hem Sp or HemSelect; Fujirebio, Tokyo, Japan) was introduced in Japan in 1986 and evaluated by case-controlled studies that showed colorectal cancer mortality reductions of up to 80% [31–33]. In Japan, 6 million people, representing 17% of the eligible population, have been screened with immunochemical tests [34]. The positivity rate was 7.1% (N = 430,000). Sixty percent of test positives complied with the diagnostic protocol, which consisted of colonoscopy, or flexible sigmoidoscopy and double contrast barium enema. The colorectal cancer detection rate was 1.6 per 1000 population, with 69% of cancers being Dukes A and 14% being Dukes B, suggesting that the program worked well in detecting early cancer. In a cohort of more than 40,000 men and women in Japan, colorectal cancer mortality was reduced by 72% and colorectal cancer incidence was reduced by 59% in subjects screened with an immunochemical test compared with unscreened controls [35].

Other countries that have evaluated immunochemical tests, such as Korea, China, Israel, Australia, and Italy, have generally concluded that these tests perform better than guaiac tests [22,36–42]. The Scottish Bowel Screening Program adopted a two-tiered screening program using an immunochemical test on guaiac-positive patients that seemed to reduce the number of colonoscopies and the overall cost of screening [43].

The Multisociety Task Force on Colorectal Cancer recommends annual screening using a guaiac test with dietary restrictions or an immunochemical test without dietary restrictions [44]. The American Cancer Society has a similar recommendation, but advises that immunochemical tests are more acceptable to patients and are likely to perform as well or better than guaiac tests [12]. The available data indicate that immunochemical tests perform better than guaiac tests, but cost more.

OTHER MARKERS
DNA in Stool and Blood
Fearon and Vogelstein [45] described early DNA mutations in colorectal cancer, such as K-ras and APC mutations, and later mutations, such as p53 and BAT-26 mutations. Mutations detected in stool DNA have been investigated as a biologic marker for colorectal cancer, but this involves separating minute amounts of abnormal human DNA from normal human DNA and bacterial DNA in stool, amplifying them, and then testing for and detecting the correct genetic molecular markers [46]. Advances in techniques, such as polymerase chain reaction (PCR), assist in this detection. Advantages of stool DNA include that the DNA is shed continuously and can be detected in minute amounts by PCR. Early results were promising. In a pilot study of stored frozen stool from 22 patients who had colorectal cancer, 11 patients who had adenoma, and 28 patients who had normal colons, Ahlquist and colleagues [47] reported a sensitivity of 91% for cancer and 82% for adenomas using an array of DNA markers. These results were not reproduced in subsequent studies; the

sensitivity using all the markers was 50% to 60% for cancer and even lower for adenomas [48–51]. Imperiale and colleagues [50] using a DNA panel of 21 mutations detected only 52% of cancers and 13% of advanced adenomas. Because of a relatively high cost, cumbersome collection process, and relatively low sensitivity, stool DNA cannot be recommended for population-based screening [52,53]. Further work is needed to improve the collection method and develop the best panel of markers to improve test sensitivity.

A recent study by Itzkowitz and colleagues [54] showed considerable improvement using improved DNA stabilization and isolation techniques to better preserve and purify the stool DNA and an improved promoter methylation marker; they reported an 87.5% sensitivity and 82% specificity for cancer regardless of cancer stage or location. Other studies involving small numbers of patients and using blood rather than stool have shown similar promising results, but confirmation is needed in larger clinical studies to develop an appropriate strategy for DNA testing for colorectal cancer and adenomas [55–58].

FLEXIBLE SIGMOIDOSCOPY

Flexible sigmoidoscopy every 5 years with or without annual fecal occult blood testing beginning at age 50 is recommended despite the absence of an RCT demonstrating effectiveness [12,44,59]. Arguments favoring this strategy are based largely on the biology of colorectal cancer and a few observational studies, but such studies generally provide biased estimates of the screening effect [60]. The biology is based on removing adenomas that are the usual precursors of colorectal cancer [61–65]. The reduction in incidence and mortality is unknown. The Prostate, Lung, Colorectal and Ovarian Screening Trial (PLCO), an RCT in which two flexible sigmoidoscopies at baseline and either 3- or 5-year intervals were offered to those in the screened group, should provide data on the mortality reduction from this mode of screening [66]. Only adenomas and early cancers within reach of the sigmoidoscope and synchronous lesions can be detected; this includes only one half to three quarters of all adenomas and cancers in the colon [67–70].

Estimates of the benefit of flexible sigmoidoscopy have come largely from case-control studies [71–74]. Selby and colleagues [71] found screening sigmoidoscopy reduced colorectal cancer by 59% in the descending colon, whereas Newcombe and colleagues [72] reported a reduction of 70% in the incidence of distal cancers in patients reporting a single flexible sigmoidoscopy and of 76% in those who had one or more flexible sigmoidoscopies. Two studies suggest that about half of significant lesions may be missed by flexible sigmoidoscopy screening. In a study of colonoscopy in 3121 adults, 52% of patients who had advanced proximal lesions would have been missed if they had been screened by flexible sigmoidoscopy alone [69]. Imperiale and colleagues [70] in a colonoscopy study of 1994 adults found that about half of patients who had significant proximal lesions had no distal polyps.

No RCTs have analyzed colorectal cancer mortality reduction from flexible sigmoidoscopy combined with FOBT. One study reported a somewhat larger reduction in colon cancer with rigid (not flexible) sigmoidoscopy and guaiac FOBT as compared with rigid sigmoidoscopy alone [75]. Two RCTs found that combined flexible sigmoidoscopy and FOBT detected four to five times more large polyps and cancers than FOBT alone [76,77]. In another trial, however, more polyps and cancers were not diagnosed in patients who had both FOBT and flexible sigmoidoscopy versus only flexible sigmoidoscopy [78]. Hendon and DiPalma [79] found that the detection of advanced neoplasia by flexible sigmoidoscopy alone was 70%, but the detection rate increased to 76% with the addition of FOBT because of identification of proximal lesions.

Flexible sigmoidoscopy screening, if proven effective in reducing colorectal cancer mortality, has some advantages over colonoscopy. It can be performed by primary care physicians and possibly nurse endoscopists in addition to gastroenterologists or other specialists [80]. Based on an American survey, Brown and colleagues [81] found that 65% of sigmoidoscopy procedures were performed by primary care physicians, 25% by gastroenterologists, and 10% by general surgeons. In a recent Canadian study, nurses capably performed flexible sigmoidoscopies to screen about 1800 asymptomatic men and women older than 50 years of age [82]. Positive results were followed by colonoscopy performed by gastroenterologists. In the PLCO Trial some centers used nurse endoscopists to perform flexible sigmoidoscopy with good results based on quality assurance parameters [66].

Flexible sigmoidoscopy screening should reduce colorectal cancer mortality but the magnitude of the reduction remains to be determined from ongoing trials. This screening method does, however, miss some proximal lesions in individuals who have no index distal lesion to warrant colonoscopy [69]. Results vary according to several factors, including gender and ethnicity. Miss rates were higher in women than men [83–85]. Francois and colleagues [86] on follow-up of individuals who had a positive flexible sigmoidoscopy found neoplasms in the proximal colon in 64% of Caucasians, 60% of African Americans, 67% of Hispanics, and 26% of Asians. Asians had a much higher rate of distal lesions compared with the other ethnic groups.

Quality control is essential. In the Norwegian Colorectal Cancer Prevention Study, a randomized controlled trial of one-time flexible sigmoidoscopy, detection rates varied among endoscopists from 36.4% to 65.5% for any polyp, from 12.7% to 21.2% for any adenoma, and from 2.9% to 5.0% for advanced lesions [87].

In a Markov model to simulate the progression of a cohort of asymptomatic average-risk individuals 55 to 64 years of age, flexible sigmoidoscopy screening was more efficient in cost per life-year saved than either FOBT or colonoscopy [88]. In the absence of good data, however, assumptions must be made about the benefit. This model was based on data from a nonrandomized, uncontrolled, community-based flexible sigmoidoscopy screening program. Furthermore, the various models of cost effectiveness are different and none have adequately measured the true costs of a screening program [89]. These studies should be interpreted cautiously pending a better understanding of the effectiveness of flexible sigmoidoscopy screening. Another consideration is the increasing incidence of right-sided lesions with increasing age [90–92].

COLONOSCOPY

The modest increase in colorectal cancer screening between 2000 and 2003 is largely attributable to increased use of colonoscopy for screening that was significant among all populations except for low-income, insured patients without Medicare coverage [93]. Despite no RCTs of colonoscopy screening, colonoscopy was proposed years ago as either a one-time or periodic screening test [84,94–97]. The National Polyp Study in 1993 demonstrated the importance of polypectomy in preventing colorectal cancer. This study showed a 76% to 90% reduction in the incidence of cancer in patients who had one or more adenomas removed [61]. Recently this group reported a 69% reduction in colorectal cancer mortality over the expected mortality in the adenoma group [98].

Evidence of effectiveness of colonoscopy screening is provided by the FOBT trials that used colonoscopy as the diagnostic test and by cohort studies, such as the National Polyp Study and the Italian Multicenter Study, that showed reductions in colorectal cancer incidence among patients who had adenomas detected and removed [61,99]. In a mathematical model of life expectancy with screening, the estimated extension of life by colonoscopy screening is two times longer than that with flexible sigmoidoscopy and three times longer than that with FOBT [100].

Screening by colonoscopy has negative aspects. Even though it is the gold standard, colonoscopy can miss lesions, particularly from incomplete procedures [101–106]. Factors associated with incomplete colonoscopy include increased patient age, female gender, and procedure performance in a private office [105].

In a review of studies of tandem or back-to-back colonoscopies, on average 21% of adenomas were missed [107]. Of these adenomas, 26% were 1 to 5 mm and 2% were 10 mm or more. In a study of 7882 colonoscopies performed by 12 experienced gastroenterologists, including 25% that were first-time screening examinations, the mean withdrawal time was related to detection rates [108]. Colonoscopies with withdrawal times of 6 minutes or more had a more than twofold higher detection rate than colonoscopies with withdrawal times less than 6 minutes (28.3% versus 11.8% for all neoplasms, and 6.4% versus 2.6% for advanced neoplasms). Furthermore, the yield varied greatly among the 12 gastroenterologists, suggesting that some gastroenterologists missed up to half of the lesions, including larger ones.

The highly variable performance of screening colonoscopy by gastroenterologists could be reduced through improvements in technology, such as chromoendoscopy, autofluorescence, Third-Eye Retroscope, and wide-angle colonoscopy, but the time and costs of colonoscopy would increase [109]. For optimal colonoscopy, the colonoscopist should obtain an effective and safe bowel preparation and be sufficiently slow and careful during colonoscopic withdrawal to identify all adenomas. Rex [110] provides an excellent review of studies on colonoscopy outcomes and suggests that suboptimal technique is a significant contributor to missed lesions.

Trecca and colleagues [111] showed that chromoendoscopy detected lesions with advanced histology that were missed by conventional colonoscopy, particularly nonpolypoid, flat lesions. They recommended selection of chromoendoscopy when optical colonoscopy provides clues of nonpolypoid lesions. Stergiou and colleagues [112] showed that zoom chromoendoscopy increased the detection rate of polyps at the cost of longer retrieval time.

Because the lifetime prevalence of colorectal cancer is about 6%, the vast majority (94%) of people who receive a screening colonoscopy do not need it. They incur the cost and risks of the procedure, including anesthesia risks, hemorrhage, and perforation, with no direct benefit. Lieberman and colleagues [69] reported that 0.3% (10 out of 3121) patients had major complications, including bleeding, myocardial infarction, and stroke [113]. Three patients died within 1 month of the procedure. Imperiale and colleagues [70] reported that 1 (0.05%) of 1994 people undergoing screening colonoscopy had a perforation that did not require surgery and 3 (0.15%) had bleeding that required treatment in an emergency department. Dafnis and colleagues [114] found that 0.4% of 6066 colonoscopies resulted in a complication, mainly bleeding and perforation. No deaths were attributed to the procedure. The overall complication rate is between 1 and 3 per 1000 colonoscopies [5,115–123]. Postpolypectomy bleeding and delayed bleeding are probably underreported [124]. In a study of more than 16,000 patients older than age 40 undergoing colonoscopy, mostly not for screening, the serious overall complication rate (procedure-related event leading to hospitalization) was 5.0 per 1000 colonoscopies, with a higher rate for colonoscopies with biopsy or polypectomy compared with colonoscopies without biopsy or polypectomy (7.0 versus 0.8 per 1000) [125].

The benefit from colonoscopic screening is unknown. Initially believed to be substantial [61,99], recent data have indicated that the benefit may be less than originally believed [73,103,104]. Problems of incomplete colonoscopies and frequently missed lesions raise concerns and prompt calls for quality improvement. Chromoendoscopy might help improve the quality of colonoscopy but it increases procedure time and cost. Wide-angle colonoscopy has not yet been shown to improve detection rates [126,127]. Preliminary data on computer-assisted colonoscopy (NeoGuide Endoscopy System) based on 11 patients showed some promise, but more data are needed to determine whether this method reduces colonic looping, improves safety, and enhances detection rates [128].

CT COLONOGRAPHY (VIRTUAL COLONOSCOPY)

CT colonography is a noninvasive imaging procedure that creates a three-dimensional image of the colon by combining multiple helical CT scans with the help of a computer program [27]. Patients found to have a significant lesion must be referred for colonoscopy. CT colonography did not perform well, particularly for smaller lesions, in early studies [129], but a subsequent well-designed study showed it can be excellent if performed under optimal circumstances [130]. This study using three-dimensional imaging reported sensitivities of 93.8% for polyps at least 10 mm in diameter, 93.9% for polyps at least 8 mm, and 88.7% for polyps at least 6 mm. These sensitivities were somewhat greater than those for colonoscopy for the two groups of larger-diameter polyps. The specificities were 96.0%, 92.2%, and 79.6% for the three groups of polyps, respectively. This study showed that CT colonography was an accurate method for detecting adenomatous polyps. An accompanying editorial identified factors unique to this study that could account for the unusually good performance of CT colonography [131]. Cotton and colleagues [132], however, presented results indicating that CT colonography was not ready for widespread use. In this study, the sensitivities were 39% and 55% and specificities were 90.5% and 96% for lesions at least 6 mm and 10 mm in diameter, respectively. Conventional colonoscopy performed much better than CT colonography, with sensitivities of 99% and 100% for the different lesion sizes. These two studies show the potential of CT colonography as a useful screening tool if done under ideal circumstances but expose the significant deficiencies of the test when performed under general practice conditions.

Patients who have significant lesions on CT colonography must undergo optical colonoscopy. Ideally, performing optical colonoscopy following a positive CT colonography on the same day would avoid the patient's taking a second colonic preparation. This plan, however, requires considerable coordination and is not generally done in screening programs.

A meta-analysis of 24 studies involving 4181 patients found high and consistent sensitivities and specificities for polyps 1 cm or larger, but much lower values for smaller polyps [133]. CT colonography detected 96% of colorectal cancers. A meta-analysis of 33 studies involving more than 6000 patients found wide variation in sensitivity among studies particularly related to polyp size but little variation in specificity; the authors concluded that the variability in sensitivity needs to be resolved before recommending CT colonography for mass screening [134]. In a meta-analysis of 30 CT colonography studies, the sensitivity was higher for larger than smaller polyps, two-dimensional and three-dimensional CT colonography performed about equally well, CT colonography was superior to air-contrast barium enema, and optical colonoscopy performed better than CT colonography for small polyps [135]. CT colonography thus performs well in identifying larger lesions, particularly those larger than 1 cm, and reasonably well for those larger than 0.6 cm. This level of performance might be sufficient because these polyps are the more clinically significant ones [136].

The rate of complications is relatively small [137]. Based on data from 50 centers in the United Kingdom representing 17,067 CT colonographic examinations, potentially serious events occurred in 0.08% of the symptomatic patients, with no deaths. Vijan and colleagues [138] reported that CT colonography was cost effective compared with no screen but was more expensive and less effective than optical colonoscopy. Pickhardt and colleagues [139] found that CT colonography with a 6-mm threshold was more cost effective than flexible sigmoidoscopy or optical colonoscopy.

CAPSULE ENDOSCOPY

Capsule endoscopy (CE), a wireless capsule containing a miniaturized camera, a light source, and a wireless circuit for acquiring and transmitting signals, provides about two pictures per second for up to 8 hours after swallowing as it travels through the small intestine [27]. It is an outpatient procedure that can be used to detect lesions in the small intestine, but it cannot take biopsies or perform therapeutic procedures [140]. Its primary use is in evaluating patients who have bleeding that remains obscure after nondiagnostic upper and lower endoscopies [141]. The capsule is typically passed per rectum in 1 to 2 days. It is generally safe, with few complications [142]. Symptomatic capsule retention occurs in less than 2% of examinations.

The interpretation time for a full 8-hour video is between 45 and 120 minutes [143]. It is primarily used to diagnose small bowel pathology, but it has been considered for colorectal cancer screening. In a pilot study, 41 patients scheduled for screening colonoscopy or colonoscopic evaluation of symptoms were also evaluated with CE [144]. CE identified 19 of the 25 patients who had positive findings, and 10 of the 13 patients who had significant findings (polyp >6 mm or three or more polyps). CE detected seven lesions in people who had a negative colonoscopy. Sensitivity of CE for significant lesions was 77%, specificity was 70%, and positive predictive value was 59%. There were no adverse events from CE. These results suggest CE may hold promise for CRC screening but more data are needed.

DOUBLE CONTRAST BARIUM ENEMA

Although double contrast barium enema (DCBE) is recommended for CRC screening, there are no randomized controlled trials of its efficacy, only observational studies [12,145–147]. Scheitel and colleagues [145] in a case-controlled study reported a 33% reduction in colorectal cancer mortality. Rex and colleagues [146] found the sensitivity of DCBE for cancer was 85% compared with 95% for colonoscopy. In a study comparing DCBE to colonoscopy, Winawer and colleagues [147] found that the sensitivity of DCBE (using colonoscopy as the standard) was only 32% for polyps less than 0.5 cm, 53% for polyps 0.6 to 1.0 cm. and 48% for polyps greater than 1 cm. DCBE was positive in 83 of 470 patients (specificity = 85%) who had no polyps found on colonoscopy. Because of its relatively poor performance, DCBE should only be used when colonoscopy is unavailable or contraindicated [148].

The risks of DCBE are relatively low [149]. Only about 1 in 10,000 examinations result in important complications, including one perforation in 25,000 examinations, and one death in 55,000 examinations [150]. Its value for screening and diagnosis has diminished as better technology has emerged. It is still occasionally used because it is a fairly inexpensive and simple test [151].

SUMMARY

Although there are several methods available for colon cancer screening, none is optimal. Colonoscopy screening for the 70 million people older than 50 years of age in the United States could cost $10 billion per annum and exceed the physician capacity to perform this procedure [152,153]. A simple, inexpensive, noninvasive, and relatively sensitive screening test is needed to identify people at risk for developing advanced adenomas or colorectal cancer who would benefit from colonoscopy. The FOBTs could accomplish this, but they are too inaccurate; hence, too many people are referred for unnecessary colonoscopy and too many are not referred for necessary colonoscopy. It is hoped that new markers will be identified that perform better. Until then we fortunately have a variety of screening strategies that do work.

References

[1] Winawer SJ. Colorectal cancer screening comes of age. N Engl J Med 1993;328: 1416–7.

[2] Centers for Disease Control and Prevention. Increased use of colorectal cancer test: United States, 2002 and 2004. MMWR Morb Mortal Wkly Rep 2006;55:308–11.

[3] Peterson NB, Murff HJ, Ness RM, et al. Colorectal cancer screening among men and women in the United States. J Womens Health (Larchmt) 2007;16:57–65.

[4] Schenck AP, Peacock S, Pignone M, et al. Increasing colorectal cancer testing: translating physician interventions into population-based practice. Health Care Financ Rev 2006;27: 25–35.

[5] Mandel JS, Bond JH, Church TR, et al. Reducing mortality from colorectal cancer by screening for fecal occult blood. N Engl J Med 1993;28:1365–71.

[6] Kronborg O, Fenger C, Olsen J, et al. Randomised study of screening for colorectal cancer with faecal-occult-blood test. Lancet 1996;348:1467–71.

[7] Hardcastle JD, Chamberlain JO, Robinson MH, et al. Randomised controlled trial of faecal-occult-blood screening for colorectal cancer. Lancet 1996;348:1472–7.

[8] Mandel JS, Church TR, Bond JH, et al. The effect of fecal occult-blood screening on the incidence of colorectal cancer. N Engl J Med 2000;343:1603–7.

[9] Jemal A, Siegel R, Ward E, et al. Cancer statistics, 2007. CA Cancer J Clin 2007;57: 43–66.

[10] Shibuya K, Mathers CD, Boschi-Pinto C, et al. Global and regional estimates of cancer mortality and incidence by site: II. Results for the global burden of disease 2000. BMC Cancer 2002;2:37–63.

[11] National Center for Health Statistics, Division of Vital Statistics, Centers for disease control. Available at: www.cdc.gov.

[12] American Cancer Society. Screening guidelines. Available at: www.cancer.org.

[13] Steele RJ. Fecal occult blood test screening in the United Kingdom. Am J Gastroenterol 2006;101:216–8.

[14] Mandel JS, Church TR, Ederer F, et al. Colorectal cancer mortality: effectiveness of biennial screening for fecal occult blood. J Natl Cancer Inst 1999;91:434–7.

[15] Jorgensen OD, Kronborg O, Fenger C. A randomised study of screening for colorectal cancer using faecal occult blood testing: results after 13 years and seven biennial screening rounds. Gut 2002;50:29–32.

[16] Kronborg O, Jorgensen OD, Fenger C, et al. Randomized study of biennial screening with a faecal occult blood test: results after nine screening rounds. Scand J Gastroenterol 2004;39:846–51.

[17] Robinson MH, Hardcastle JD, Moss SM, et al. The risks of screening: data from the Nottingham randomised controlled trial of faecal occult blood screening for colorectal cancer. Gut 1999;45:588–92.

[18] Scholefeld JH, Moss S, Sufi F, et al. Effect of faecal occult blood screening on mortality from colorectal cancer: results from a randomised controlled trial. Gut 2002;50: 840–4.

[19] Cole SR, Young GP, Esterman A, et al. A randomized trial of the impact of new faecal haemoglobin test technologies on population participation in screening for colorectal cancer. J Med Screen 2003;10:117–22.

[20] Fraser CG, Matthew CM, Mowat NA, et al. Immunochemical testing of individuals positive for guaiac faecal occult blood test in a screening programme for colorectal cancer: an observational study. Lancet Oncol 2006;7:127–31.

[21] Smith A, Young GP, Cole SR, et al. Comparison of a brush-sampling fecal immunochemical test for hemoglobin with a sensitive guaiac-based fecal occult blood test in detection of colorectal neoplasia. Cancer 2006;107:2152–9.

[22] Young GP, St John DJ, Winawer SJ, et al. Choice of fecal occult blood tests for colorectal cancer screening: recommendations based on performance characteristics in population studies. Am J Gastroenterol 2002;97:2499–507.

[23] Federici A, Rossi PG, Borgia P, et al. The immunochemical faecal occult blood test leads to higher compliance than the guaiac for colorectal cancer screening programmes: a cluster randomized controlled trial. J Med Screen 2005;12:83–8.

[24] Hewitson P, Glasziou P, Irwig L, et al. Screening for colorectal cancer using the faecal occult blood test, Hemoccult [review]. Cochrane Database Syst Rev 2007; CD001216.

[25] Kewenter J, Brevinge H, Engaras B, et al. Results of screening, rescreening, and follow-up in a prospective randomized study for detection of colorectal cancer by fecal occult blood testing. Scand J Gastroenterol 1994;29:468–73.

[26] Faivre J, Dancourt V, Lejeune C, et al. Reduction in colorectal cancer mortality by fecal occult blood screening in a French controlled study. Gastroenterology 2004;126: 1674–80.

[27] Levin B, Brooks D, Smith RA, et al. Emerging technologies in screening for colorectal cancer: CT colonography, immunochemical fecal occult blood tests and stool screening using molecular markers. CA Cancer J Clin 2003;53:44–55.

[28] St. John DJ, Young GP, Alexeyeff MA, et al. Evaluation of new occult blood tests for detection of colorectal neoplasia. Gastroenterology 1993;104:1661–8.

[29] Smith A, Young GP, Cole SR. A quantifiable fecal immunochemical test for hemoglobin facilitates balancing sensitivity with specificity when screening for colorectal cancer. Gastroenterology 2004;126:A-199.

[30] Levi Z, Rozen P, Hazazi R, et al. A quantitative immunochemical fecal occult blood test for colorectal neoplasia. Ann Intern Med 2007;146:244–55.

[31] Saito H, Soma Y, Koeda J, et al. Reduction in risk of mortality from colorectal cancer by fecal occult blood screening with immunochemical hemagglutination test. A case-control study. Int J Cancer 1995;61:465–9.

[32] Saito H, Soma M, Nakajima M, et al. A case-control study evaluating occult blood screening for colorectal cancer with Hemoccult test and immunochemical hemagglutination test. Oncol Rep 2000;7:815–9.

[33] Nakajima M, Saito H, Soma Y, et al. Prevention of advanced colorectal cancer by screening using the immunochemical faecal occult blood test: a case-control study. Br J Cancer 2003;89:23–8.

[34] Saito H. Colorectal cancer screening using immunochemical faecal occult blood testing in Japan. J Med Screen 2006;13(Suppl 1):S6–7.

[35] Lee KJ, Inoue M, Otani T, et al. Colorectal cancer screening using fecal occult blood test and subsequent risk of colorectal cancer: a prospective cohort study in Japan. Cancer Detect Prev 2007;31:3–11.

[36] Ko CW, Dominitz JA, Nguyen TD. Fecal occult blood testing in a general medical clinic: comparison between guaiac-based and immunochemical-based tests. Am J Med 2003;115:111–4.

[37] Zappa M, Castiglione G, Paci E, et al. Measuring interval cancers in population-based screening using different assays of fecal occult blood testing: the District of Florence experience. Int J Cancer 2001;92:151–4.

[38] Cole S, Smith A, Bampton P, et al. Screening for colorectal cancer: direct comparison of a brush-sampling fecal immunochemical test for hemoglobin with Hemoccult. Gastroenterology 2003;124:A80.

[39] Levi Z, Hazazi P, Rozen P, et al. A quantitative immunochemical faecal occult blood test is more efficient for detecting significant colorectal neoplasia than a sensitive guaiac test. Aliment Pharmacol Ther 2006;23:1359–64.

[40] Woo HY, Mok RS, Park YN, et al. A prospective study of a new immunochemical fecal occult blood test in Korean patients referred for colonoscopy. Clin Biochem 2005;38:395–9.

[41] Wong BC, Wong WM, Cheung KL, et al. A sensitive guaiac faecal occult blood test is less useful than an immunochemical test for colorectal cancer screening in a Chinese population. Aliment Pharmacol Ther 2003;18:941–6.

[42] Li S, Wang H, Hu J, et al. New immunochemical fecal occult blood test with two-consecutive stool sample testing is a cost-effective approach for colon cancer screening: results of a prospective multicenter study in Chinese patients. Int J Cancer 2006;118:3078–83.

[43] Fraser CG, Matthew CM, Mowat NA, et al. Evaluation of a card collection based faecal immunochemical test in screening for colorectal cancer using a two-tier reflex approach. Gut 2007;59:1415–8.

[44] Winawer S, Fletcher R, Rex D, et al. Colorectal cancer screening and surveillance: clinical guidelines and rationale—update based on new evidence. Gastroenterology 2003;124: 544–60.

[45] Fearon ER, Vogelstein B. A genetic model for colorectal tumorigenesis. Cell 1990;61: 759–67.

[46] Atkin W, Martin JP. Stool DNA-based colorectal cancer detection: finding the needle in the haystack. J Natl Cancer Inst 2001;93:858–65.

[47] Ahlquist DA, Skoletsky JE, Boynton KA, et al. Colorectal cancer screening by detection of altered human DNA stool: feasibility of a multitarget assay panel. Gastroenterology 2000;119:1219–27.

[48] Tagore KS, Lawson MJ, Yucatis JA, et al. Sensitivity and specificity of a stool DNA multitarget assay panel for the detection of advanced colorectal neoplasia. Clin Colorectal Cancer 2003;3:47–53.

[49] Calistri D, Rengucci C, Bocchini R, et al. Fecal multiple molecular tests to detect colorectal cancer in stool. Clin Gastroenterol Hepatol 2003;1:377–83.

[50] Imperiale TF, Ransohoff DF, Turnbull BA, et al. Fecal DNA versus fecal occult blood for colorectal cancer screening in average risk population. N Engl J Med 2004;351:2704–14.

[51] Syngal S, Stoffel E, Chung D, et al. Detection of stool DNA mutations before and after treatment of colorectal neoplasia. Cancer 2006;106:277–83.

[52] Song K, Fendrick AM, Ladabaum U. Fecal DNA testing compared with conventional colorectal cancer screening methods: a decision analysis. Gastroenterology 2004;126: 1270–9.

[53] Wu GH, Wang YM, Yen AM, et al. Cost-effectiveness analysis of colorectal cancer screening with stool DNA testing in intermediate-incidence countries. BMC Cancer 2006;6: 136–47.

[54] Itzkowitz SH, Jandork L, Brand R, et al. Improved fecal DNA test for colorectal cancer screening. Clin Gastroenterol Hepatol 2007;5:111–7.

[55] Model F, Osborn N, Ahlquist D, et al. Identification and validation of colorectal neoplasia—specific methylation markers for accurate classification of disease. Molecular Cancer Research 2007;5:153–63.

[56] Lees NP, Harrison KL, Hall CN, et al. Human colorectal mucosal O^6-alkylguanine DNA-alkyltransferase activity and DNA-N7-methylguanine levels in colorectal adenoma cases and matched referents. Gut 2007;56:318–20.

[57] Huang ZH, Li LH, Wang JF. Detection of aberrant methylation in fecal DNA as a molecular screening tool for colorectal cancer and precancerous lesions. World J Gastroenterol 2007;13:950–4.

[58] Abbaszadegan MR, Tavasoli A, Velayati A, et al. Stool-based DNA testing, a new noninvasive method for colorectal cancer screening, the first report from Iran. World J Gastroenterol 2007;13:1528–33.

[59] US Preventive Services Task Force. The guide to clinical preventive services 2006. Available at: www.ahcpr.gov/clinic/pocketgd.

[60] Church TR. A novel form of ascertainment bias in case-control studies of cancer screening. J Clin Epidemiol 1999;52:837–47.

[61] Winawer SJ, Zauber AG, Ho MN, et al. Prevention of colorectal cancer by colonoscopic polypectomy. N Engl J Med 1993;329.1977–81.

[62] Muto T, Bussey HJ, Morson BC. The evolution of cancer of the colon and rectum. Cancer 1975;36:2251–70.

[63] Spencer RJ, Melton LJ, Ready RL, et al. Treatment of small colorectal polyps: a population-based study of the risk of subsequent carcinoma. Mayo Clin Proc 1984;59:305–10.

[64] Atkin WS, Morson BC, Cuzick J. Long-term risk of colorectal cancer after excision of rectosigmoid adenomas. N Engl J Med 1992;326:658–62.

[65] Saitoh Y, Waxman I, West AB, et al. Prevalence and distinctive biologic features of flat colorectal adenomas in North American populations. Gastroenterology 2001;120:1657–65.

[66] Prorok PC, Andriole GL, Bresalier RS, et al. Design of the Prostate, Lung, Colorectal and Ovarian (PLCO) Cancer Screening Trial. Control Clin Trials 2000;21:273S–309S.

[67] Cajucom CC, Barrios GC, Cruz L, et al. Prevalence of colorectal polyps in Filipinos. An autopsy study. Dis Colon Rectum 1992;35:676–80.

[68] Eide TJ. The age-, sex- and site-specific occurrence of adenomas and carcinomas of the large intestine within a defined population. Scand J Gastroenterol 1986;21:1083–8.

[69] Lieberman DA, Weiss DG, Bond JH, et al. Use of colonoscopy to screen asymptomatic adults for colorectal cancer. Veterans Affairs Cooperative Study Group. N Engl J Med 2000;343:162–8.

[70] Imperiale TF, Wagner DR, Lin CY, et al. Risk of advanced proximal neoplasms in asymptomatic adults according to the distal colorectal findings. N Engl I Med 2000;343:169–74.

[71] Selby JV, Friedman GD, Quesenberry CP Jr, et al. A case-control study of screening sigmoidoscopy and mortality from colorectal cancer. N Engl J Med 1992;326:653–7.

[72] Newcombe PA, Norfleet RG, Storer BE, et al. Screening sigmoidoscopy and colorectal cancer mortality. J Natl Cancer Inst 1992;84:1572–5.

[73] Muller AD, Sonnenberg A. Protection by endoscopy against death from colorectal cancer. A case-control study among veterans. Arch Intern Med 1995;155:1741–8.

[74] Kavanaugh AM, Giaovannucci EL, Fuchs CS, et al. Screening endoscopy and risk of colorectal cancer in United States men. Cancer Causes Control 1998;9:455–62.

[75] Winawer SJ, Flehinger BJ, Schottenfeld D, et al. Screening for colorectal cancer with fecal occult blood testing and sigmoidoscopy. J Natl Cancer Inst 1993;85:1311–8.

[76] Berry DP, Clarke P, Hardcastle JD, et al. Randomized trial of the addition of flexible sigmoidoscopy to fecal occult blood testing for colorectal neoplasia population screening. Br J Surg 1997;84:1274–6.

[77] Rasmussen M, Kronborg O, Fenger C, et al. Possible advantages and drawbacks of adding flexible sigmoidoscopy to Hemoccult-II in screening for colorectal cancer. Scand J Gastroenterol 1999;34:73–8.

[78] Verne JE, Aubrey R, Love SB, et al. Population based randomized study of uptake and yield of screening by flexible sigmoidoscopy compared with screening by faecal occult blood testing. BMJ 1998;317:182–5.

[79] Hendon SH, DiPalma JA. US practices for colon cancer screening. Keio J Med 2005;54: 179–83.

[80] American Society for Gastrointestinal Endoscopy. Guidelines for training non-specialists in screening flexible sigmoidoscopy. Gastrointest Endosc 2000;51:783–5.

[81] Brown ML, Klabunde CN, Mysliwiec P. Current capacity for endoscopic colorectal cancer screening in the United States: data from the National Cancer Institute survey of colorectal cancer screening practices. Am J Med 2003;115:129–33.

[82] Shapero TF, Hoover J, Paszat LF, et al. Colorectal cancer screening with nurse-performed flexible sigmoidoscopy: results from a Canadian community-based program. Gastrointest Endosc 2007;65:640–5.

[83] Wolf JL. Uniquely women's issues in colorectal cancer screening. Am J Gastroenterol 2006;101:S625–9.

[84] Lieberman DA, Weiss DG. One-time screening for colorectal cancer with combined fecal occult-blood testing and examination of the distal colon. N Engl J Med 2001;345: 555–60.

[85] Schoenfeld P, Cash B, Flood A, et al. Colonoscopic screening of average-risk women for colorectal neoplasia. N Engl J Med 2005;352:2061–8.

[86] Francois F, Park J, Bini EJ. Colon pathology detected after a positive screening flexible sigmoidoscopy: a prospective study in an ethnically diverse cohort. Am J Gastroenterol 2006;101:823–30.

[87] Bretthauer M, Skovlund E, Grotmol T, et al. Inter-endoscopist variation in polyp and neoplasia pick-up rates in flexible sigmoidoscopy screening for colorectal cancer. Scand J Gastroenterol 2003;38:1268–74.

[88] O'Leary BA, Olynyk JK, Neville AM, et al. Cost-effectiveness of colorectal cancer screening: comparison of a community-based flexible sigmoidoscopy with fecal occult blood testing and colonoscopy. J Gastroenterol Hepatol 2004;19:38–47.

[89] Pignone M. Is population screening for colorectal cancer cost effective? Nat Clin Pract Gastroenterol Hepatol 2005;2:288–9.

[90] Cooper GS, Yuan Z, Landefeld CS, et al. A national population based study of incidence of colorectal cancer and age. Implications for screening in older Americans. Cancer 1995;75:775–81.

[91] Gonzlalez EC, Roetzheirm RG, Ferrante JM, et al. Predictors of proximal vs. distal colorectal cancers. Dis Colon Rectum 2001;44:251–8.

[92] Yamji Y, Mitsushima T, Ikuma H, et al. Right-sided shift of colorectal adenomas with aging. Gastrointest Endosc 2006;63:453–8.

[93] Phillips KA, Liang SY, Ladabaum U, et al. Trends in colonoscopy for colorectal cancer screening. Med Care 2007;45:160–7.

[94] Lieberman DA, Smith FW. Screening for colon malignancy with colonoscopy. Am J Gastroenterol 1991;86:946–51.

[95] Rex DK, Cummings OW, Helper DJ, et al. 5-year incidence of adenomas after negative colonoscopy in asymptomatic average-risk persons. Gastroenterology 1996;111: 1178–81.

[96] Lieberman DA. Endoscopic colon screening: is less more? Gastroenterology 1996;111: 1385–7.

[97] Rogge JD, Elmore MF, Mahoney SJ, et al. Low-cost office-based screening colonoscopy. Am J Gastroenterol 1994;89:1775–80.

[98] Zauber A, Winawer SJ, O'Brien MJ, et al. Significant long term reduction in colorectal cancer mortality with colonoscopic polypectomy. Gastroenterology 2007;132:A-50.

[99] Citarda F, Tomaselli G, Capocaccia R, et al. Efficacy in standard clinical practice of colonoscopic polypectomy in reducing colorectal cancer incidence. Gut 2001;48:812–5.

[100] Inadomi JM, Sonnenberg A. The impact of colorectal cancer screening on life expectancy. Gastrointest Endosc 2000;51:517–23.

[101] Haseman JH, Lemmel GT, Rahmani EY, et al. Failure of colonoscopy to detect colorectal cancer: evaluation of 47 cases in 20 hospitals. Gastrointest Endosc 1997;45:451–5.

[102] Pabby A, Schoen RE, Weissfeld JL, et al. Analysis of colorectal cancer occurrence during surveillance colonoscopy in the dietary Polyp Prevention Trial. Gastrointest Endosc 2005;61:385–9.

[103] Robertseon DJ, Greenber ER, Beach M, et al. Colorectal cancer in patients under close surveillance. Gastroenterology 2005;129:34–41.

[104] Singh H, Turner D, Xue L, et al. Risk of developing colorectal cancer following a negative colonoscopy. JAMA 2006;131:1700–5.

[105] Shah HA, Paszat LF, Saskin R, et al. Factors associated with incomplete colonoscopy: a population-based study. Gastroenterology 2007;132:2297–303.

[106] Bressler B, Paszat LF, Chen Z, et al. Rates of new or missed colorectal cancers after colonoscopy and their risk factors: a population-based analysis. Gastroenterology 2007;132: 96–102.

[107] van Rijn JC, Reitsma JB, Stoker J, et al. Polyp miss rate determined by tandem colonoscopy: a systematic review. Am J Gastroenterol 2006;101:343–50.

[108] Barclay RL, Vicari JJ, Doughty AS, et al. Colonoscopic withdrawal times and adenoma detection during screening colonoscopy. N Engl J Med 2006;355:2533–41.

[109] Rex D. Who is the best colonoscopist? Gastroenterol Endosc 2007;65:145–50.

[110] Rex D. Maximizing detection of adenomas and cancers during colonoscopy. Am J Gastroenterol 2006;101:2866–77.

[111] Trecca A, Gaj F, DiLorenzo GP, et al. Improved detection of colorectal neoplasms with selective use of chromoendoscopy in 2005 consecutive patients. Tech Coloproctol 2006;10: 339–44.

[112] Stergiou N, Frenz MB, Menke D, et al. Reduction of miss rate of colonic adenomas by zoom chromoendoscopy. Int J Colorectal Dis 2006;21:560–5.

[113] Nelson DB, McQuaid KR, Bond JH, et al. Procedural success and complications of large-scale screening colonoscopy. Gastrointest Endosc 2002;55:307–14.

[114] Dafnis G, Ekbom A, Pahlman L, et al. Complications of diagnostic and therapeutic colonoscopy within a defined population in Sweden. Gastrointest Endosc 2001;54:302–9.

[115] Anderson ML, Pasha TM, Leighton JA. Endoscopic perforation of the colon: lessons from a 10-year study. Am J Gastroenterol 2000;95:3418–22.

[116] Eckardt VF, Kanzler G, Schmitt T, et al. Complications and adverse effects of colonoscopy with selective sedation. Gastrointest Endosc 1999;49:560–5.

[117] Wexner SD, Forde KA, Sellers G, et al. How well can surgeons perform colonoscopy? Surg Endosc 1998;12:1410–4.

[118] Ure T, Dehghan K, Vernava AM, et al. Colonoscopy in the elderly. Low risk, high yield. Surg Endosc 1995;9:505–8.

[119] Zubarik R, Fleischer DE, Mastropietro C, et al. Prospective analysis of complications 30 days after outpatient colonoscopy. Gastrointest Endosc 1999;50:322–8.

[120] Lo AY, Beaton HL. Selective management of colonoscopic perforations. J Am Coll Surg 1994;179:333–7.

[121] Webb WA, McDaniel L, Jones L. Experience with 1000 colonoscopic polypectomies. Ann Surg 1985;201:626–32.

[122] Cobb WS, Heniford BT, Sigmon LB, et al. Colonoscopic perforations: incidence, management, and outcomes. Am Surg 2004;70:750–7.

[123] Korman LY, Overholt BF, Box T, et al. Perforations during colonoscopy in endoscopic ambulatory surgical centers. Gastrointest Endosc 2003;58:554–7.

[124] Pignone M, Rich M, Teutscch SM, et al. Screening for colorectal cancer in adults at average risk: a summary of the evidence for the U.S. Preventive Services Task Force. Ann Intern Med 2002;137:132–41.

[125] Levin TR, Zhao W, Conell C, et al. Complications of colonoscopy in an integrated health care delivery system. Ann Intern Med 2006;145:880–6.

[126] Rex DK, Chadalawada V, Helper DJ. Wide angle colonoscopy with a prototype instrument: impact on miss rates and efficiency determined by back-to-back colonoscopies. Am J Gastroenterol 2003;98:2000–5.

[127] Deenadayalu VP, Chadalawada V, Rex DK. 170 degrees wide-angle colonoscope: effect on efficiency and miss rates. Am J Gastroenterol 2004;99:2138–42.

[128] Eickhoff A, Van Dam J, Jakobs R, et al. Computer-assisted colonoscopy (the NeoGuide Endoscopy System): results of the first human clinical trial ("PACE Study"). Am J Gastroenterol 2007;102:261–6.

[129] Rex DK, Vining MD, Kopecky K. An initial experience with screening for colon polyps using spiral CT with and without CT colography (virtual colonoscopy). Gastrointest Endosc 1999;50:309–13.

[130] Pickhardt PJ, Choi JR, Hwang I, et al. Computed tomographic virtual colonoscopy to screen for colorectal neoplasia in asymptomatic adults. N Engl J Med 2003;349:2191–200.

[131] Morrin MM, LaMont T. Screening virtual colonoscopy—ready for prime time? N Engl J Med 2003;349:2261–4.

[132] Cotton PB, Durkalski VL, Pineau BC, et al. Computed tomographic colonography (virtual colonoscopy): a multicenter comparison with standard colonoscopy for detection of colorectal neoplasia. JAMA 2004;291:1713–9.

[133] Halligan S, Altman DG, Taylor SA, et al. CT colonography in the detection of colorectal polyps and cancer: systematic review, meta-analysis, and proposed minimum data set for study level reporting. Radiology 2005;237:893–904.

[134] Mulhall BP, Veerappan GR, Jackson JL. Meta-analysis: computed tomographic colonography. Ann Intern Med 2005;142:635–50.

[135] Rosman AS, Korsten MA. Meta-analysis comparing CT colonography, air contrast barium enema, and colonoscopy. Am J Med 2007;120:203–10.

[136] Kim DH, Pickhardt PJ, Taylor AJ. Characteristics of advanced adenomas detected at CT colonographic screening: implications for appropriate polyp size thresholds for polypectomy versus surveillance. AJR Am J Roentgenol 2007;188:940–4.

[137] Burling D, Halligan S, Slater A, et al. Potentially serious adverse events at CT colonography in symptomatic patients: national survey of the United Kingdom. Radiology 2006;239:464–71.

[138] Vijan S, Hwang I, Inadomi J, et al. The cost-effectiveness of CT colonography in screening for colorectal neoplasia. Am J Gastroenterol 2007;102:380–90.

[139] Pickhardt PJ, Hassan C, Laghi A, et al. Cost-effectiveness of colorectal cancer screening with computed tomography colonography: the impact of not reporting diminutive lesions. Cancer 2007;109:2213–21.

[140] Pennazio M. Capsule endoscopy: where are we after 6 years of clinical use? Dig Liver Dis 2006;38:867–78.

[141] Mazzarolo S, Brady P. Small bowel capsule endoscopy: a systematic review. South Med J 2007;100:274–80.

[142] Ho KK, Joyce AM. Complications of capsule endoscopy. Gastrointest Endosc Clin N Am 2007;17:169–78.

[143] Yagi Y, Vu H, Echigo T, et al. A diagnosis support system for capsule endoscopy. Inflammopharmacology 2007;15:78–83.

[144] Schoofs N, Deviere J, Van Gossum A. PillCam colon capsule endoscopy compared with colonoscopy for colorectal tumor diagnosis: a prospective study. Endoscopy 2006;38:971–7.

[145] Scheitel SM, Ahlquist DA, Wollan PC, et al. Colorectal cancer screening: a community case-control study of proctosigmoidoscopy, barium enema radiography and fecal occult blood test efficacy. Mayo Clin Proc 1999;74:1207–13.

[146] Rex DK, Rahmani EY, Haseman JH, et al. Relative sensitivity of colonoscopy and barium enema for detection of colorectal cancer in clinical practice. Gastroenterology 1997;112:17–23.

[147] Winawer SJ, Stewart ET, Zauber AG, et al. A comparison of colonoscopy and double-contrast barium enema for surveillance after polypectomy. National Polyp Work Group. N Engl J Med 2000;342:1766–72.

[148] Fletcher RH. The end of barium enema? N Engl J Med 2000;342:1823–5.

[149] Kewenter J, Brevinge H. Endoscopic and surgical complications of work-up in screening for colorectal cancer. Dis Colon Rectum 1996;39:676–80.

[150] Blakeborough A, Sheridan MB, Chapman AH. Complications of barium enema examinations: a survey of UK Consultant Radiologists 1992 to 1994. Clin Radiol 1997;52:142–8.

[151] Rollandi G, Biscaldi E, DeCicco E. Double contrast barium enema: technique, indications, results and limitations of a conventional imaging methodology in the MDCT virtual endoscopy era. Eur J Radiol 2007;61:382–7.

[152] Ludabaum U, Song K. Projected national impact of colorectal cancer screening on clinical and economic outcomes and health services demand. Gastroenterology 2005;129: 1151–62.

[153] Levin TR. Colonoscopy capacity: can we build it? Will they come? Gastroenterology 2004;127:1841–4.

Gastroenterol Clin N Am 37 (2008) 117–128

GASTROENTEROLOGY CLINICS
OF NORTH AMERICA

Implementation of Colonoscopy for Mass Screening for Colon Cancer and Colonic Polyps: Efficiency with High Quality of Care

Susan L. Mihalko, BAS, CGRN, RN

Endoscopy Center, William Beaumont Hospital, 3601 W. 13 Mile Road, Royal Oak, MI 48073, USA

As awareness of colon cancer by the public continues to increase, screening colonoscopy procedures will proportionately increase. There is much written on the design of new ambulatory gastroenterology clinics, but little practical information about high-volume, mass colonoscopic screening of patients in the hospital outpatient setting. Many institutions struggle with inefficient endoscopy units that cannot always meet the dual needs of high quality and efficient performance of screening endoscopy. The patient undergoing screening colonoscopy seeks an efficient unit with state-of-the-art equipment, highly skilled physicians, highly competent staff, accurate case documentation, comfortable surroundings, and consumer-friendly follow-through of care. Optimizing these factors in existing spaces may require revision of an endoscopy unit's operations and, possibly, renovation of the endoscopy suite.

This article is based on our practical experience in a 10–procedure room endoscopy unit, located in a nearly 1100 bed teaching hospital that performs about 23,000 endoscopies annually. Although in this endoscopy unit multiple specialties use the endoscopy suite and various different endoscopic procedures are performed, this article focuses on screening colonoscopy. Standard practices within an endoscopy unit should enhance the efficiency of mass screening colonoscopy, whereas deviations from these standards can decrease the quality or efficiency of the service.

COLON CANCER SCREENING

An estimated 112,000 cases of colon cancer and 41,000 cases of rectal cancer were expected to occur in 2007. Screening is used to detect colorectal cancer at an early stage when it is more likely to be curable. Screening can also result in the detection and removal of colorectal polyps before they become cancerous

E-mail address: smihalko@beaumonthospitals.com

0889-8553/08/$ – see front matter
doi:10.1016/j.gtc.2007.12.011

and can thereby prevent colon cancer. Both of these effects can decrease the overall mortality from colon cancer [1].

Men and women at average risk for developing colorectal cancer should begin screening at age 50. Personal risk for colon cancer varies along with the best screening method for individuals. The American Cancer Society recommends one of the five following screening methods for adults at average risk beginning at age 50:

- Annual fecal occult blood test (FOBT)
- Flexible sigmoidoscopy every 5 years
- Annual FOBT and flexible sigmoidoscopy every 5 years
- Double contrast barium enema every 5 years
- Colonoscopy every 10 years [1].

Colonoscopy has become the most important method of screening because of a high diagnostic sensitivity and specificity, the ability to procure tissue from identified lesions for histologic analysis, and the ability to completely remove polyps during the procedure.

PRACTICAL CONSIDERATIONS IN HIGH-VOLUME UNITS
Scheduling

Scheduling, or boarding, involves several considerations. For maximal efficiency, open dates and times should be immediately available when scheduling. The boarding office should have software that links patient data (medical record number, date of birth, and so forth) with physician and room availability. Blockboarding schedules built into software grids streamline the process, allowing individual physicians or their office staff to schedule procedures many weeks ahead at designated times. These blocks should be periodically monitored for use, usually targeted at 75% to 80% use, and the blocked times adjusted to accommodate the physician's volume. Open blocks of time should be available to accommodate urgent procedures or cases performed by physicians not using blocked time. Having 100% blocked times, with a release date to automatically open up the blocked time 3 to 7 days before the procedure date, provides for efficient usage but is problematic for endoscopic physicians who do not block board. A mixture of 80% blocked time and 20% unblocked time is a reasonable compromise. The ability of a physician or office personnel to directly access the hospital's scheduling system to schedule a procedure in the predetermined blocked time requires safeguards to protect patient confidentially. Faxing and phoning directly to the boarding office are alternatives.

The scheduling of procedures has many variations. Procedure length varies according to case complexity and individual physician performance patterns. To minimize delays, the average time of a procedure should be considered when scheduling boarding times for procedures, which is simply determined by averaging the time for the last 50 procedures for the particular physician. Average screening colonoscopy times vary from 30 to 45 minutes. Extra time must be added if the colonoscopy is combined with an upper endoscopy or if the patient has multiple comorbidities. In a teaching hospital, fellows and residents often accompany the attending physician during the procedure, which can increase the average procedure time.

After a procedure is scheduled, patients should receive instructions that include the procedure date and time, designated area of arrival, and colonoscopy preparation directions. The patient may also be given a simple educational pamphlet about screening colonoscopy, to better inform the patient and to enhance the procedural experience. Directing the patient to arrive 45 to 60 minutes before the procedure provides ample time for them to arrive, register, and be assessed by the nursing staff. This amount of time provides a safety margin for late arrivals. If a patient is tardy, the next patient can be selected ahead of time. If the patient arrives prepped on the wrong day, every attempt should be made to accommodate him. Adding them after the end of a block of time may be feasible, but this may require starting some initial steps, such as intravenous infusion, during the waiting period.

No-show patients impact the flow and efficiency of the daily schedule. If this occurs frequently, the communication processes with the patient should be reviewed. The following steps are recommended to ensure communication of the correct date and time:

1. Hospital scheduler and physician's office scheduler verify correct information at the time of boarding and reconfirm the schedule 1 week before the scheduled procedure.
2. Patient is mailed a confirmation letter from the hospital 1 week before the procedure, providing an opportunity to instruct the patient to complete an updated medication list for medication reconciliation.
3. Patient is called 24 to 48 hours before the scheduled procedure as a reminder. If the patient does not answer but an answering machine is on, a message should be left with an accessible number to be called back to confirm or cancel the procedure.

These measures should greatly reduce the no-show rate. Timeliness of the procedures also requires physician punctuality. The first procedure of the day should start on time. A delay in this procedure impacts on the remainder of the daily schedule and does a disservice to the following patients and physicians. Restricting a chronically tardy endoscopist to cases later in the day may solve the problem.

Computerization

Computerization of the endoscopy unit improves the efficiency of communication. Linking the patient data, at the time of boarding, with registration services expedites the patient processing at the time of the endoscopy. If appropriately interfaced, the data will link and prefill the demographics to the hospital's on-line reporting pieces, such as documented care, endoscopy reports, pathology reports, and discharge instructions. Oral dictation, with reports being subsequently transcribed and downloaded to the patient's on-line chart, should be available for when the computer system is down, or for endoscopists who are unable to use computers.

Credentialing

Credentialing for procedures is based on established hospital criteria. New physicians apply for privileges determined by their past experience and training. A review by the appropriate service chief, an expert in the specialty, ensures maintenance of quality. If the established criteria are not met, however, a mentoring process is followed to guide the endoscopist to the expected level of performance.

Consent

Informed consent requires the patient to understand the risk for complications. Information given to the patient, in the form of a handout that provides procedure-specific facts, can supplement the physician's discussion with the patient [2]. This handout can promote efficiency in the preprocedure area by reducing the need for addressing questions by the patient. Obtaining consent for inpatients at the bedside allows the patient or staff sufficient time to inform family members who may desire to be present at the procedure and can decrease delays from questions and answers at the time of service. Mentally incompetent patients require a legal guardian's consent for an elective procedure. In an emergency, the endoscopist can notify and obtain concurrence for the procedure from the appropriate service chief, when the legal guardian is unavailable.

Open Access

In open access, patients referred for screening colonoscopy do not meet their endoscopist until the time of service. This method eliminates one visit for the patient and the endoscopist, but may impact the flow if required information is not in place before the procedure. A preassessment patient profile provides the necessary information to formulate a plan of care for the patient, a requirement of the Joint Commission on Accreditation of Healthcare Organizations [2]. To avoid another office visit for the patient, referring physicians should complete this profile when the referral is made and forward it to the appropriate office for submission to the endoscopy suite. The attending physician does not need to meet the patient before the procedure if all this was correctly performed.

Patients Requiring Special Care

The preassessment profile alerts endoscopy staff of the special needs of particular patients. Staff, such as nurse clinicians, should screen the patient profiles at least 24 hours before the procedure and initiate an action plan to address these alerts. Potential actions include arranging for turning cardiac defibrillators off and on, administration of prophylactic antibiotics, or ordering special equipment for handicapped patients or large patients. Interpreters, located by a hospital database or supplied by an outside agency, can be prearranged to accommodate non-English speaking or hearing impaired patients when necessary.

Patients on anticoagulants require special instructions for discontinuance of their medications before the procedure. Compliance is crucial in the event of polypectomy during endoscopy. The instructions are best provided in advance of the procedure at the office visit to the internist or the endoscopist. Patients who have communicable diseases, such as tuberculosis, require special handling. Ideally, the procedure should be performed at the bedside for inpatients to reduce the exposure of other patients. For outpatients, planning for a mask to be presented to them at their arrival and limiting their contact with others throughout the visit is important.

Unstable or extremely ill patients, with an American Society of Anesthesiologists class rating of IV, are at an increased risk for adverse sedation reactions and should be closely monitored by an anesthesiologist. This arrangement allows the endoscopist and staff to focus on the procedure. Untoward medication reactions must be quickly addressed. Procedure rooms need intercoms or telephones to call for cardiopulmonary resuscitation (CPR) if necessary. A readily available in-house team offers support for these emergencies. An unstable patient is best served with mobile endoscopy at the bedside in the emergency room or the intensive care unit. These areas are staffed and equipped to address the needs of unstable patients. A colonoscopy in a pregnant woman who has strong procedure indications requires additional safety measures regarding awareness of medication effects, including bowel preparation, on the fetus. Obstetric consultation is required [3,4].

Patients who undergo an unsuccessful colonoscopy have several options, including a barium enema or a virtual colonoscopy. Both of these diagnostic tools need to be coordinated with the radiology department. They may possibly be performed immediately following the failed colonoscopy for the patient's convenience.

Equipment

Colonoscopes are manufactured to meet the varied preferences among endoscopists. Recent models offer features such as variable stiffness, forward water-jet channels with a flushing pump, and different diameters and lengths. Recent models offer greater flexibility and visual fields of 180 degrees for better visualization of colonic mucosa. The newest generation colonoscopes also offer enhanced optics, such as narrow band or high-definition imaging. For fast turnaround, three colonoscopes should be in service per an endoscopist who performs screening colonoscopies within 30 minutes. If the blocked schedule alternates between upper and lower endoscopic procedures, two colonoscopes may be sufficient.

Technical support and backup are important to maintain endoscopes. Rapid turnaround time for repairs depends on efficient processes for sending a malfunctioning endoscope from the facility to the repair shop, promptly repairing the endoscope, and promptly returning it to the facility. Providing accurate information to the repair facility concerning the malfunction expedites the repair. Dealing with the original endoscope manufacturer guarantees correct parts are used in the service repair, which often extends the life of the endoscope. The life expectancy of an endoscope used in a teaching hospital staffed with residents and training fellows is decidedly less than otherwise expected. In a large endoscopy suite that performs about 23,000 procedures per year, the average life expectancy of an endoscope is about 1 year. To extend endoscope life, an endoscope can have major overhauls up to the $7000 range. These costly repairs have to be weighed against the enhancements that occur approximately every 3 years as new generations of colonoscopes are manufactured. Providing state-of-the-art endoscopes versus repairing outdated endoscopes that do not provide the highest quality of screening is the dilemma. On average, one major overhaul repair should be budgeted annually for frequently used endoscopes.

Mobile carts, for on-call and bedside colonoscopy procedures, and typical procedure room carts should be equipped with the following:

- Colonoscope with processor, light source, monitor, heater probe unit, cautery, and grounding pads
- Sterile water, lubricant, and appropriate gowns, gloves, and masks
- Snares of various size and shape, such as rotatable, small, hexagonal, and oval with spiral wire barbs, suitable for sessile polyps; and forceps, regular or large capacity
- Cytology brushes, sclerotherapy needles, sclerosant solutions, retrieval baskets, nets, and specimen traps
- Polyp injection solutions (usually saline) used before polypectomy
- Sterile ink for injection to tattoo a polyp or lesion before surgery
- Ligating devices, such as detachable loops and clips of different lengths
- Epinephrine to deal with postpolypectomy bleeding and an argon plasma coagulator on stand-by for surface cautery
- Specimen jars and preservative

The endoscopy unit should have a CPR cart equipped with an automatic defibrillator, oxygen, suction, and resuscitation supplies.

An enhancement to the endoscopy unit is rigid endoscopic ultrasound probes for measuring intramural depth of rectal polyps or cancer in preparation for surgery. Cautery must be used cautiously. An increasing number of patients are presenting with automatic defibrillators that must be turned off temporarily during colonoscopy if polypectomy is possible. Identifying this type of patient ahead of time and notifying appropriate cardiologic staff in advance reduces delays. An increasing number of patients have a metal prosthesis, which requires careful placement of the cautery ground pad preferably on the flank side closest to the polyp site and away from the prosthesis.

ENDOSCOPY SUITE DESIGN

The flow of five entities must be considered in the design of an endoscopy suite. Patients, physicians, staff, mobile equipment, and material deliveries are traffic that must enter, merge, and exit without blockages (Fig. 1). First, outpatient throughput requires an easy way to find the unit, including signs

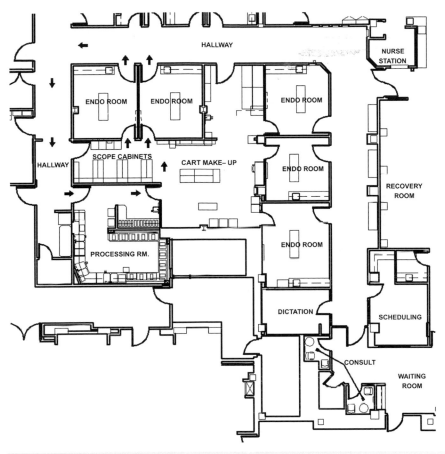

Fig. 1. Endoscopy procedure rooms.

and instructions; large, comfortable waiting areas; restroom accommodations; private preprocedure areas; and recovery areas with easy discharge access. The suite should be preferably located on the ground floor of the facility. Inpatients brought to the endoscopy suite have similar needs as the outpatient. Combining inpatients with outpatients in the same preprocedure area is not aesthetically pleasing because of the higher acuity level or medical interventions possibly needed for inpatients; this may be alarming to healthy outpatients who expect a different environment. Ideally, separate areas should be used. Companions or drivers who accompany the patient need comfortable accommodations, private areas to speak to the physician about the results of the procedure, access to staff for updates, and areas to use personal electronic devices.

Second, physicians need a designated room near the boarding office and the waiting room. This room should contain dictation equipment, computer software, phones, printers, a coat closet, personal storage area, intercom, and beverage station. The room should be large enough for attendings and fellows to collaborate and interact to promote the quality and efficiency of patient care. Third, endoscopy staff needs access to a locker room, lounge, and a time clock within the suite for record keeping. Support areas include a library or conference room, central administrative offices, scheduling/business office with fax and computers, and a nursing station equipped with computers and phones. A pneumatic tube system is useful to quickly receive paperwork or medication from the registration desk or hospital pharmacy.

Fourth, equipment should flow unidirectionally from soiled to clean (see Fig. 1). Soiled endoscopes and accessories are brought from the procedure room to the processing area to be cleaned and disinfected at a high level or to be cold sterilized in glutaraldehyde, the most commonly used disinfectant/sterilant for reprocessing gastrointestinal endoscopes [5]. Endoscopes are then taken to a preparation area to have medical air blown through the inner channels. Endoscopes are then hung vertically in ventilated cupboards in a clean storage area. Personnel remove endoscopes from these clean supplies to prepare for the next case. Ideally, two access areas to a procedure room (one for clean entry and one for soiled exit) optimize the unidirectional flow of soiled to clean. Fifth, materials, such as linen and supplies, delivered or picked up daily, need to enter or exit at nonpublic points adjacent to the storage areas to improve efficiency and minimize disruption.

The size of endoscopy rooms is regulated by codes that may differ in various locales. The room should be sufficiently large to be able to turn the stretcher containing a patient within the room. A room with 220 sq ft is adequate. The room should have a sink for hand washing, a documentation/computer area, a specimen preparation area, and a mobile procedure cart. Ceiling-mounted procedure monitors free up valuable floor space and minimize hazards from tripping on cables. Mobile equipment carts simplify transforming a room for different procedures. The endoscopy room should be arranged to provide unidirectional flow from soiled to clean to optimize the efficiency of equipment preparation.

Patients may bring more than one companion to the endoscopy suite. Measures must be considered for child-friendly areas, television viewing or soft overhead music, wireless access, nourishment, and comfortable seating arrangements. Plants, end tables, and adequate lighting for reading are also recommended. Nearby restrooms, with an infant changing area, are advisable. Encouraging the companion to remain in this area will keep them accessible to the physician for discussing procedure results, if the patient has given consent for this discussion. For a volume of about 100 procedures per day, it is advisable to have at least 30 chairs in the waiting room.

Having patients rest on a well-padded, adjustable-height stretcher before the procedure reduces the time of transferring them to the procedure room and then to the postprocedure areas. These stretchers can be equipped with intravenous poles and vinyl pillows that are permanently attached, and storage shelves for personal belongings. Adjustable head and foot lifts add comfort for the patient. Wheels that have steer locking capability make the stretcher easier to handle. A 10-room endoscopy unit requires about 30 stretcher spaces to accommodate pre- and postprocedure patients, with a storage bay that holds 5 more stretchers.

Separate pre- and postprocedure rooms are ideal. Separate pre- and postprocedure areas can be created in one room, however, provided the room is sufficiently large. A screen or other barrier should separate these two areas as much as possible. An ebb–flow design of these areas promotes the best use. If use of a preprocedure area begins to subside by the afternoon, the postprocedure area can be expanded. All spaces need to address patient confidentiality. In older pre/post areas, spaces are usually divided by curtains. This type of barrier does not offer much privacy to patients during confidential discussion. These areas are often too small to accommodate family members at the bedside. Walls are better than curtains for separating cubicles.

A consultation room for physicians to discuss the procedure results with the patient companions should accommodate a small table and two or three chairs. This room should be about 64 sq ft large and should have a door to provide privacy. A glass window on the door is a nice amenity that provides openness. The room should contain educational devices, such as anatomic diagrams and educational material.

The endoscope processing room is a major hub of activity in the endoscopy suite. It should be designed ergonomically. Endoscopes are received in a designated dirty area where they are manually washed, disinfected, and prepared for use or storage. The unilateral dirty-to-clean flow principle applies to this room. Three or four washing stations with at least 18 disinfecting machines that accommodate two endoscopes simultaneously are needed to handle a volume of 100 procedures per day. Stainless steel sinks and counters, although costly, require little maintenance, last many years, and are cleaned and disinfected easily. Disinfectors should be installed close to the washing sinks at a height and location for easy access by staff. Floor mats and other amenities, such as a radio or CD access, are appreciated by staff working in this physically demanding area. Two doors, one to enter with soiled equipment and one to exit with clean equipment to the cart make-up area, are recommended for a unidirectional dirty-to-clean flow. Proper ventilation with room air exchange is essential for staff safety [5]. A hand washing and eye splash station should be available in this area.

PERSONNEL/STAFFING

Staffing models vary based on the acuity and complexity of the caseload. A 1100-bed teaching hospital with a mix of 20% inpatients and 80% outpatients in an endoscopy unit that operates from 6:00 AM until 6:30 PM Monday through Saturday can expect to be challenged each day with different needs. Daily staff coverage for 10 procedure rooms with separate pre- and postprocedure areas, and ancillary areas, such as the waiting room, may require

19 registered nurses (RNs), including one charge nurse;

4 licensed practical nurses (LPNs), working under the direction of an RN or certified registered nurse anesthetist (CRNA);

14 technicians who provide technical assistance in the procedure rooms and work in the processing area to clean and disinfect the equipment;

4 nursing assistants (NAs) for the pre- and postprocedure areas; and

4 scheduling clerks who are cross-trained to board cases, prepare daily schedules, and do billing.

According to the guidelines for moderate sedation promulgated by the American Society for Gastrointestinal Endoscopy and the Society of Gastroenterology Nurses and Associates, an RN must be present in a procedure room to monitor the patient and a second staff member must be present to assist the physician with technical tasks, such as endoscopic biopsy [6,7].

Other support includes administrative staff, a departmental secretary cross-trained to perform payroll duties, and a medical director. Service chiefs of the various specialties that use the endoscopy center are included in decision making and in quality improvement reviews by attending a monthly meeting chaired by the medical director. This endoscopy-specific committee should also have representation from nursing, including a nursing administrator, the endoscopy suite nursing manager, and the assistant nursing manager. Guests from the hospital pharmacy, anesthesia department, or biomedical unit are invited as needed. Complications or quality issues that are deemed severe errors in practice or behavior are referred to a specialty-specific mortality and morbidity committee or the hospital quality assurance committee. Each specialty performs its own mortality and morbidity reviews and refers applicable reviewed cases to the hospital-wide committee for further determination for quality improvement. This process meets the requirements of regulatory or accrediting bodies. Minutes are prepared and distributed to all physicians who have endoscopy privileges to expedite communication of information and decisions of the endoscopy committee.

Clinical education is highly important in the endoscopy suite. The large number of staff members should be kept current on new equipment, regulatory mandates, and hospital-mandated training. These duties are fulfilled by two full-time equivalent nurse clinicians, who serve as physician and patient liaisons, screen outpatient preassessment forms, oversee orientation of new personnel, and can fill in for staffing shortages.

Occasionally, an emergent endoscopy must be performed at night or on the weekend when the endoscopy suite is closed. This requires an on-call arrangement, whereby members of the nursing staff are paged or called. An established set of criteria for on-call nursing assistance, agreed on by all the services using the endoscopy suite, ensures uniform adherence to this service.

Procedures such as endoscopic retrograde cholangiopancreatography and complex endoscopic ultrasound cases involve extra staff training. Maintaining competency of skills is difficult if a large group of staff occasionally rotates through these complex cases. It is better to assign specific staff members for these procedures.

ANESTHESIA

Endoscopy units may provide anesthesia services for all or selected endoscopic procedures. Without an anesthesiologist, the endoscopist administers and monitors the moderate sedation. It is our practice to provide 4 out of our 10 endoscopy rooms with anesthesia personnel. Three of these 4 rooms are reserved for outpatients and the fourth room is used for inpatients and urgent outpatients requiring deeper sedation. This fourth room addresses the increasing severity of disease of inpatients and the increasingly more complex endoscopic procedures. Routine sedation, with benzodiazepines and narcotics, has been traditionally used for endoscopic procedures. Propofol has advantages as a sedative because of deeper sedation and more rapid recovery. It is currently primarily administered by anesthesia staff in the United States but has been safely administered by non-anesthesiologists [8]. This controversy is increasingly relevant as endoscopy units examine cost effectiveness because of the substantial additional costs of an anesthesiologist.

SAFETY MEASURES

Throughput of a large volume of patients requires safety measures throughout the process. Correct patient identification is essential from the initial boarding to the time of arrival and at every point of hand-off between personnel throughout the patient visit. At least two patient identifiers are needed to ensure a correct match. The name, birth date and medical record number are the most commonly used identifiers. All patients need to wear wristbands, placed by the registration personnel, that contain this correct data. A safety check verification of the patient's name, procedure, equipment needed, patient position and physician (time out) needs to be performed by the staff, including the endoscopist, before administering sedation.

The risk for falls is a major concern in the hospital, especially with sedated, unstable, or frail patients. Maintaining areas free of cords, using side rails appropriately, and providing nurse-call devices at the bedside and in restrooms or changing booths reduce the risks for patient falls.

POSTPROCEDURE AND DISCHARGE

Patients recover differently from sedation, the rigors of bowel preparation, and the stress of the endoscopic procedure. An established set of discharge criteria, including alertness, vital signs, comfort, and activity, ensures consistent discharge practices. These criteria should be approved by the medical staff. Supportive measures, such as additional intravenous fluids, may be initiated to stabilize the patient. Thirty minutes is the accepted minimal recovery time for moderate sedation. Toleration of oral fluids, dangling of the feet over the bedside, and a steady gait should be observed and documented by the nursing staff before discharge. A wheelchair is the safest means of discharge, especially if the distance to the hospital exit and parked car is long. Volunteers can enhance the flow by accompanying a patient to his companion and his vehicle.

Written discharge instructions help assure follow-up of care. In the preprocedure setting, before sedation, the patient may receive general postprocedure instructions. The patient should be advised not to drive for 24 hours, to watch for excessive bleeding, and to maintain appropriate temporary dietary restrictions. After sedation wears off, the questions usually concern the physician's findings, resumption of eating, and the next scheduled endoscopic procedure. If the patient agrees, reiterating these instructions with the companion further ensures understanding and compliance. The procedure report, if documented on computerized software and a printed copy is made available, provides the patient a record for subsequent follow-up appointments or procedures.

SUMMARY

Service, efficiency, quality, safety, and successful outcomes are the lofty demands placed on endoscopy units, whether freestanding or hospital-based. With procedural volumes expected to continue to increase for screening for colon cancer, endoscopy units need to review their practices, concentrate on the appropriate flow of patients and equipment, and frequently evaluate important quality indicators to measure their success. High efficiency of volume with high quality of performance is based on high standards that are promulgated, communicated to all participants, consistently performed, and periodically monitored.

Acknowledgments
Appreciation is expressed to Dr. Donald Barkel, Nancy Gdowski, Nancy Gursin and Jack Mihalko for their helpful review of this manuscript.

References

[1] American Cancer Society. Cancer facts and figures 2007. Atlanta (GA): American Cancer Society; 2007.
[2] The Joint Commission on Accreditation of Healthcare Organization. Comprehensive accreditation manual for hospitals: the official handbook. Oakbrook Terrace (IL): The Joint Commission on Accreditation of Healthcare Organization; 2007.
[3] Cappell MS. The fetal safety and clinical efficacy of gastrointestinal disorders during pregnancy. Gastroenterol Clin North Am 2003;32:123–79.
[4] Siddiqui U, Proctor DD. Flexible sigmoidoscopy and colonoscopy during pregnancy. Gastrointest Endosc Clin N Am 2006;16:66–7.
[5] SGNA Guidelines: Guidelines for the use of high-level disinfectants and sterilants for reprocessing of flexible gastrointestinal endoscopes. Gastroenterol Nurs 2004;27:198–206.
[6] SGNA Position Statement on Minimal Registered Nurse Staffing for Patient Care in the Endoscopy Unit: May, 2002: Society of Gastroenterology Nurses and Associates' Practice Committee.
[7] Society of Gastroenterology Nurses and Associates, Inc. ASGE/SGNA role of GI registered nurses in the management of patients undergoing sedated procedures [position statement]. Chicago: Society of Gastroenterology Nurses and Associates, Inc; 2004. Available at: http://www.sgna.org/Resources/ASGESGNAPOSITIONSTATEMENT0613047.pdf. Accessed February 13, 2008.
[8] Rex DK, Heuss LT, Walker JA, et al. Trained registered nurses/endoscopy teams can administer propofol safely for endoscopy. Gastroenterology 2005;129:1384–91.

Gastroenterol Clin N Am 37 (2008) 129–160

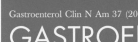

GASTROENTEROLOGY CLINICS
OF NORTH AMERICA

Reducing the Incidence and Mortality of Colon Cancer: Mass Screening and Colonoscopic Polypectomy

Mitchell S. Cappell, MD, PhD

Division of Gastroenterology, William Beaumont Hospital, MOB 233, 3601 West
Thirteen Mile Road, Royal Oak, MI 48073, USA

C olorectal cancer afflicts about 150,000 Americans annually, about 50,000 of whom die from the disease [1]. Established screening and surveillance colonoscopy regimens, as recommended by American and international medical societies [2,3], largely can prevent this mortality by detecting and removing premalignant colonic polyps and by detecting colon cancer at an early and curable stage [4–6]. Yet, nearly half of eligible United States patients have not undergone any form of screening for colon cancer [7,8]. Patients refuse screening because of embarrassment, fear of potential complications, reluctance to undergo invasive tests when asymptomatic, denial, and potential economic costs. Patients will become progressively harder to recruit for colon cancer screening tests as the more compliant patients have already undergone screening. The residual unscreened patients tend to be poor or ethnic minorities who have limited access to health care [9].

Although mostly because of patient factors, noncompliance also stems from physician factors. For example, most United States primary care physicians do not offer any form of colon cancer screening to eligible indigent patients [9]. This problem is not confined to America, but occurs throughout the world [10]. In a recent survey, only about one-quarter of 700 Italian general practitioners properly referred their patients for colon cancer screening, with both frequent over-referral and under-referral [11]. Under-referral results in thousands of preventable deaths in Italy per year [12]. Over-referral, such as referral for colonoscopy of average-risk patients less than 5 years after a negative screening colonoscopy, results in excessive costs without demonstrable benefits. To save patient lives and minimize costs, physicians in the United States and throughout the world must educate themselves to appropriately advocate screening colonoscopy, to answer patient misgivings about undergoing colonoscopy [13], and to follow practice guidelines [10]. Patient education by educated physicians moreover, should help eliminate patient barriers to mass screening [10].

E-mail address: mscappell@yahoo.com

0889-8553/08/$ – see front matter
doi:10.1016/j.gtc.2007.12.003

A review of the natural history of premalignant colonic polyps and the benefits of colorectal cancer screening is important and timely. This field is changing rapidly because of breakthroughs in the pathophysiology of colon cancer and in the technology for colon cancer screening and therapy. This article reviews colon cancer with a focus on the natural history, detection, and therapy of colonic polyps, the precursor lesions of colon cancer, to help the clinician and the gastroenterologist appropriately screen and treat patients to reduce colon cancer mortality.

PATHOPHYSIOLOGY

Histopathogenesis

Colon cancer arises from mucosal colonic polyps. Polyp histology is critical for determining malignant potential. The two common histologic types are hyperplastic and adenomatous. Histologically, hyperplastic polyps contain an increased number of glandular cells with decreased cytoplasmic mucus, but lack nuclear hyperchromatism, stratification, or atypia [14]. Adenomatous nuclei are usually hyperchromatic, enlarged, cigar-shaped, and crowded together in a palisade pattern. Adenomas are classified as tubular or villous. Histologically, tubular adenomas are composed of branched tubules, whereas villous adenomas contain digitiform villi arranged in a frond. Tubulovillous adenomas contain both elements.

Most colon cancers arise from conventional adenomas (conventional adenoma-to-carcinoma sequence) as demonstrated by epidemiologic, clinical, pathologic, and molecular genetic findings [15]. Although many hyperplastic polyps have little or no association with colon cancer [2], some hyperplastic polyps are associated with colon cancer [16]. Hyperplastic polyps appear to be linked to colon cancer by means of the recently reclassified (sessile) serrated adenoma (serrated adenoma-to-carcinoma theory), which previously was characterized as a hyperplastic polyp [17]. The pathophysiology of colon cancer, including its pathogenesis from conventional adenomas and serrated adenomas, is considered in detail in accompanying articles by Cappell, and East and Jass.

EPIDEMIOLOGY OF CONVENTIONAL ADENOMAS

Adenomas are somewhat more common in men than in women. Their incidence increases with patient age. They are rare in patients younger than 40 years old, except in patients who have genetic syndromes. Classically, about 15% to 25% of asymptomatic patients age 50 or older have adenomas detected at screening colonoscopy. A higher rate is, however, found at autopsy. For example, in a prospective necropsy study of 365 patients, 121 (33%) had colonic polyps [18]. The incidence rose to 50% in patients more than 70 years old.

CLINICAL PRESENTATION OF CONVENTIONAL ADENOMAS

Symptoms and signs are common when colon cancer is advanced and most likely incurable. They are less common when colon cancer is early and highly curable, and they are relatively uncommon with adenomatous polyps. This phenomenon renders adenomas or early colon cancer difficult to detect by clinical presentation and provides the rationale for mass screening of the general population before symptoms or signs occur to detect colon cancer at an early stage and to detect and remove premalignant colonic polyps to prevent their malignant transformation.

In a review of 800 patients who had colorectal polyps, about two-thirds were asymptomatic, and many of the others had symptoms that were likely coincidental and not caused by the polyps [19]. For example, rectal bleeding in a patient who has a small colonic polyp is more likely caused by other conditions, especially hemorrhoids [20]. Polyps more than 1 cm in diameter are more likely to produce symptoms, and polyps less than 0.5 cm rarely produce symptoms [21]. The most common symptoms attributable to polyps are rectal bleeding, abdominal pain, and change in bowel habits. A large polyp rarely forms the leading edge of a colonic intussusception.

Physical findings and laboratory abnormalities are uncommon with adenomatous polyps. A rectal polyp may be palpable by digital rectal examination. Much less than half of adenomas cause fecal occult blood [22]. Large adenomas are much more likely than small adenomas to cause fecal occult blood [21]. A benign colonic polyp rarely causes iron deficiency anemia; iron deficiency anemia is much more common with a malignant polyp because of greater chronic blood loss.

Small adenomas are believed to grow very slowly, unless they undergo malignant transformation. Perhaps, only 1 in 20 adenomas progresses to colon cancer. Advanced adenomas with significant dysplasia, diameter greater than 1 cm, or villous features, are more likely to progress to colon cancer.

CLINICAL PRESENTATION OF SERRATED ADENOMAS

Serrated adenomas are relatively uncommon. In a pioneering pathologic study of 18,000 colonic polyps published in 1990, only 0.6% were serrated adenomas [23]. In another study, about 18% of removed polyps originally classified as hyperplastic were reclassified as serrated adenomas using the revised histologic criteria [24]. Serrated adenomas frequently are right-sided and sessile. They may be flat and therefore difficult to identify at conventional colonoscopy using white light. The clinical presentation of serrated adenomas is largely unstudied and unknown. It is likely that most serrated adenomas are asymptomatic and do not produce fecal occult blood. For example, in a prospective study, only 10 of 276 hyperplastic polyps identified by colonoscopy and characterized pathologically after colonoscopic polypectomy had produced guaiac positive stool [22]. This study, and other studies, however, did not stratify and differentiate serrated adenomas from ordinary hyperplastic polyps. Large clinical studies are needed with sufficient follow-up to ascertain the clinical presentation and natural history of serrated adenomas.

SCREENING AND DIAGNOSTIC TESTS FOR COLONIC LESIONS

Screening of Average-risk Patients

Fecal occult blood: guaiac testing

Fecal occult blood testing (FOBT) was the traditional mainstay of screening for colon cancer and colonic polyps. It is tested most commonly by a colorimetric assay of a guaiac-based reaction catalyzed by the pseudoperoxidase present in blood. It is based on increased microscopic rectal bleeding in patients who have colon cancer compared with patients without colonic disease. Patients who have colon cancer, however, have a range of microscopic bleeding with considerable overlap with normal controls [21]. This overlap results in moderate test specificity. Specificity is increased by avoiding ingestion of broccoli, cauliflower, or red meats and by discontinuing aspirin therapy for 3 days before the test. Whether iron causes a falsely positive FOBT is controversial, but withholding iron therapy for several days before the test is prudent because of possible test interference. Even in ideal research studies, only 5% to 10% of patients who have fecal occult blood have colon cancer, and another 20% to 30% have colonic adenomatous polyps [25]. Although true-positive tests can lead to early colon cancer detection and cure, false-positive tests result in a large number of expensive and unnecessary colonoscopies.

FOBT is, moreover, only moderately sensitive. Sensitivity is improved by:

Performing stool tests on three different occasions, because colon cancer typically bleeds intermittently
Avoiding ascorbic acid for several days before the test, because ascorbic acid inhibits the guaiac reaction
Performing the test on fresh stool

Nevertheless, the sensitivity of FOBT for colon cancer using ideal techniques under the ideal circumstances of a research study is only about 85% [26]. The sensitivity for detecting adenomas is much less than 50%, because colonic adenomas bleed less frequently than colon cancer [22]. The sensitivity is particularly low for adenomas that are small or are located in the proximal colon.

Despite these flaws, FOBT was a traditional screening test because of test safety, simplicity, noninvasiveness, and low cost. Mandel and colleagues [27] demonstrated that annual screening by FOBT, with referral for colonoscopy if the test was positive, reduced mortality from colon cancer in a study of 46,551 patients. Study patients who had annual screening by FOBT had a 5.88 per 1000 cumulative mortality from colon cancer compared with an 8.83 per 1000 cumulative mortality in control subjects not undergoing such screening. Unexplained fecal occult blood mandates further evaluation of the colon to exclude colon cancer or polyps in any patient more than 40 years old [28].

Fecal occult blood: immunochemical testing
The Japanese have developed and extensively tested the fecal immunochemical test (FIT), in which antibodies are used to detect the globin protein within human hemoglobin in stool. These tests are more specific than guaiac tests, because they:

Do not react with food that contains peroxidase activity, such as broccoli
Do not react with food that contains nonhuman hemoglobin, such as (cow) steak
Do not register a positive result with upper gastrointestinal bleeding, because the globin protein in blood is degraded during intestinal transit by intestinal enzymes

Patient participation in FIT is simple because of the absence of dietary restrictions and the ease of procuring a sample by merely swishing a brush within the toilet bowl after defection.

FIT is significantly more sensitive than guaiac testing [29]. For example, in a colonoscopic study of 2512 patients, the FIT detected 87.5% of cancers versus 54.2% for guaiac testing, and detected 42.6% of advanced adenomas versus 23.0% for guaiac testing [30]. FIT has been used to screen more than six million people for colon cancer in Japan [31]. Screening with FIT, followed by colonoscopy if the screening test is positive, substantially reduces colon cancer mortality. In a study of 42,150 Japanese patients followed for 13 years, the mortality from colon cancer decreased by nearly 70% in patients screened by FIT compared with unscreened controls [32]. Other studies have confirmed this finding [31]. FIT, however, requires processing by a centralized laboratory and costs substantially more than guaiac tests.

Screening colonoscopy is superceding FIT . Although the 42.6% sensitivity of FIT for advanced adenomas is superior to that for guaiac testing, this rate is much lower than the 90% or higher sensitivity of screening colonoscopy. FIT may, however, play a subsidiary role for targeted screening of certain populations at mildly increased risk of colon cancer, such as asymptomatic African Americans aged 45 to 50 years.

Barium enema

Barium enema was a historically important alternative to colonoscopy, but its role is being superceded by virtual colonoscopy (CT colonography). It is only about 80% sensitive at detecting colon cancer and is much less sensitive at detecting colonic polyps [33]. In a study of 580 patients undergoing both barium enema and colonoscopy, barium enema detected only 32% of colonic polyps less than 6 mm in diameter, and only about 50% of larger (at least 6 mm) colonic polyps [34]. Barium enema also does not permit histologic characterization of an identified lesion because of an inability to perform biopsies, and it does not permit therapeutic removal of polyps. Thus detection of a moderate or large polyp at barium enema necessitates follow-up colonoscopy for polypectomy.

Flexible sigmoidoscopy

Flexible sigmoidoscopy every 3 to 5 years with annual FOBT has been recommended for screening [35]. Sigmoidoscopy decreases mortality from rectosigmoid colon cancer. Selby and colleagues [36] reported a 59% reduction of rectosigmoid cancer in patients undergoing one or more rigid sigmoidoscopies in the prior decade compared with unscreened controls matched for age and sex. In a retrospective case-controlled study by Newcomb and colleagues [37], 66 patients who died from colon cancer had a much lower frequency of having undergone screening flexible sigmoidoscopy than age- and sex-matched controls without colon cancer during a 13-year study period (10% versus 30% rate, $P<.05$).

Flexible sigmoidoscopy is, however, playing an increasingly limited role in screening. It is relatively insensitive at colon cancer and colon polyp detection, because the proximal half of the colon, where up to one-half of lesions are located, is not visualized endoscopically [38]. Even a screening strategy that calls for colonoscopy when a patient has a distal colonic polyp detected by sigmoidoscopy misses most proximal lesions, because proximal lesions usually do not have synchronous distal lesions [39]. Flexible sigmoidoscopy results in negligible prevention of right-sided colon cancer. For example, in the study by Newcomb and colleagues [37] cited previously, the observed reduction in colon cancer mortality was limited to left-sided cancers. Sigmoidoscopy is also an inadequate test for patients who have distal colon cancer, because 3% to 5% of these patients have a synchronous proximal cancer [15].

Diagnostic colonoscopy

Colonoscopy is recommended for screening of patients more than 50 years old at average risk for colon cancer or colonic polyps [35]. Colonoscopy is highly sensitive at detecting large (greater than 1 cm) colonic polyps, with a miss rate of only 6%, and it is moderately sensitive at detecting diminutive (less than 0.6 cm) polyps, with a miss rate of about 27% as reported in a study published in 1997 [40]. Recent data, however, suggest that the miss rate may be higher than previously appreciated. Colon cancers rarely are missed at colonoscopy, because they tend to be larger than adenomatous polyps. Colonoscopy is a highly specific test. At colonoscopy, polyps are removed and masses biopsied for a pathologic diagnosis.

The adenoma-to-carcinoma sequence strongly suggests that screening colonoscopy with polypectomy of adenomas should prevent colon cancer substantially. This is supported strongly by clinical trials. For example, in the National Polyp Study, 699 patients underwent surveillance colonoscopy at 1, 3, and every 2 subsequent years after detecting at least one adenomatous polyp at an index colonoscopy [41]. The 699 patients had a 76% to 90% decline in the incidence of colon cancer compared with historical reference groups. All the cancers were detected early. More recent studies have suggested a somewhat smaller reduction in colon cancer mortality.

Colonoscopy, however, has disadvantages as a screening test, because it is resource intensive, expensive, somewhat invasive, and uncomfortable, and entails a small, but significant, risk of serious complications. It requires a team, including a technician, nurse, and highly trained colonoscopist. Colonic preparation and dietary restrictions are necessary for 24 hours before the test. Diagnostic colonoscopy has about a 0.4% complication rate [42]. The most common major complications are gastrointestinal (GI) bleeding and colonic perforation.

Current Screening Guidelines

The relative benefits of the various screening tests are summarized in Table 1. Because of the importance of high sensitivity and relative specificity of a screening test to prevent cancer, colonoscopy has emerged as the screening test of choice [43]. Ironically, colonoscopy is both the screening test for polyp detection, the diagnostic test (gold standard) for polyp detection, and the therapeutic

Table 1

A comparison of the relative benefits of the various screening tests for colon cancer and colonic polyps

Beneficial screening characteristics	Fecal guaiac test	Fecal immunochemical Test	Flexible sigmoidoscopy	Barium enema	Colonoscopy	Virtual colonoscopy
Low cost	++++	+++	++	++	+	+
Convenient	++++	++	++	++	++	+
Easily accessible	++++	+++ [a]	+++	+++	++	+
Noninvasive	++++	++–+	++	++	+	++
Safe	++++	++++	++	++	+	++ [b]
High sensitivity	+	++	+++	+++	++++	+++
Relatively specific	+	++	+++	++	++++	++
Beneficial diagnostic or therapeutic characteristics						
Does not require a second (diagnostic) test if positive	+	+	++	+	++++	+
Therapeutic	+	+	++	+	++++	+

The above relative scale ranges from poor (+) to excellent (++++).

[a] Accessibility varies among countries depending upon commercial availability. The fecal immunochemical test is used routinely and is widely available in Japan, but is used rarely and is not readily available in America.

[b] Serious concerns have been raised about radiation risks to asymptomatic patients from mass screening of the general population.

technique for polyp removal. Because of the several disadvantages of colonoscopy as a screening test (see Table 1), alternative screening tests have been approved by multiple professional organizations (Table 2) [44]. Professional organizations generally have not endorsed virtual colonoscopy (CT colonography) for colon cancer screening because of highly variable and conflicting data about test sensitivity [45].

Surveillance of High-risk Patients and Diagnostic Testing of Patients Who Have Strong Clinical Indications

Patients at average risk for colonic adenomatous polyps or cancer undergo screening colonoscopy every 10 years, or alternative screening tests at periodic intervals. Patients who are members of high-risk groups undergo periodic surveillance more frequently, with colonoscopy as the recommended test. The age of beginning surveillance and the frequency of surveillance depend upon the age of onset of the increased cancer risk and the quantitative risk of cancer [46]. This topic is reviewed in detail in accompanying articles by Konda and Duffy for nonsyndromic colon cancer, and by Desai and Barkel for syndromic colon cancer. Aside from periodic screening or surveillance, patients require colonoscopy to exclude colon cancer, adenomatous polyps, or other colonic diseases for specific indications, as listed in Boxes 1 and 2.

Improving Polyp Detection at Colonoscopy: Conventional Techniques

The primary benefit of screening colonoscopy in preventing colon cancer lies in the removal of premalignant polyps, which is predicated upon polyp identification. Identification of premalignant or potentially malignant polyps has become more complicated recently with the realization that serrated adenomas, which are often flat and inconspicuous, have a risk of malignant transformation equivalent to, or potentially greater than, that of conventional adenomas [22], and

Table 2	
Recommendations by the American Cancer Society for screening for colon cancer in average-risk asymptomatic individuals beginning at age 50 years	
Recommended tests or procedures	**Frequency**
1. Fecal occult blood test (FOBT) or fecal immunochemical test (FIT)[a]	Annually Annually
2. Flexible sigmoidoscopy[a]	Every five years
3. Fecal occult blood test (FOBT) and flexible sigmoidoscopy	Annual FOBT and flexible sigmoidoscopy every five years
4. Double contrast barium enema	Every five years
5. Colonoscopy	Every 10 years

[a]The American Cancer Society recommends "Flexible sigmoidoscopy together with FOBT is preferred compared with FOBT or flexible sigmoidoscopy alone." The author feels strongly that only FOBT (option 1) or only flexible sigmoidoscopy (option 2) should be eliminated as acceptable screening tests because of insufficient sensitivity of these tests, and that these tests only should be used in combination (option 3). For example, FOBT may fail to detect up to 87% of colonic adenomas [22].

Data from Smith RA, Cokkinides V, Eyre HJ. Cancer screening in the United States: a review of current guidelines, practices, and prospects. CA Cancer J Clin 2007;57:90–104.

Box 1: Indications for colonoscopic surveillance for colon cancer

Personal history
Prior colonic adenomatous polyps
Prior colon cancer
Peutz-Jeghers syndrome
Hereditary nonpolyposis colon cancer (Lynch syndrome)
Juvenile polyposis syndrome
Chronic ulcerative colitis
Chronic Crohn's colitis

Family history
Colon cancer
Colonic adenomatous polyps
Hereditary nonpolyposis colon cancer (Lynch syndrome)
Familial adenomatous polyposis

the realization that conventional colonoscopy frequently misses colonic polyps. In a study of 26 colonoscopists, the miss rates of adenomas ranged from 17% to 28%, as determined by a second tandem colonoscopy performed immediately after the index colonoscopy [40]. Moreover, the detection rate of adenomas varies greatly among experienced colonoscopists. For example, the rate of

Box 2: Acute indications for colonoscopy to exclude colonic adenomas, colon cancer, or other colonic diseases

Fecal occult blood
Iron deficiency anemia
Hematochezia
Melena with a nondiagnostic esophagogastroduodenoscopy (EGD)
Streptococcus bovis bacteremia
Finding of colonic polyps at sigmoidoscopy
Adenocarcinoma metastatic to the liver with an unknown primary
Change in bowel habits in the elderly
Follow-up after colonoscopic removal of a large sessile proximal colonic polyp
Abnormal radiologic study (barium enema, virtual colonoscopy) suggestive of colon cancer
Colonic stricture
Dye injection to label a malignant polyp for subsequent surgical removal
Intraoperative colonoscopy to localize a lesion for surgical removal

adenoma detection varied tenfold among 12 experienced colonoscopists in private practice in Rockford, Illinois [47], and varied threefold among academic colonoscopists at the Mayo Clinic [48]. Although colonoscopy tends to be quite sensitive at detecting large polyps, which are more likely to be malignant or advanced adenomas, colonoscopy occasionally can miss even these polyps [47]. Furthermore, small polyps, which are missed frequently, occasionally exhibit advanced histology or even harbor frank cancer. For example, in a study of 1933 small (5 to 10 mm) or diminutive (1 to 4 mm) adenomatous polyps detected in 3291 consecutive colonoscopies, 10.1% of small polyps exhibited cancer or advanced adenomatous histology, and 1.7% of diminutive polyps exhibited these histologic findings [49]. In another study of 5047 consecutive small or diminutive polyps, 15.6% of small polyps and 4.4% of diminutive polyps exhibited advanced histology [50]. Even small, flat serrated adenomas have a malignant potential [51].

Several colonoscopic techniques are recommended to increase the detection of colonic polyps. First, a properly prepared colon is essential for colonoscopy. Polyps can and are missed in areas containing stool. An unclean colon also renders colonoscopic intubation and colonoscopic polypectomy technically more difficult and potentially more dangerous. A dirty colon usually is caused by failure of the patient to follow the proper directions for colonic preparation. When scheduling a colonoscopy, the colonoscopist should review the colonic preparation with the patient and stress the importance of the patient taking the whole colonic preparation and drinking only clear liquids the day before the procedure. The polyethylene glycol (PEG) electrolyte solution requires drinking 4 L of liquid in about 4 hours. Some patients fail to drink the entire amount. Administration of a PEG electrolyte solution on the day of colonoscopy or in divided doses, with one half the night before and one half on the day of the procedure, may improve the quality of the colonic preparation [52]. Fleet's phospho-soda is a useful alternative preparation, but the patient must drink plenty of fluids when taking this preparation. It should be used with extreme caution in patients who have even mild renal insufficiency. This preparation can precipitate renal failure or electrolyte disturbances [53,54].

Second, adequate sedation is a prerequisite for colonoscopy. Highly anxious patients, patients who failed a prior attempt at colonoscopy because of pain or anxiety, and uncooperative patients may require the assistance of an anesthesiologist for adequate sedation. Propofol provides deeper sedation and a faster recovery time than conventional sedation with benzodiazepines and opiates, highly attractive attributes for outpatient screening colonoscopy [55]. In many endoscopy units, propofol is administered exclusively by anesthesiologists because of concerns about its toxicity, mostly hypoventilation, caused by a low therapeutic index. This practice is controversial, however. Participation of an anesthesiologist at colonoscopy substantially increases the procedural costs. A very large colonoscopic study has shown gastroenterologists and nurses can administer propofol safely [56].

Third, confirmation of cecal intubation is essential at colonoscopy. Mischaracterization of an incomplete colonoscopy as complete because of mistaken identification of the cecum can result in missing clinically significant right-sided colonic lesions, including cancers. Missed polyps that are not removed at an index incomplete screening colonoscopy may continue to grow without colonoscopic intervention for 10 years until the next recommended screening colonoscopy. This phenomenon may be a common reason for early interval cancers after an index colonoscopy purportedly devoid of polyps [57]. For example, in a retrospective analysis of 35,975 colonoscopies in Manitoba, Canada, the rate of colon cancer was reduced markedly for the first 5 years after an index colonoscopy, but an unusually large proportion of the early cancers detected during these 5 years were right-sided, presumably because of right-sided lesions missed at the index colonoscopy [58].

Deep colonoscopic intubation, as indicated by the centimeter ruler markings on the colonoscope shaft, does not indicate cecal intubation reliably, because the colonoscope could be looped within the colon. Several cecal landmarks reliably confirm cecal intubation. The appendix is visualized as a slit-like, semi-lunar, or ovoid opening near the caput of the cecum on the (medial) colonic wall closest to the middle of the ileocecal valve. The ileocecal valve is a characteristic round, smooth, soft, homogeneous mound lying on a prominent fold on the medial colonic wall just distal to the caput of the cecum. Occasionally, air or stool is seen exiting by means of the ileocecal valve into the colon. The ileocecal valve may contain a central dimple above its opening, and may appear yellowish due to fatty infiltration. The valve opening is not seen directly, because it is perpendicular to the colon, but may be intubated blindly. Such intubation also confirms ileocecal valve identification. Documentation of cecal landmarks by a videophotograph during colonoscopy may help avoid malpractice litigation concerning missed colonic lesions because of incomplete colonoscopy [59].

Other colonic landmarks suggest but do not prove cecal intubation. A combination of landmarks may be convincing. The cecum is a wide saccular organ that ends blindly. Other colonic regions, particularly the hepatic flexure, may be confused with the cecum, because the lumen may appear to end blindly at a sharp colonic turn. The merger of the three teniae coli at the cecal base produces a characteristic appearance resembling a crow's foot or the "Mercedes Benz" car symbol. Transillumination with the colonoscopic light source during cecal intubation may demonstrate light visible in the deep right lower quadrant of the abdomen. External manual compression in the same abdominal region may reveal discrete one-for-one indentation of the colonic lumen in the cecum. Colonoscopic passage through the hepatic flexure usually is indicated by visualization of a purplish-blue macular patch on one side of the colonic wall at an acute colonic turn due to the adjacent liver. A similar finding occasionally can be seen at the splenic flexure caused by the adjacent spleen.

Fourth, if a screening colonoscopy is incomplete, another colonic examination is indicated. If it was incomplete because of poor colonic preparation, the colonoscopy should be repeated after a more vigorous colonic preparation. Repeating the colonoscopy on the next day is advantageous, because the patient can be prepared further to supplement the prior partial, but inadequate, preparation. If the colonoscopy was incomplete because the patient was uncooperative or experienced too much pain, it should be repeated with an anesthesiologist in attendance. If it was incomplete because of technical difficulty, such as diverticular disease or excessive colonic looping, virtual colonoscopy should be considered instead of colonoscopy. The previous recommendations pertain when the ileocecal valve was not visualized at the initial colonoscopy. In this situation, the colonoscopist does not know how much of the colon was not intubated and not visualized. If the colonoscopy was complete except for visualization of the last few centimeters beyond the ileocecal valve–whether because of stool in the caput of the cecum, spasm of the caput, or excessive looping–and the colonoscopy was otherwise free of polyps, the situation should be explained to the patient. The patient may in this situation elect to forgo the rigors of another colonoscopy because of the small likelihood of missing a polyp in the cecum.

Several colonoscopic maneuvers aid in colonoscopic intubation beyond the ileocecal valve into the cecum, including:

Colonic decompression by aspiration of air
Manual external compression of the abdomen by the endoscopic assistant to prevent colonic looping during colonic intubation
Colonic aspiration to hold the colonoscope against the cecal wall while withdrawing the colonoscope a few centimeters
Jiggling the colonoscope back and forth over a short distance to reduce colonic loops
Turning the patient
Partial withdrawal of the colonoscope shaft to reduce colonic loops before attempting cecal intubation

In a variable stiffness colonoscope, the colonoscope should be set on maximal stiffness to minimize colonic looping during cecal intubation.

Fifth, a withdrawal time of at least 6 min is recommended to ensure adequate colonic examination and to maximize the detection of adenomas [60]. In an initial study of 10,159 diagnostic colonoscopies among 31 colonoscopists, the detection rate of polyps was correlated directly with the mean time of colonoscopy [48]. In a subsequent study, these data were refined by analyzing only colonoscopic withdrawal time to more accurately measure the time spent searching for colonic polyps. Colonoscopists generally search for polyps during colonoscopic withdrawal as they focus on finding the colonic lumen for safe colonoscopic advancement during colonic intubation. The author's practice is to examine for colonic polyps during colonoscopic withdrawal by holding the colonoscope in the center of the colonic lumen and circling around toward the periphery as necessary. In a prospective study of 7882 colonoscopies among 12 colonoscopists, colonoscopists who had a mean withdrawal time greater than 6 min had, compared with colonoscopists who had a shorter withdrawal time, a significantly higher detection rate of neoplastic polyps (28.3% versus 11.8%, $P<.001$), and of advanced neoplasia (6.4% versus 2.6%, $P<.005$; [47]).

Sixth, colonoscopic maneuvers can improve polyp detection. Colonic polyps may be missed around sharp turns, especially the hepatic and sigmoid flexures; at areas of colonic spasm, especially in the sigmoid colon or with severe diverticulosis; and behind large folds. During withdrawal, the colonoscope may fly rapidly around a turn so that one side or that entire area is not visualized. If this occurs, the colon should be reintubated beyond the poorly visualized area. The missed area around the turn should be inspected during the second intubation and the second withdrawal. This maneuver may be repeated until this area is inspected satisfactorily. The colonoscope also can rapidly fly around colonic areas occasionally because of reduction of a loop during extubation. This phenomenon is best prevented by avoiding colonic loops.

Colonic spasm is avoided by not irritating the colon by meticulous colonoscopic technique that avoids excessive colonic air insufflation, colonic loops, and traumatic intubation. Trauma is avoided by identifying proximal lumen before colonoscope advancement, with minimal, judicious use of the slide-by technique. Colonic spasm is usually more apparent during colonic intubation than extubation. Colonic spasm is often troublesome in areas of severe colonic diverticulosis, particularly in the sigmoid colon where the lumen is relatively narrow even without diverticulosis. Colonic spasm may be addressed by gentle air insufflation to distend the spastic area. Paradoxically, withdrawal of air from other colonic areas not suffering from spasm may decrease colonic irritability and decrease the spasm in the area being examined. Instillation of warm water may be more effective than insufflation of air to address colonic spasm, because water is less irritating to the colon than air [61]. The author suspects that the conscious sensation of pain during colonoscopy may increase colonic spasm, and that adequate sedation and analgesia may reduce colonic spasm. Although intravenous glucagon can help reverse colonic spasm, this agent should be used rarely and sparingly. If colonic visualization is limited in a small colonic segment because of the presence of liquid stool, the area can be irrigated and aspirated to remove the stool and to improve visibility. This approach is not feasible if most of the colon is contaminated heavily with stool, particularly if the stool is solid.

Areas behind a fold not visualized with the colonoscope in the orthograde (unretroflexed) position can be viewed by retroflexing the colonoscope. A colonoscope with variable shaft stiffness should be set on minimal shaft stiffness during colonic retroflexion. Retroflexion can be performed safely by an experienced colonoscopist in the ascending colon, where the colonic lumen is sufficiently wide to permit this maneuver. This maneuver:

Should not be attempted by inexperienced colonoscopists
Should be avoided in areas where the colon is narrow, such as the sigmoid
Should be avoided in areas of diverticulosis
Should be avoided in areas where the colon is weakened by disease

The author is aware of two cases of colonic perforation due to colonoscopic retroflexion, one performed in an area of ischemic colitis, where the colonic wall integrity was weakened by the colonic ischemia, and one performed in an area of colonic diverticulosis, in which a diverticulum was intubated inadvertently during colonoscopic retroflexion.

The Third Eye Retroscope (Avantis Medical Systems, Sunnyvale, California) is an auxiliary viewing lens that is passed through the instrument channel and positioned several centimeters beyond the tip of a standard colonoscope to provide a retrograde view behind colonic folds. The Third Eye Retroscope permitted identification of significantly more simulated colonic polyps, placed behind a fold, than a standard colonoscope (81% versus 12%, $P<.0001$) in a commercially available anatomic model of the colon [62]. This device has not been tested in people and is currently experimental. Conventional colonoscopes with a 140° angle of view are being replaced with new-generation colonoscopes with a 170° angle of view. These wide-angle colonoscopes may render colonic intubation more efficient, as measured by a shorter intubation time, because of better visualization of colonic lumen around sharp turns, but they have not resulted in a greater detection rate of colonic polyps by visualizing polyps behind folds [63]. A small area not visualized behind a single large fold usually can be visualized by pressing a closed biopsy forceps against the fold to efface it. This technique is useful to visualize a polyp behind a fold for forceps biopsy or snare polypectomy, but it is time-consuming and impractical to apply to the entire colon or even a large colonic segment.

Improving Colonic Polyp Detection at Colonoscopy: Advanced Techniques

New technologies can enhance the detection rate of colonic polyps, particularly chromoendoscopy and narrow band imaging. In chromoendoscopy a vital dye, either methylene blue or indigo carmine, is sprayed on the colon to highlight areas of abnormal mucosa before the area of the colon is examined. This technique requires insertion of a special catheter through the instrument channel to completely spray and uniformly cover colonic mucosa. In a colonoscopic study of 259 patients randomly assigned to chromoendoscopy versus standard colonoscopy, chromoendoscopy was associated with a trend toward greater detection of adenomas, which was statistically significant only for diminutive (less than 5 mm) adenomas (89 versus 37 $P=.026$; [64]). In another colonoscopic study, 260 patients were randomized to receive either panchromoendoscopy, performed throughout the colon, versus targeted chromoendoscopy, performed only at the site of potential lesions [65]. Panchromoendoscopy detected significantly more adenomas than targeted chromoendoscopy (66% versus 33%, $P<.05$), including detection of significantly more diminutive (less than 5 mm wide) adenomas. Flat adenomas are important because of a potentially significant risk of high-grade dysplasia. They are difficult to detect and often missed at conventional colonoscopy. These lesions are identified better by high magnification colonoscopy with either chromoendoscopy or narrow-band imaging [66].

Although chromoendoscopy increases the detection of small polyps and flat adenomas, the clinical significance of this improved detection is uncertain.

Chromoendoscopy is not indicated for routine screening colonoscopy in average-risk patients, because it greatly prolongs procedure time, leading to significantly greater costs [67]. A recent study suggests that an expert colonoscopist may detect as many colonic polyps using ordinary white light, with a new-generation high-definition colonoscope, as when using expensive, advanced technology, such as narrow band imaging. In this colonoscopic study of 434 patients, the colonoscopist detected 1 or more adenomas in 67% of patients with white light versus 65% of patients with narrow band imaging ($P=.61$; [68]). This study suggests that advanced, expensive colonoscopic technologies may be unnecessary, and may be replaced by introduction of the new-generation high-definition colonoscopes and by further education of colonoscopists to recognize subtle colonoscopic features of small or inconspicuous adenomas. Methylene blue use for chromoendoscopy recently has been associated with DNA damage to colonocytes [69].

The enhanced detection rate of advanced technologies, such as chromoendoscopy, however, may be beneficial for high-risk patients, such as patients who have the Lynch syndrome [70,71]. It also may permit targeted biopsies of suspicious areas in patients who have ulcerative colitis, as opposed to the standard clinical practice of random nontargeted biopsies [72].

Finally, even under ideal circumstances and even with excellent colonoscopic technique, significant colonic lesions are missed. In one colonoscopic study of 5055 colonoscopies, 17 (5.9%) of 286 cancers were missed by an initial colonoscopy [73]. Missed lesions at colonoscopy are a potential source of medical malpractice litigation [74]. It is recommended that the colonoscopist inform the patient of this potential complication of colonoscopy when obtaining informed consent for the procedure. Also, if a patient presents with symptoms or signs highly suggestive of colon cancer after a recent negative colonoscopy, the colonoscopist should consider repeating the colonoscopy [73].

HISTOLOGIC CLASSIFICATION OF COLONIC POLYPS AT COLONOSCOPY: CONVENTIONAL TECHNIQUES

It is impossible to accurately determine polyp histology solely by colonoscopic criteria. Even diminutive polyps or flat lesions can be conventional adenomas or serrated adenomas, respectively, with a potential for malignant transformation. This phenomenon has led to a general policy of removing all polyps detected at colonoscopy. Colonoscopic polypectomy entails some risk, however, including the risk of colonic perforation, the postpolypectomy syndrome [75], and postpolypectomy hemorrhage [76]. The number of identified polyps is increasing rapidly because of the increasing performance of colonoscopy for screening, slower colonoscopic withdrawal [47], introduction of new generation high-definition colonoscopes [68], and application of novel technologies for better polyp detection, such as chromoendoscopy [77] or narrow band imaging [78]. This phenomenon may result in potentially more frequent postpolypectomy complications.

Progress is being made in determining polyp histology based solely on colonoscopic criteria. The goal is to rationally decide on colonoscopic removal versus nonremoval of individual polyps based on accurate histologic classification by colonoscopic criteria (ie, to remove polyps classified as an adenoma, whether conventional or serrated, and to not remove a polyp classified as a conventional hyperplastic polyp). This strategy would eliminate polypectomy and its attendant risks for polyps with a histology that has no known malignant potential. The success of this strategy depends on accurate determination of polyp histology based solely on colonoscopic criteria, and excellent data on the natural history of all types of colonic polyps. Neither of these prerequisites is satisfied. A polyp currently cannot be classified definitively as a serrated adenoma solely based on colonoscopic criteria, and the natural history of small adenomas, including biologic predictors of malignant transformation, are characterized poorly.

Conventional colonoscopy, using white light, provides useful data concerning polyp histology but this characterization is somewhat inaccurate (Table 3; [15,28,79–81]). Polyps are characterized at colonoscopy according to size, color, number, segmental location, intramural location (mucosal versus submucosal), presence or absence of a stalk (pedunculated versus sessile), and superficial appearance. Polyp characteristics at colonoscopy provide important clues concerning polyp histology and malignant potential that influence colonoscopic management. Hyperplastic polyps are usually small, pale, and unilobular, and are located in the rectum [28]. Adenomas are larger, redder, and more multilobular, and are distributed throughout the colon. Villous adenomas tend to be large, bulky, sessile, shaggy, soft, velvety, and friable [28]. Flat adenomas tend to be small, discoid, and erythematous plaques. Colonoscopic appearance, however, only moderately correlates with polyp histology. Pathologic examination of a colonoscopic biopsy provides an indication of polyp histology, but is subject to sampling error. A polyp is definitively classified by pathologic examination of the entire polyp after polypectomy. Colonoscopic polypectomy is diagnostic and therapeutic for noncancerous adenomatous polyps.

The differential diagnosis of numerous polypoid colonic masses detected at colonoscopy includes familial adenomatous polyposis (FAP), attenuated FAP, hyperplastic polyposis, juvenile polyposis, Peutz-Jeghers syndrome, pseudopolyposis, diffuse colonic hemangiomatosis, and pneumatosis coli. These conditions are differentiated by clinical, radiologic, colonoscopic, and histologic findings. In patients with FAP, the colonic mucosa is carpeted by hundreds or thousands of adenomatous polyps. In patients with attenuated FAP, only about thirty adenomatous polyps are present. These polyps are usually located in the proximal colon, and tend to be flat growths because of intramural, rather than intraluminal, growth. Classic and attenuated FAP are both caused by *APC* mutations. In attenuated FAP, *APC* mutations occur at certain sites, particularly the extreme proximal or distal ends of the *APC* gene [46]. Patients with FAP must undergo prophylactic colectomy after puberty to prevent colon cancer [46]. Hyperplastic polyposis is characterized by 30 or more polyps in the colon, a predominantly right-sided polyp distribution, and a positive family history [82]. Juvenile polyposis is characterized by a family history of juvenile

Type of polyp	Typical endoscopic appearance	References
Common mucosal polyps		
Simple hyperplastic	Small, pale, homogeneous surface, unilobular, minimally elevated, may flatten with air insufflation, nonpedunculated, located in rectum, often multiple when present	[28,79]
Sessile serrated adenomas	Flat or sessile, coating of brown adherent mucus, often in right colon, indistinct margins, wrinkles develop with snaring	[79]
Tubular adenomas	Reddish, quite vascular, typically > 5mm, homogenous surface, typically pedunculated, typically unilobular	[28]
Villous adenomas	Large, bulky, sessile, multinodular, shaggy, soft, velvety, and friable	[15]
Frank cancer	Large size (mass), inhomogeneous surface, possible superficial ulceration, often hard, multinodular	
Invasive cancer	Findings of frank cancer together with "non-lift" sign during submucosal injection	[81]
Other polyps		
Lipomas	Submucosal location with normal overlying mucosa, smooth surface, homogeneous yellow color, usually not pedunculated, rounded shape, naked fat sign, pillow sign	[28]
Inverted diverticulum	Characteristic ovoid shape, smooth surface, margins of mass continuous with adjoining mucosa, very soft, compressible (indents) when probed with a closed biopsy forceps, may recede into bowel wall with air insufflation, homogenous pink color that resembles normal mucosa, typically in distal colon, near haustral folds, typically in a patient with numerous true diverticuli, minimally elevated, nonpedunculated	[80] & current report
Pseudopolyps	Filiform appearance or pedunculated, usually multiple, characteristically associated with inflammatory bowel disease and occurring in colonic areas affected by the colitis, mucus adherent to the apex of the polyp	

polyposis, more than five juvenile polyps in the colon, multiple juvenile polyps throughout the rest of the GI tract, and polyp development at a young age [83]. This syndrome is associated with a greatly increased risk of colon cancer. In Peutz-Jeghers syndrome, multiple hamartomatous polyps, which characteristically contain abundant branching smooth muscle, occur throughout the GI tract. Patients characteristically have perioral and oral hyperpigmentation caused by melanin deposition [46]. This syndrome is associated with a greatly increased risk of colon cancer [84]. Pseudopolyps represent islands of variably inflamed residual mucosa surrounded by a background of previously sloughed off mucosa. It is associated most commonly with ulcerative colitis. Other colonoscopic findings of ulcerative colitis, including mucosal erythema, granularity, blunting of the normal vascular pattern, friability, mucopus, mucosal hemorrhage, and superficial ulcerations may be present. At colonoscopy, hemangiomas often appear as multiple, violet-blue, sessile, polypoid lesions [28]. They are associated with characteristic dermatologic lesions in the blue rubber bleb nevus syndrome. In pneumatosis coli, multiple air-filled cysts are present in the colonic submucosa. Colonoscopy reveals multiple, pale, cystic, round polypoid masses with overlying intact mucosa [28].

Early colon cancer may occur in an adenomatous polyp and therefore may be difficult to distinguish by colonoscopy from a nonmalignant adenomatous polyp. For example, a 2 cm wide villous adenoma has an approximately 40% chance of harboring cancer [28]. Polyp risk factors for malignancy include villous rather than tubular histology, large size, sessile morphology, superficial ulceration, multinodularity, depressed lesions, and increasing number of colonic polyps [28]. The colonoscopic nonlift sign is associated with infiltrative malignancy. Advanced colon cancer typically appears as a large, exophytic mass because of intraluminal growth, or as a colonic stricture because of circumferential growth. A colonic stricture may, however, be benign. Malignancy is suggested when a colonic stricture is ulcerated, indurated, asymmetric, and friable, and has irregular or overhanging margins. The colonoscopic appearance is not definitive. Pathologic examination of multiple colonic biopsies and cytologic analysis of stricture brushings are usually diagnostic.

In exceptional circumstances, the colonoscopic appearance provides sufficiently accurate information to permit polyp nonremoval. When a patient has numerous pale, diminutive polyps in the rectum and sigmoid that bear the classic colonoscopic appearance of hyperplastic polyps, it is unnecessary and inadvisable to remove all of them to avoid the extra risks and costs of their removal. The author's practice is to remove the largest and most atypical-appearing of these polyps and to sample several others by biopsies. Right-sided flat lesions, even when multiple, should be removed aggressively, however, because they may be serrated adenomas. Lipomas should not be removed, unless their identification is uncertain, because of their harmless nature and the risk associated with removing a submucosal lesion. In a patient who has known inflammatory bowel disease, typical inflammatory polyps in an affected colonic area may be sampled by biopsies, but it is unnecessary to remove these polyps if they are characteristic in colonoscopic appearance. Atypical polyps or flat lesions should be treated aggressively, however, to exclude a dysplasia-associated lesion or mass (DALM). Polypectomy should not be performed on a lesion exhibiting the characteristic findings of an inverted diverticulum because of the risk of colonic perforation [85].

Large polyps that are likely or obviously malignant should be sampled extensively by multiple biopsies to increase the diagnostic yield, but not removed in toto by polypectomy at an initial colonoscopy to avoid the extra risks of poly-pectomy when cancer surgery likely will be required subsequently [86]. This permits a rational approach to the polyp based on histologic analysis of the biopsies, and a planned approach based on discussion of the therapeutic alter-natives with the patient.

HISTOLOGIC CHARACTERIZATION OF COLONIC POLYPS AT COLONOSCOPY: ADVANCED TECHNOLOGY

Advanced colonoscopic accessories increasingly have been applied to classify polyps according to histology at colonoscopy. The most experience has accumu-lated with high magnification chromoendoscopy. This method combines chro-moendoscopy with an advanced colonoscope that provides zoom optics with up to 100 times magnification. Chromoendoscopic spraying highlights the colonic pits because of their retention of the dye. The high magnification then permits detailed analysis of the anatomy of the superficial colonic pits. Kudo has classified six colonic pit patterns, labeled 1, 11, 111 s, 111 1, IV, and V [87]. Type I pits are round in size and resemble that of normal colonic mucosa, while type II pits are stellate or papillary in shape. These two patterns are characteristic of ordinary hyperplastic polyps. Type III s pits are tiny and round, while type III l pits are large and tubular. Type IV pits resemble the sulci or gyri on the surface of the cerebral cortex. Adenomas typically exhibit type III l or type IV pits. Type V pits are typical of advanced neoplasia. Several studies have shown that pit pattern analysis is quite reliable at histologic classification of colonic polyps. For example, in a study of 905 colonic polyps, prediction of neoplasia by pit analysis had a sen-sitivity of 90.8% and specificity of 72.7% [88]. In another study of 110 colonic polyps in 78 patients, the prediction of neoplasia based on pit analysis had a sen-sitivity of 95.7% and specificity of 87.5% [89]. This reported sensitivity and specificity are much higher than that reported for conventional colonoscopy. Other techniques for histologic characterization of polyps at colonoscopy include narrow band imaging, autofluorescence, and confocal laser microscopy. These techniques and technologies show promise for clinical applications, but have not yet been adapted into general gastroenterologic practice. For clinical use, these technologies must be nearly 100% accurate to avoid nonremoval of advanced adenomas that are falsely characterized as non-neoplastic.

STRATEGIES TO REDUCE THE RISKS OF COLONOSCOPIC POLYPECTOMY

Several strategies are recommended to reduce the risks of colonoscopic poly-pectomy. First, less invasive and less risky techniques are recommended to remove low-risk small polyps. Colonic polyps less than 0.8 cm in diameter usually are removed by hot biopsy, especially when sessile, whereas polyps that are larger than 0.8 cm in diameter usually are removed by snare polypec-tomy, especially when pedunculated [28]. Hot biopsy is performed cautiously in the cecum using a low amplitude and brief duration of current, because the colonic wall is thinnest and most vulnerable to transmural necrosis in this region [28]. Diminutive polyps that are less than 6 mm in diameter and sessile may be removed by cold snare polypectomy, wherein the polyp is snared and transected in guillotine fashion without electrocautery. Cold snare polypectomy may be preferred to hot snare or hot biopsy polypectomy for diminutive polyps because of less polypectomy risks. Cold snare polypectomy is very safe. It has a low risk of postpolypectomy hemorrhage [90]. It does not cause the postpolypectomy syndrome and exceedingly rarely causes colonic perforation because of the absence of thermal injury. Ultradiminutive (less than 4 mm) polyps may be removed by repeated cold biopsies without electrocautery. Cold snare or cold biopsy polypectomy avoids diathermy artifact in the resected specimen, but entails a theoretic risk of incomplete removal of neoplastic tissue. Electrocautery, in contrast, theoretically destroys residual neoplastic tissue in the unremoved stump. Even electrocautery, however, can leave residual unremoved neoplastic tissue. For example, after hot biopsy removal of 62 diminutive polyps, 11 (17%) had residual viable polyp remnants on flexible sigmoidoscopy performed 2 weeks after the initial polyp removal [91].

Second, adjunctive techniques are being applied to remove high-risk polyps to increase the safety of their removal. Deep submucosal injection of normal saline is applied to larger polyps before colonoscopic polypectomy to thicken the colonic wall and decrease the risk of a transmural burn. For example, sessile polyps between 2 and 3 cm in diameter may be removed by snare polypectomy after creating a pseudopedicle by injecting normal saline or another solution into the polyp base [90]. This technique is discussed later under endoscopic mucosal resection. Sessile polyps more than 3 cm in diameter may not be amenable to conventional snare polypectomy, but may be removed by sequential piecewise polypectomy during several colonoscopic sessions. Pedunculated polyps more than 5 cm in diameter or occluding the lumen may not be amenable to conventional colonoscopic polypectomy because of the technical difficulty of looping a snare around these polyps. These polyps may require surgical resection even when benign.

Third, minimally invasive colonoscopic management of postpolypectomy complications is often effective. The complication rate of therapeutic colonoscopy is about 1.4% [42]. Common major postpolypectomy complications include GI bleeding, colonic perforation, and the postpolypectomy syndrome. Significant postpolypectomy bleeding can occur immediately after polypectomy or be delayed. Bleeding occurs after about 1% of polypectomies [76]. Most immediate postpolypectomy bleeding is capillary and minor. Significant immediate postpolypectomy bleeding is usually arterial and arises from failure to thermocoagulate or electrocoagulate the feeding artery during polypectomy. This bleeding should be managed immediately at the index colonoscopy. The polyp remnant should be resnared and held taut for about 5 minutes, without applying current, to compress the bleeding vessel and promote thrombostasis [76]. After 5 minutes, the snare should be loosened but not removed around the stalk base to check if the polyp is still bleeding. If bleeding recurs, the snare should be tightened again immediately around the stalk and held taught for another 10 minutes.

Delayed significant postpolypectomy hemorrhage also is managed initially by colonoscopy. Active bleeding from the polypectomy site usually is managed by injection of epinephrine at a concentration of 1:10,000 using a sclerotherapy needle, by short bursts of electrocoagulation or thermocoagulation at the bleeding site, or by painting the site with argon plasma coagulation. These treatments are not mutually exclusive. Epinephrine may be injected first to reduce the bleeding, and then electrocoagulation applied for definitive hemostasis. Detachable clips also can be deployed at the bleeding site to compress the bleeding vessel and arrest the bleeding [92]. Detachable clips or detachable snares can be placed proximally on the stalk of a pedunculated polyp before conventional snare polypectomy to prevent postpolypectomy bleeding.

Perforation after polypectomy results from thermal injury to the colonic wall during electrocoagulation with snare polypectomy. Occasionally adjacent mucosa may be caught up in the snare and ligated during polypectomy resulting in perforation. Cecal polyps must be removed carefully by a hot snare with a low current setting because of the thinner colonic wall and consequently increased risk of colonic perforation at the cecum. Suspected colonic perforation requires abdominal roentgenograms and, often, abdominal CT to exclude pneumoperitoneum. The patient who has colonic perforation initially should be managed by nothing per os, intravenous antibiotics, repletion of fluid losses, and correction of electrolyte imbalances. Hospitalization and prompt surgical consultation is required. Perforations that are large, accompanied by sepsis, exhibit progressive peritoneal signs, or occur in a dirty, poorly prepared colon usually require surgical repair. Detachable clips can be deployed at colonoscopy to close off a colonic perforation and obviate the need for surgery. This has been successfully performed numerous times in a porcine model [93], and scattered cases have been reported in people [94,95]. This technically demanding, experimental technique only should be attempted by expert colonoscopists with surgical backup.

The postpolypectomy syndrome is caused by nearly transmural extension of the cautery burn, without true colonic perforation. Patients present with pyrexia, abdominal pain, leukocytosis, and localized peritoneal irritation within several hours to several days postpolypectomy [96]. Frank peritoneal signs are generally absent. Abdominal imaging studies do not demonstrate pneumoperitoneum. This syndrome is managed medically with nothing per os, intravenous antibiotics, and close monitoring in hospital with surgical backup. Colonoscopy should not be performed because of the risk of inducing a true, transmural, perforation. Patients usually can be managed medically without surgery [75].

Endomucosectomy

Endomucosectomy, or endoscopic mucosal resection (EMR), is being used increasingly to remove colorectal lesions, particularly large adenomas. Endomucosectomy adapts the classic principles of conventional snare polypectomy combined with submucosal injection to cut through the middle or deep submucosa to remove lesions lying in the deep mucosa or in the submucosa. It provides an alternative to surgery for deeper superficial lesions without evident penetration of the deep muscle layer, regional lymph nodes, or distant metastases. Sessile villous adenomas, adenomas with carcinoma in situ (T0 lesions), and early (T1N0M0) cancers invading the submucosa are candidates for endomucosectomy. Usually the tumor is characterized by endoscopy, sampled by endoscopic biopsy, and locally staged by endosonography before considering endomucosectomy. Patients are evaluated for the suitability of endomucosectomy based on tumor size, endoscopic appearance, pathology of the initial endoscopic biopsy, and the estimated depth of tumor penetration (T stage). Endomucosectomy usually is applied to polypoid (protruding) lesions, but sometimes can be applied to flat or even minimally depressed lesions provided the previously cited criteria are satisfied. Endomucosectomy has an advantage over endoscopic ablative therapy—using argon plasma coagulation or photodynamic therapy—because the entire treated specimen is removed and available for histologic analysis and pathologic staging. Endomucosectomy has advantages over the alternative of surgical resection of less procedure morbidity and mortality.

The basic technique of endomucosectomy is deep submucosal injection of normal saline or another solution to thicken the colonic wall at the polypectomy site to permit deep resection of the submucosa without causing a transmural burn or colonic perforation. This injection also tamponades the feeding artery to reduce postpolypectomy bleeding, promotes vasospasm, and increases tissue liquidity and electrical conductivity at the polyp base to facilitate electrocautery. The effect of submucosal injection is observed carefully during endoscopy. A lesion that lifts during submucosal injection is amenable to endomucosectomy; a lesion that partly lifts may be amenable to endomucosectomy after due consideration. A lesion that fails to lift (nonlift sign) is not amenable to endomucosectomy because of a high risk of invasive carcinoma [81]. Deep carcinomatous invasion causes adherence of submucosa to deep muscle manifested by the nonlift sign. Failure to lift also increases the risk of endomucosectomy because of poorly defined tissue planes for endoscopic resection.

The tumor then may be resected deeply using conventional snare polypectomy. Adjunctive equipment used for deeper endoscopic resection include:

A special shark tooth snare with small hooks along the wire loop—the hooks dig into the lesion to prevent slippage of the lesion during snare closure.

A transparent cap inserted at the tip of the endoscope—the cap contains an internal rim at the tip in which an open snare is prepositioned; After the lesion is sucked into the cap using endoscopic suction, the snare is closed on the suctioned tissue (neopolyp), and electrocautery is applied to resect deeper tissue

A double channel endoscope with a biopsy forceps and a snare advanced through separate channels and with the snare loop opened around the biopsy forceps—the lesion is grasped and lifted by the biopsy forceps, and the snare is closed around the lifted submucosal tissue

Complications of endomucosectomy include abdominal pain, bleeding, perforation, and stricture formation. The risk of bleeding varies from 1.5% to 24%, depending on the size and type of the lesion and the definition of bleeding [81]. Endoscopic hemostasis frequently is required during endomucosectomy because of transection of submucosal vessels. The endoscopist must be experienced and highly competent at endoscopic hemostasis to promptly achieve hemostasis. The simplest technique of hemostasis is endoscopic clipping.

Endomucosectomy is insufficient therapy for locally extensive or metastatic disease. Endosonography much more frequently understages lesions reported as stage T1 than lesions reported as T0. About 10% of apparently T1N0 lesions turn out to be more deeply invasive cancers, including about 5% with residual cancer in the bowel wall and about 5% with undetected nodal metastases [97]. Such patients usually require cancer surgery for cure following endomucosectomy.

NEW AND EVOLVING TECHNOLOGY

Colon cancer incidence and survival has improved only moderately during the past two decades despite the manifest efficacy of colonoscopic polypectomy at cancer prevention [98]. This failure is caused by insufficient implementation of colonoscopy screening partly because of the expense, invasiveness, discomfort, and risks of colonoscopy. New simpler, less invasive, and safer tests are being designed to overcome these barriers to universal screening for colon cancer.

Stool Genetic Markers

DNA from colon cancer is shed into the fecal stream in greater quantities than DNA from normal colonic mucosa. Cancerous DNA is degraded only slowly with time or by contiguity with stool during colonic passage. Much as guaiac can detect minute quantities of blood in stool, the polymerase chain reaction (PCR) amplification can detect minute quantities of cancerous DNA in stool specimens. Among several trials of multiarray DNA assays, the sensitivity for detecting colon cancer ranged from 52% [22] to 91% [99]. Detected cases tend to have histologically advanced and clinically symptomatic colon cancer; an ideal screening test also should detect early asymptomatic and potentially curable colon cancer and adenomas [100]. The sensitivity of detecting adenomas is much lower than that for colon cancer [22,101]. For example, only 13% of adenomas were detected in a large prospective colonoscopic study [22]. Genetic stool screening has the potential test advantages of noninvasiveness and user friendliness, but needs further refinement in technique and testing in large clinical trials. Incorporation of additional molecular markers and other technical improvements may improve test sensitivity and specificity. Recently, Itzkowitz and colleagues [102] reported a 72.5% sensitivity of detecting colon cancer using an improved assay containing two new promoter methylation markers and a buffer to better preserve DNA samples. Colorectal cancer also can be detected in the serum using molecular markers. Preliminary, small studies so far have demonstrated low test sensitivity [103].

With further technical refinements, these molecular, noninvasive approaches could become highly useful for screening for colon cancer. The key criterion for test applicability for colon cancer screening is a high sensitivity in detecting adenomas. In the future, molecular genetics may play other important roles in managing sporadic colon cancer, including:

Cancer prognostication
Choice of chemotherapeutic agents
Monitoring cancer response to therapy
Detecting cancer recurrence
Development of novel biologic agents that interfere with specific molecular mechanisms of carcinogenesis [84]

Virtual Colonoscopy

Virtual colonoscopy avoids many of the undesirable features of colonoscopy of test invasiveness, patient discomfort, and need for sedation and analgesia, and entails fewer risks. In virtual colonoscopy, CT images are obtained in the prone and supine positions during a prolonged breath hold. The CT images are reformatted into two-dimensional images in the three orthogonal (axial, sagittal, and coronal) planes, or reconstructed into three-dimensional endoluminal (virtual colonoscopy) images that simulate the conventional colonoscopic view [104]. Like colonoscopy, virtual colonoscopy generally requires colonic preparation with oral laxatives. Application of digital subtraction technology to stool and administration of oral contrast to tag stool, however, may obviate the need for oral laxatives [105].

CT colonography is relatively safe [106]. The risk of colonic perforation from colonic insufflation with air is small but significant. Seven colonic perforations occurred among 11,870 CT colongraphies, yielding a rate of 1 per 1700 studies [107]. A telephone survey of all radiology departments in the United Kingdom encompassing 16,500 examinations reported a similar rate of 1 per 1650 procedures [108]. Some of these perforations were small and incomplete (intramural) or retroperitoneal and were managed conservatively without surgery, but many of the perforations were complete and intraperitoneal and required surgery. Risk factors for colonic perforation include:

Colonic overinflation with air
Pre-existing colonic diseases such as ulcerative colitis that weaken the colonic wall
Colonic diverticulosis, which leads to a focally thinned colonic wall
Anatomic conditions blocking free flow of the insufflated air such as colonic obstruction or hernias that result in increased localized pressure

A single CT colonography, using the most modern machines and a low-dose radiation protocol, exposes the patient to about half the radiation dose of a conventional barium enema [109]. The risks from such a single exposure to radiation are characterized incompletely. One study estimated that the cumulative mortality from radiation-induced cancer from a single prone and supine CT colonographic scan was 0.14% for a 50-year-old patient, the typical age for initiating colon cancer screening [110].

Unlike colonoscopy, virtual colonoscopy can visualize extracolonic intra-abdominal organs. It therefore can provide cancer staging simultaneous with colon cancer detection and can visualize intra-abdominal abnormalities such as extracolonic malignancies and aneurysms [111]. Detection of true major asymptomatic abnormalities can be beneficial by instituting earlier therapy. In a meta-analysis of 3488 patients among 17 CT studies, extracolonic cancers were detected in 2.7% of patients and aortic aneurysms in 0.9% [112]. From 69% to 80% of putatively clinically significant abnormalities detected at CT colonography prove to be clinically unimportant following thorough evaluation, however [111].

The accuracy of virtual colonoscopy is controversial, with conflicting data [45]. For example, Pickhardt and colleagues [106] reported in 2003 that CT colonography had a sensitivity of 94% for polyps at least 10 mm in diameter, 94% for polyps at least 8 mm in diameter, and 89% for polyps at least 6 mm in diameter. In this study, CT colonography was an excellent screening test for colonic polyps with high sensitivity and specificity. Contrariwise, Cotton and colleagues reported in 2004 in a study of 600 patients undergoing both CT colonography and colonoscopy that the sensitivity of CT colonography was only 39% for lesions less than 6 mm in diameter, and only 55% for lesions more than 10 mm in diameter [113]. In this study, CT colonography was poorly sensitive and specific and not useful as a screening test. The wide discrepancy between various studies may be because of different CT technology, especially use of four- versus 16-slice scanners, use of supine versus supine and prone views, different computerized software for colonic fly-through endoluminal views, different levels of radiologist expertise, and administration of dual oral contrast versus single oral contrast versus no oral contrast for tagging stool [104].

The accuracy of virtual colonoscopy is a function of polyp size. It is much more accurate for lesions larger than 10 mm than for lesions less than 5 mm [106]. It is, therefore, more accurate at detecting cancers than adenomas, because cancers tend to be larger than adenomas [114]. An important disadvantage of virtual colonoscopy is the inability to remove polyps for definitive therapy, the inability to biopsy masses for histologic classification, and the inability to apply other therapies such as injection or ablation that are available by means of colonoscopy. Detection of a polyp or mass at virtual colonoscopy currently requires follow-up colonoscopy for polypectomy or biopsy.

Videocapsule Endoscopy

The videocapsule is delivered orally to the small intestine by peristalsis to provide wireless endoscopy by radiofrequency transmission. The videocapsule then moves passively from proximal to distal by GI peristalsis. The videocapsule

Table 4
Current technical problems with application of videocapsule technology for endoscopic examination of the colon for colon cancer screening

Deficiency	Technical reason
Poor sensitivity in the presence of stool	Inability to wash away, aspirate, or navigate around stool
Misses sides of bowel wall	Lacks steering capability
Cannot determine lesion histology	Lacks biopsy capability
Cannot examine entire colon	Videocapsule telecommunications last for only about 8 hours because of the short battery half-life
No therapeutic capabilities of injection, decompression, ablation, or polypectomy	Instrument lacks a therapeutic channel
Poor vision of lesions	Weak illumination is inadequate for the wide-caliber large intestine
Poor visualization of collapsed colon	Lacks insufflation capability

contains a miniaturized image capturing system, battery, light source, and transmitter, all of which are contained within an 11×30 mm capsule. Videocapsule endoscopy has developed a niche in the evaluation of jejunoileal bleeding [115]. It is theoretically attractive as a screening test for colon cancer because of examination simplicity, noninvasiveness, minimal patient discomfort, and apparent relative safety. The test has serious practical disadvantages for colonic examination (Table 4). A major limitation is that the videocapsule battery lasts only about 8 hours; this time is insufficient to view the entire colon after battery ingestion. New prototype videocapsules that correct some of these deficiencies are being tested [116]. Ideally, if these deficiencies are corrected, videocapsule endoscopy could provide an initial screening examination of the colon. A lesion detected by this examination would prompt colonoscopy to confirm the diagnosis, to determine the histology of the lesion by colonoscopic biopsy, and potentially to remove the lesion by colonoscopic polypectomy [117]. In a pilot study, in which 41 patients underwent both capsule endoscopy and colonoscopy, capsule endoscopy had a sensitivity of 77% and specificity of 70%, using colonoscopy as the gold standard [118].

SUMMARY

With improved education of physicians resulting in effective and appropriate implementation of screening colonoscopy guidelines, and with improved technology, equipment, and training, colon cancer should be virtually eradicated like cholera or other infectious scourges of yore.

References
[1] Jamal A, Siegel R, Ward E, et al. Cancer statistics, 2007. CA Cancer J Clin 2007;57: 43–66.

[2] Winawer SJ, Zauber AG, Fletcher RH, et al. Guidelines for colonoscopy surveillance after polypectomy: a consensus update by the US Multi-Society Task Force on Colorectal Cancer and the American Cancer Society. Gastroenterology 2006;130:1872–85.

[3] Levin B, Barthel JS, Burt RW, et al. Colorectal cancer screening clinical practice guidelines. J Natl Compr Canc Netw 2006;4:384–420.

[4] Cappell MS, Goldberg ES. The relationship between the clinical presentation and spread of colon cancer in 315 consecutive patients: a significant trend of earlier cancer detection from 1982 through 1988 at a university hospital. J Clin Gastroenterol 1992;14:227–35.

[5] Levine JS, Ahnen DJ. Adenomatous polyps of the colon. N Engl J Med 2006;355:2551–7.

[6] Pignone M, Rich M, Teutsch SM, et al. Screening for colorectal cancer in adults at average risk: a summary of the evidence for the US Preventive Services Task Force. Ann Intern Med 2002;137:132–41.

[7] Khankari K, Eder M, Osborn CY, et al. Improving colorectal cancer screening among the medically underserved: a pilot study within a federally qualified health center. J Gen Intern Med 2007;22:1410–4.

[8] Balluz L, Ahluwalia IB, Murphy W, et al. Surveillance for certain behaviors among selected local areas: United States. Behavioral risk factor surveillance system, 2002. Morb Mort Wkly Rep 2004;53(5).1–100.

[9] Wolf MS, Satterlee M, Calhoun EA, et al. Colorectal cancer screening among the medically underserved. J Health Care Poor Underserved 2006;17:46–54.

[10] Taylor ML, Anderson R. Colorectal cancer screening: physician attitudes and practices. WMJ 2002;101:39–43.

[11] Federici A, Giorgi Rossi P, Bartolozzi F, et al. Survey on colon cancer screening knowledge, attitudes, and practices of general practice physicians in Lazio, Italy. Prev Med 2005;41:30–5.

[12] Grassini M, Verna C, Niola P, et al. Appropriateness of colonoscopy: diagnostic yield and safety in guidelines. World J Gastroenterol 2007;13:1816–9.

[13] Harewood GC, Wiersma MJ, Melton LJ 3rd. A prospective, controlled assessment of factors influencing acceptance of screening colonoscopy. Am J Gastroenterol 2002;97:3186–94.

[14] Tsai CJ, Lu DK. Small colorectal polyps: histopathology and clinical significance. Am J Gastroenterol 1995;90:988–94.

[15] Cappell MS. From colonic polyps to colon cancer: pathophysiology, clinical presentation, and diagnosis. Clin Lab Med 2005;25:135–77.

[16] Jass JR. Hyperplastic polyps and colorectal cancer: is there a link? Clin Gastroenterol Hepatol 2004;2:1–8.

[17] Higuchi T, Jass JR. My approach to serrated polyps of the colorectum. J Clin Pathol 2004;57:682–6.

[18] Williams AR, Balasooriya BA, Day DW. Polyps and cancer of the large bowel: a necropsy study in Liverpool. Gut 1982;23:835–42.

[19] Rex DK. Colonoscopy: a review of its yield for cancers and adenomas by indication. Am J Gastroenterol 1995;90:353–65.

[20] Ransohoff DF, Lang CA. Small adenomas detected during fecal occult blood test screening for colorectal cancer: the impact of serendipity. JAMA 1990;264:76–8.

[21] Lieberman D. Rectal bleeding and diminutive colon polyps. Gastroenterology 2004;126:1167–74.

[22] Imperiale TF, Ransohoff DF, Itzkowitz SH, et al. Colorectal Cancer Study Group. Fecal DNA versus fecal occult blood for colorectal cancer screening in an average-risk population. N Engl J Med 2004;351:2704–14.

[23] Longacre TA, Fenoglio-Preiser CM. Mixed hyperplastic adenomatous polyps/serrated adenomas: a distinct form of colorectal neoplasia. Am J Surg Pathol 1990;14:524–37.

[24] Torlakovic E, Skovlund E, Snover DC, et al. Morphologic reappraisal of serrated colorectal polyps. Am J Surg Pathol 2003;27:65–81.

[25] Simon JB. Fecal occult blood testing: clinical value and limitations. Gastroenterologist 1998;6:66–78.

[26] Church TR, Ederer F, Mandel JS. Fecal occult blood screening in the Minnesota Study: sensitivity of the screening test. J Natl Cancer Inst 1997;89:1440–8.

[27] Mandel JS, Bond JH, Church TR, et al. Reducing mortality from colorectal cancer by screening for fecal occult blood: Minnesota Colon Cancer Control Study. N Engl J Med 1993;328:1365–71.

[28] Cappell MS, Friedel D. The role of sigmoidoscopy and colonoscopy in the diagnosis and management of lower gastrointestinal disorders: endoscopic findings, therapy, and complications. Med Clin North Am 2002;86:1253–88.

[29] Guittet L, Bouvier V, Mariotte N, et al. Comparison of a guaiac-based and an immunochemical fecal occult blood test in screening for colorectal cancer in a general average-risk population. Gut 2007;56:210–4.

[30] Smith A, Young GP, Cole SR, et al. Comparison of a brush-sampling fecal immunochemical test for hemoglobin with a sensitive guaiac-based occult blood test in detection of colorectal neoplasia. Cancer 2006;107:2152–9.

[31] Saito H. Colorectal cancer screening using immunochemical faecal occult blood testing in Japan. J Med Screen 2006;13(Suppl 1):S6–7.

[32] Lee KJ, Inoue M, Otani T, et al. Colorectal cancer screening using fecal occult blood test and subsequent risk of colorectal cancer: a prospective cohort study in Japan. Cancer Detect Prev 2007;31:3–11.

[33] Rex DK, Rahmani EV, Haseman JH, et al. Relative sensitivity of colonoscopy and barium enema for detection of colorectal cancer in clinical practice. Gastroenterology 1997;112:17–23.

[34] Winawer SJ, Stewart ET, Zauber AG, et al. A comparison of colonoscopy and double-contrast barium enema for surveillance after polypectomy: National Polyp Work Group. N Engl J Med 2000;342:1766–72.

[35] Winawer S, Fletcher R, Rex D, et al. Colorectal cancer screening and surveillance: clinical guidelines and rationale—update based on new evidence. Gastroenterology 2003;124: 544–60.

[36] Selby JV, Friedman GD, Quesenberry CP Jr, et al. A case-control study of screening sigmoidoscopy and mortality from colorectal cancer. N Engl J Med 1992;326: 653–7.

[37] Newcomb PA, Norfleet RG, Storer BE, et al. Screening sigmoidoscopy and colorectal cancer mortality. J Natl Cancer Inst 1992;84:1572–5.

[38] McCallion K, Mitchell RM, Wilson RH, et al. Flexible sigmoidoscopy and the changing distribution of colorectal cancer: implications for screening. Gut 2001;48:522–5.

[39] Anderson JC, Alpern Z, Messina CR, et al. Predictors of proximal neoplasia in patients without distal adenomatous pathology. Am J Gastroenterol 2004;99:472–7.

[40] Rex DK, Cutler CS, Lemmel GT, et al. Colonoscopic miss rates of adenomas determined by back-to-back colonoscopies. Gastroenterology 1997;112:24–8.

[41] Winawer SJ, Zauber AG, Ho MN, et al. Prevention of colorectal cancer by colonoscopic polypectomy. N Engl J Med 1993;329:1977–81.

[42] Cappell MS. The pathophysiology, clinical presentation, and diagnosis of colon cancer and adenomatous polyps. Med Clin North Am 2005;89:1–42.

[43] Rex DK. Colonoscopy: the dominant and preferred colorectal cancer screening strategy in the United States. Mayo Clin Proc 2007;82:662–4.

[44] Smith RA, Cokkinides V, Eyre HJ. Cancer screening in the United States: a review of current guidelines, practices, and prospects. CA Cancer J Clin 2007;57:90–104.

[45] Rex DK, Lieberman D. ACG colorectal cancer prevention action plan: update on CT colonography. Am J Gastroenterol 2006;101:1410–3.

[46] Syngal S, Bandipalliam P, Boland R. Surveillance of patients at high risk for colorectal cancer. Med Clin North Am 2005;89:61–84.

[47] Barclay RL, Vicari JJ, Doughty AS, et al. Colonoscopic withdrawal times and adenoma detection during screening colonoscopy. N Engl J Med 2006;355:2533–41.

[48] Sanchez W, Harewood GC, Petersen BT. Evaluation of polyp detection in relation to procedure time of screening or surveillance colonoscopy. Am J Gastroenterol 2004;99: 1941–5.

[49] Butterly LF, Chase MP, Pohl H, et al. Prevalence of clinically important histology in small adenomas. Clin Gastroenterol Hepatol 2006;4:343–8.

[50] Church JM. Clinical significance of small colorectal polyps. Dis Colon Rectum 2004;47: 481–5.

[51] Gualco G, Reissenweber N, Cliché I, et al. Flat elevated lesions of the colon and rectum: a spectrum of neoplastic and non-neoplastic entities. Ann Diagn Pathol 2006;10:333–8.

[52] Parra-Blanco A, Nicolas-Perez D, Gimeno-Garcia A, et al. The timing of bowel preparation before colonoscopy determines the quality of cleansing, and is a significant factor contributing to the detection of flat lesions: a randomized study. World J Gastroenterol 2006;14: 6161–6.

[53] Vukasin P, Weston LA, Beart RW. Oral Fleet phospho-soda laxative-induced hyperphosphatemia and hypocalcemic tetany in an adult: report of a case. Dis Colon Rectum 1997;40:497–9.

[54] Ullah N, Yeh R, Ehrinpreis M. Fatal hyperphosphatemia from a phospho-soda bowel preparation. J Clin Gastroenterol 2002;34:457–8.

[55] Vargo JJ, Bramley T, Meyer K, et al. Practice efficiency and economics: the case for rapid recovery sedation agents for colonoscopy in a screening population. J Clin Gastroenterol 2007;41:591–8.

[56] Rex DK. Review article: moderate sedation for endoscopy—sedation regimens for nonanesthesiologists. Aliment Pharmacol Ther 2006;24:163–71.

[57] Bressler B, Paszat LF, Chen Z, et al. Rates of new or missed colorectal cancers after colonoscopy and their risk factors: a population-based analysis. Gastroenterology 2007;132: 96–102.

[58] Singh H, Turner D, Xue L, et al. Risk of developing colorectal cancer following a negative colonoscopy: evidence for a 10-year interval between colonoscopies. JAMA 2006;295: 2366–73.

[59] Rex DK, Bond JH, Feld AD. Medical–legal risks of incident cancers after clearing colonoscopy. Am J Gastroenterol 2001;96:952–7.

[60] Rex DK, Bond JH, Winawer S, et al. Quality in the technical performance of colonoscopy and the continuous quality improvement process for colonoscopy: recommendations of the US Multi-Society Task Force on Colorectal Cancer. Am J Gastroenterol 2002;97: 1296–308.

[61] Church JM. Warm water irrigation for dealing with spasm during colonoscopy: simple, inexpensive, and effective. Gastrointest Endosc 2002;56:672–4.

[62] Triadifilopoulos G, Watts HD, Higgins J, et al. A novel retrograde-viewing auxiliary imaging device (Third Eye Retroscope) improves the detection of simulated polyps in anatomic models of the colon. Gastrointest Endosc 2007;65:139–44.

[63] Deenadayalu VP, Chadalawada V, Rex DK. 170 degrees wide-angle colonoscope: effect on efficiency and miss rates. Am J Gastroenterol 2004;99:138–42.

[64] Brooker J, Saunders B, Shah S, et al. Total colonic dye-spray increases the detection of diminutive adenomas during routine colonoscopy: a randomized controlled trial. Gastrointest Endosc 2002;56:333–8.

[65] Hurlstone DP, Cross SS, Slater R, et al. Detecting diminutive colorectal lesions at colonoscopy: a randomized controlled trial of pan-colonic versus targeted chromoscopy. Gut 2004;53:376–80.

[66] Chiu HM, Chang CY, Chen CC, et al. A prospective comparative study of narrow-band imaging, chromoendoscopy, and conventional colonoscopy in the diagnosis of colorectal neoplasia. Gut 2007;56:373–9.

[67] Johanson JF. Practicality of high-resolution chromoendoscopy during routine screening colonoscopy. Gastrointest Endosc 2006;63:829–30.

[68] Rex DK, Helbig CC. High yields of small and flat adenomas with high-definition colonoscopes using either white light or narrow band imaging. Gastroenterology 2007;133: 42–7.

[69] Davies J, Burke D, Olliver JR, et al. Methylene blue but not indigo carmine causes DNA damage to colonocytes in vitro and in vivo at concentrations used in clinical chromoendoscopy. Gut 2007;56:155–6.

[70] Hurlstone DP, Karajeh M, Cross SC, et al. The role of high-magnification chromoscopic colonoscopy in hereditary nonpolyposis colorectal cancer screening: a prospective "back-to-back" endoscopic study. Am J Gastroenterol 2005;100:2167–73.

[71] Lecomte T, Cellier C, Meatchi T, et al. Chromoendoscopic colonoscopy for detecting preneoplastic lesions in hereditary nonpolyposis colorectal cancer syndrome. Clin Gastroenterol Hepatol 2005;3:897–902.

[72] Kiesslich R, Goetz M, Lammersdorf K, et al. Chromoscopy-guided endomicroscopy increases the diagnostic yield of intraepithelial neoplasia in ulcerative colitis. Gastroenterology 2007;132:874–82.

[73] Leaper M, Johnston MJ, Barclay M, et al. Reasons for failure to diagnose colorectal carcinoma at colonoscopy. Endoscopy 2004;36:499–503.

[74] Feld AD. Medicolegal implications of colon cancer screening. Gastrointest Endosc Clin N Am 2002;12:171–9.

[75] Fatima H, Rex DK. Minimizing endoscopic complications: colonoscopic polypectomy. Gastrointest Endosc Clin N Am 2007;17:145–56.

[76] Cappell MS, Abdullah M. Management of gastrointestinal bleeding induced by gastrointestinal endoscopy. Gastroenterol Clin North Am 2000;29:125–67.

[77] Hurlstone DP, Fujii T. Practical uses of chromoendoscopy and magnification at colonoscopy. Gastrointest Endosc Clin N Am 2005;15:687–702.

[78] Adler A, Pohl H, Papanikolaou IS, et al. A prospective randomized study on narrow-band imaging versus conventional colonoscopy for adenoma detection: does narrow-band imaging induce a learning effect? Gut 2008;57:59–64.

[79] Rex DK, Ulbright TM. Step section histology of proximal colon polyps that appear hyperplastic by endoscopy. Am J Gastroenterol 2002;97:1530–4.

[80] Yusuf SI, Grant C. Inverted colonic diverticulum: a rare finding in a common condition? Gastrointest Endosc 2000;52:111–5.

[81] Soetikno RM, Gotoda T, Nakanishi Y, et al. Endoscopic mucosal resection. Gastrointest Endosc 2003;57:567–79.

[82] Jeevaratnam P, Cottier DS, Browett PJ, et al. Familial giant hyperplastic polyposis predisposing to colon cancer: a new hereditary bowel cancer syndrome. J Pathol 1996;179:20–5.

[83] Desai DC, Neale KF, Talbot IC, et al. Juvenile polyposis. Br J Surg 1995;82:14–7.

[84] Gryfe R. Clinical implications of our advancing knowledge of colorectal cancer genetics: inherited syndromes, prognosis, prevention, screening, and therapeutics. Surg Clin North Am 2006;86:787–817.

[85] Ladas SD, Prigouris SP, Pantelidaki C, et al. Endoscopic removal of inverted sigmoid diverticulum: is it a dangerous procedure? Endoscopy 1989;21:243–4.

[86] Williams CB, Saunders BP, Talbot IC. Endoscopic management of polypoid early colon cancer. World J Surg 2000;24:1047–51.

[87] Rex DK. Maximizing detection of adenomas and cancers during colonoscopy. Am J Gastroenterol 2006;101:2866–77.

[88] Liu HH, Kudo SE, Juch JP. Pit pattern analysis by magnifying chromoendoscopy for the diagnosis of colorectal polyps. J Formos Med Assoc 2003;102:178–82.

[89] Su MY, Hsu CM, Ho YP, et al. Comparative study of conventional colonoscopy, chromoendoscopy, and narrow-band imaging systems in differential diagnosis of neoplastic and nonneoplastic colonic polyps. Am J Gastroenterol 2006;101:2711–6.

[90] Deenadayalu VP, Rex DK. Colon polyp retrieval after cold snaring. Gastrointest Endosc 2005;62:253–6.

[91] Peluso F, Goldner F. Follow-up hot biopsy forceps treatment of diminutive colonic polyps. Gastrointest Endosc 1991;37:604–6.

[92] Letard JC, Kaffy F, Rousseau D, et al. Postpolypectomy colonic arterial hemorrhage can be treated by hemoclipping. Gastroenterol Clin Biol 2001;25:323–4.

[93] Raju GS, Ahmed I, Shibukawa G, et al. Endoluminal clip closure of a circular full-thickness colon resection in a porcine model (with videos). Gastrointest Endosc 2007;65:503–9.

[94] Barbagallo F, Castello G, Latteri S, et al. Successful endoscopic repair of an unusual colonic perforation following polypectomy using an endoclip device. World J Gastroenterol 2007;13:2889–91.

[95] Dhalla SS. Endoscopic repair of a colonic perforation following polypectomy using an endoclip. Can J Gastroenterol 2004;18:105–6.

[96] Waye JD, Kahn O, Auerbach ME. Complications of colonoscopy and flexible sigmoidoscopy. Gastrointest Endosc Clin N Am 1996;6:343–77.

[97] Muto T, Oya M. Recent advances in diagnosis and treatment of colorectal T1 carcinoma. Dis Colon Rectum 2003;46(Suppl):S89–93.

[98] Cress RD, Morris CR, Wolfe BM. Cancer of the colon and rectum in California: trends in incidence by race/ethnicity, stage, and subsite. Prev Med 2000;31:447–53.

[99] Ahlquist DA, Skoletsky JE, Boynton KA, et al. Colorectal cancer screening by detection of altered human DNA in stool: feasibility of a multitarget assay panel. Gastroenterology 2000;119:1219–27.

[100] Atkin W, Martin JP. Stool DNA-based colorectal cancer detection: finding the needle in the haystack (editorial). J Natl Cancer Inst 2001;93:798–9.

[101] Agrawal J, Syngal S. Colon cancer screening strategies. Curr Opin Gastroenterol 2005;21:59–63.

[102] Itzkowitz SH, Jandorf L, Brand R, et al. Improved fecal DNA test for colorectal cancer screening. Clin Gastroenterol Hepatol 2007;5:111–7.

[103] Lauschke H, Caspari R, Friedl W, et al. Detection of APC and k-ras mutations in the serum of patients with colorectal cancer. Cancer Detect Prev 2001;25:55–61.

[104] Lefkovitz Z, Shapiro R, Koch S, et al. The emerging role of virtual colonoscopy. Med Clin North Am 2005;89:111–38.

[105] Zalis ME, Hahn PF. Digital subtraction bowel cleansing in CT colonography. AJR Am J Roentgenol 2001;176:646–8.

[106] Pickhardt PJ, Choi JR, Hwang I, et al. Computed tomographic virtual colonoscopy to screen for colorectal neoplasia in asymptomatic adults. N Engl J Med 2003;349:2191–200.

[107] Sosna J, Sella T, Bar-Zvi J, et al. Perforation of the colon and rectum: A newly recognized complication of CT colonography. Semin Ultrasound CT MR 2006;27:161–5.

[108] Burling D, Halligan S, Slater A, et al. Potentially serious adverse events associated with CT colonography performed in symptomatic patients: a national survey of the UK. Presented at the 91st Annual Meeting of the Radiological Society of North America, Chicago (IL), November 27–December 2, 2005.

[109] Barish MA, Rocha TC. Multislice CT colonography: current status and limitations. Radiol Clin North Am 2005;43:1049–62.

[110] Brenner DJ, Georgsson MA. Mass screening with CT colonography: should the radiation exposure be of concern? Gastroenterology 2005;129:328–37.

[111] Hara AK, Johnson CD, MacCarty RL, et al. Incidental extracolonic findings at CT colonography. Radiology 2000;215:353–7.

[112] Xiong T, Richardson M, Woodroffe R, et al. Incidental lesions found on CT colonography: their nature and frequency. Br J Radiol 2005;78:22–9.

[113] Cotton PB, Durkalski VL, Pineau BC, et al. Computed tomographic colonography (virtual colonoscopy): a multicenter comparison with standard colonoscopy for detection of colorectal neoplasia. JAMA 2004;29:1713–9.

[114] Royster AP, Fenlon HM, Clarke PD, et al. CT colonoscopy of colorectal neoplasms: two-dimensional and three-dimensional virtual reality techniques with colonoscopic correlation. AJR Am J Roentgenol 1997;169:1237–42.

[115] Appleyard M, Glukhovsky A, Swain P. Wireless capsule diagnostic endoscopy for recurrent small-bowel bleeding. N Engl J Med 2001;344:232–3.

[116] Cotton PB, Barkun A, Ginsberg G, et al. Diagnostic endoscopy: 2020 vision. Gastrointest Endosc 2006;64:395–8.

[117] Fireman Z, Kopelman Y. The colon: the latest terrain for capsule endoscopy. Dig Liver Dis 2007;39:895–9.

[118] Schoofs N, Deviere J, van Gossum A. PillCam colon capsule endoscopy compared with colonoscopy for colorectal tumor diagnosis: a prospective study. Endoscopy 2006;38: 971–7.

Gastroenterol Clin N Am 37 (2008) 161–189

GASTROENTEROLOGY CLINICS
OF NORTH AMERICA

CT Colonography: Current Status and Future Promise

Susan Summerton, MD[a,b,]*, Elizabeth Little, MD[a],
Mitchell S. Cappell, MD, PhD[c]

[a]Department of Radiology, Albert Einstein Medical Center, 5501 Old York Road, Philadelphia,
PA 19141, USA
[b]Jefferson Medical College, Thomas Jefferson University, Philadelphia, PA, USA
[c]Division of Gastroenterology, MOB 233, William Beaumont Hospital, 3601 W. Thirteen Mile
Road, Royal Oak, MI 48073, USA

Colorectal cancer is one of the most commonly diagnosed cancers in the world with approximately 1 million new cases diagnosed annually and approximately half a million annual deaths [1]. The highest incidence occurs in North America and Europe [2]. Colon cancer is the second most common cause of mortality from cancer in the United States, causing more than 52,000 deaths in 2006 [1]. The lifetime risk of colon cancer in America is about 1 in 17 [3]. Colon cancer characteristically begins as slow-growing premalignant polyps that take approximately 10 years to progress to carcinoma [4]. It therefore is believed that colon cancer is largely preventable by mass screening to detect and then remove such polyps [5]. Only one half of the average-risk population in the United States undergoes any of the currently available screening tests for colorectal cancer, however [6,7], because of safety concerns, test invasiveness, inconvenience, costs, embarrassment, and lack of education concerning colon cancer screening [8].

CT colonography (virtual colonoscopy, CTC) is an innovative technology that entails CT examination of the entire colon and computerized processing of the raw data after colon cleansing and colonic distention. CTC currently is under intense analysis as a screening test that potentially could increase the screening rate for colon cancer because of its relative safety, relatively low expense, and greater patient acceptance as compared with other current screening methods. Its role in mass colon cancer screening is controversial, however, because of its highly variable reported sensitivity, concerns about specificity because of the inability to sample polyps for histologic analysis, and lack of therapeutic capabilities.

*Corresponding author. Department of Radiology, Albert Einstein Medical Center,
5501 Old York Road, Philadelphia, PA 19141. E-mail address: summertons@einstein.edu
(S. Summerton).

0889-8553/08/$ – see front matter
doi:10.1016/j.gtc.2007.12.016

A review of this topic is both timely and important because CTC is evolving rapidly due to improvements in methodology and computerized technology as well as new clinical data. To help clinicians optimize colon cancer screening for their patients, this article reviews the exponentially expanding literature on CTC, including imaging techniques, adjunctive techniques, radiologic interpretation, procedure indications, contraindications, risks, sensitivity, interpretation pitfalls, and controversies.

PATHOGENESIS OF COLON CANCER
Colon cancer arises from mucosal polyps. The critical polyp characteristic in terms of malignant potential is histology. The two most common histologic types are hyperplastic and adenomatous. According to the traditional adenoma-to-carcinoma sequence, nearly all colon cancers arise from adenomatous polyps, as demonstrated by epidemiologic, clinical, pathologic, and genetic data. About one third of operative specimens with colon cancer contain one or more synchronous adenomas, a significantly higher rate than in age-matched controls without colon cancer [9]. The risk of colon cancer increases markedly with increasing number of adenomatous polyps [10]. Adenomatous tissue frequently is found contiguous to frank carcinoma [11,12]. Patients who refuse polypectomy for colonic adenomas develop colon cancer at a rate of about 4% after 5 years and 14% after 10 years [13]. Patients who have familial adenomatous polyposis, who have hundreds or thousands of adenomatous colonic polyps, inevitably develop colon cancer if prophylactic colectomy is not performed [14]. Patients who have sporadic adenomas have genetic mutations in the same *APC* gene as patients who have syndromic colon cancer from familial adenomatous polyposis [15,16].

Hyperplastic polyps traditionally were believed to have negligible or no malignant potential [17], but findings of mixed hyperplastic-adenomatous polyps [18,19], clustering of adenomas and colon cancers adjacent to hyperplastic polyps [20], and a high risk of colon cancer in patients who have syndromic hyperplastic polyposis [21] provided evidence that some hyperplastic polyps may increase the risk of colon cancer. A distinct histologic subset of colonic polyps previously classified as hyperplastic recently has been shown to have a significant risk of progressing to colon cancer and has been reclassified as serrated adenomas (see the article by East and Jass, elsewhere in this issue). The genetic basis of this cancer risk is being elucidated currently [22].

Benign premalignant colonic polyps occur through at least three distinct genetic mechanisms: mutation of the *APC* gene leading to adenomatous polyps, genetic changes associated with serrated adenomas, and mutations in several mismatch repair genes leading to sessile adenomatous polyps [23]. Further mutations result in malignant transformation.

PRINCIPLES OF COLON CANCER SCREENING
Application of a screening test to the general population is predicated on (1) the disease to be screened being sufficiently prevalent in the population to justify

the cost and effort of mass screening, (2) the disease being easily treatable and curable when detected early or in a precursor phase but highly fatal or otherwise severe when detected late or in an advanced stage, and (3) the availability of a second diagnostic or reference test to be performed on patients who have a positive screening test. Colon cancer satisfies all three criteria. It is (1) extremely common in American patients over 50 years old, with 150,000 cases diagnosed per annum [1], (2) highly lethal when advanced (Dukes stage D) but reliably curable by surgery when detected very early (Dukes stage A) and preventable by colonoscopic polypectomy when detected as a premalignant adenomatous polyp [24], and (3) has colonoscopy available as a reference or diagnostic standard to confirm the existence of polyps or cancer and to remove detected polyps for histologic characterization and prevention of colon cancer. Colon cancer screening therefore is highly desirable and important for public health.

A screening test, for colon cancer or for any other disease, ideally should be (1) relatively inexpensive, because it must be performed on so many patients (eg, for colon cancer screening, the approximately 77,000,000 Americans ≥ 50 years old [25]); (2) very safe, because so many patients will be subjected to the test; (3) relatively noninvasive and acceptable to the general population so that few patients will refuse to undergo screening; and (4) highly sensitive so as not to miss patients who have the condition (false negatives). A screening test need be only moderately specific; however, poor specificity would result in an unacceptably large number of patients (false positives) required to undergo a second, diagnostic test, thereby increasing the costs and risks of mass screening.

Development of a practical screening test for colon cancer that is acceptable to the general public has proven troublesome and elusive (Table 1) [26–33]. Only about 50% of eligible Americans have undergone any form of colon cancer screening [6,7]. The requirements for a screening test have become more rigorous with the recent focus on detection of benign colonic adenomas rather than only colon cancer. For example, the sensitivity of fecal occult blood testing is several-fold lower for colonic polyps than for colon cancer [34].

CT COLONOGRAPHY

Vining and Gelfand [35] from Bowman Gray University introduced CTC and exhibited the first CTC fly-through video in 1994 at the annual meeting of the Society of Gastrointestinal Radiologists. The original test took 50 seconds for data acquisition and 8 hours for computer processing [36]. The data acquisition time now is only 15 seconds using multislice CT scanners, and the computer processing time is less than 10 minutes [37]. CTC depends on (1) an adequately cleansed colon, (2) an adequately distended colon, (3) rapid thin-section CT examination in both prone and supine positions, (4) computerized processing of the data to generate two-dimensional (2D) images in the axial, sagittal, and coronal planes or three-dimensional (3D) virtual colonoscopy images, and (5) study interpretation by a well trained and experienced reader.

Table 1
Historical perspective on screening tests for colon cancer and colonic polyp detection

Historical test	Benefits	Major drawbacks
Fecal occult blood	Very cheap, very safe, and very noninvasive	Only moderately sensitive at detecting colon cancer. Poorly sensitive at detecting colonic polyps [26]. Poor specificity. Sensitivity of test may be markedly better for fecal immunochemical tests than for fecal guaiac tests [27].
Flexible sigmoidoscopy	Relatively cheap, much less invasive than colonoscopy.	Only examines colonic region responsible for about 60% of colon cancers or polyps [28,29].
Fecal molecular markers	Very safe and very noninvasive. Costs would decrease if widely used.	Currently experimental. Needs further research and development to improve test sensitivity [26,30].
Barium enema	Safer and cheaper than colonoscopy	Has become a secondary screening test because of poor sensitivity in detecting colonic polyps [31].
Colonoscopy	Highly sensitive and highly specific, provides diagnosis and therapy for benign polyps	Relatively expensive, somewhat invasive, some risks, and inconvenient for patients [32].
CT colonography	Safer and cheaper than colonoscopy and probably more patient friendly	Probably is less sensitive than colonoscopy for polyp detection, especially for smaller polyps. Misses many flat colonic adenomas [33]. Poor specificity because histology of polyps undetermined. Lacks therapeutic capabilities, so patients who have a positive finding of a colonic polyp must undergo subsequent colonoscopy.

Patient Preparation

Patient referral

When scheduling CTC, the referring physician and the radiology department should ascertain whether the patient has a valid indication for CTC (Box 1) without contraindications [37] and should verify that the patient has the correct prescriptions and proper directions for bowel preparation.

Relative contraindications to CTC include

Severe allergy to administered contrast (CTC can be performed without contrast)

Suspected colonic perforation or peritonitis

Walled off colonic leak/pericolonic abscess

Medically highly unstable patient (eg, unstable angina, uncontrolled sepsis)

Acute lower gastrointestinal bleeding

Pregnancy

Inability to tolerate pneumocolon

Highly uncooperative patient

Inability to undergo colonic preparation: congestive heart failure, severe electrolyte imbalances, severe dehydration

Refusal to undergo colonic preparation

Abnormal anorectal anatomy (eg, imperforate anus, tight anal stricture)

Severe colonic disease (toxic colitis, toxic megacolon, severe colonic pseudo-obstruction)

Acute colonic infection (acute diverticulitis, severe infectious colitis)

Complete mechanical colonic obstruction

Very recent colonic surgery (<1 week)

Colonic cleansing

Proper bowel preparation is essential. Residual fecal material can mimic or obscure polyps. A low-residue and/or clear liquid diet is instituted 24 hours before CTC. Bowel preparations include colonic lavage solutions, such as polyethylene glycol, and cathartics, such as magnesium citrate or phospho-soda (sodium phosphate). The patient should be advised to take the entire colonic preparation as prescribed. Polyethylene glycol, the standard preparation for conventional colonoscopy, leaves less residual fecal material but more residual

---

Box 1: Current generally accepted indications for CTC

Incomplete colonoscopy because an obstructing mass or stricture prevented examination of the proximal colon

Incomplete colonoscopy because of colonic tortuosity, adhesions, severe diverticular disease, or patient intolerance of colonoscopy

Inability to perform colonoscopy because of a strong requirement for anticoagulant therapy or risks of sedation

Patients who have a strong indication for diagnostic colonoscopy but who adamantly refuse to undergo colonoscopy

fluid in the colon than either magnesium citrate or sodium phosphate preparations at barium enema or CTC [38,39]. Residual fluid can be eliminated during conventional colonoscopy by colonoscopic aspiration but cannot be eliminated during CTC and can limit CTC sensitivity. Therefore, a "dry prep" with a saline laxative of phospho-soda or magnesium citrate, combined with bisacodyl tablets the night before CTC and a bisacodyl suppository the morning of CTC is recommended to eliminate residual fluid. Patients administered phospho-soda require adequate hydration. This preparation is absolutely contraindicated in patients who have renal insufficiency or congestive heart failure and is relatively contraindicated in patients who have large ascites or ileus because of potentially large fluid and electrolyte shifts or induction of renal failure [40]. Magnesium citrate is a useful alternative in such patients. The patient evacuates any residual colonic fluid just before CTC.

Oral contrast

Residual colonic fluid decreases polyp detection by obscuring the contrast (difference in attenuation) between the bowel wall and the air-filled lumen. Administration of iodinated oral contrast theoretically opacifies (increases the attenuation of) residual fluid, allowing for the detection of otherwise invisible polyps submerged in intraluminal fluid (Fig. 1). Fluid tagging has shown mixed results because of unsatisfactory fluid attenuation and inadequate polyp detection despite adequate fluid attenuation [41]. It may yield a sensitivity as low as 78% for polyps 10 mm or larger [42]. Moreover, techniques such as dual-position image acquisition can increase polyp detection significantly without

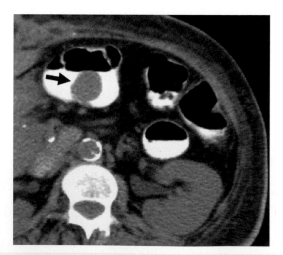

Fig. 1. Fluid tagging. In this axial 2D supine image with a soft tissue window, a large polyp (*arrow*) is demonstrated in the dependent portion of the midtransverse colon as a relatively low-density mass compared with the high-density tagged fluid.

fluid tagging [41,42]. Fluid tagging requires ingestion of substantial amounts of liquid.

Barium can be used to tag particulate stool. Small amounts of barium are ingested during several meals over several days before CTC to become incorporated into fecal material. The contrast-enhanced stool is identified easily by its high attenuation and is differentiated easily from colonic mucosa. Barium contrast with a reduced bowel preparation may yield sensitivity and specificity at least equal to that of a standard bowel preparation without barium [43,44]. Tagging of liquid or solid stool precludes colonoscopy for removal of an identified colonic polyp immediately after CTC.

Colonic distention

Adequate colonic distention is critical to increase polyp conspicuity. Air provides a low-density background to help identify medium-density colonic polyps or masses. The patient is placed in a decubitus position on the CT scanning table. A small plastic or rubber catheter is introduced into the rectum to deliver room air or carbon dioxide by either a handheld bulb pump or automated insufflator to distend the colon. Room air is inexpensive and simply administered manually. Carbon dioxide is more expensive, requires a gas tank, and is administered automatically. Automated insufflation permits control of the rate of insufflation and provides a maximal intraluminal pressure with automatic shut-off capabilities, a potential safety benefit. The adequacy of colonic distention is ascertained by a scout CT film with the patient in the supine position, and more carbon dioxide is administered as needed.

Carbon dioxide and automated insufflation improve colonic distention compared with room air [45] and manual insufflation, respectively [46]. Patient discomfort with carbon dioxide insufflation is similar to that with room air insufflation during the procedure, but there is less discomfort afterwards because of the rapid absorption of carbon dioxide from the colonic lumen [45]. Most reported colonic perforations have involved room air and manual insufflation, but several perforations have involved carbon dioxide and automated insufflation [47,48]. Colonic perforation is extremely rare (0.059%–0.08%). Risk factors for perforation include advanced age and underlying colonic pathology [47,49].

Spasmolytics

Patient discomfort can limit colonic distention and significantly reduce CTC sensitivity. Smooth muscle relaxants such as glucagon improve bowel relaxation, decrease patient discomfort, and improve colonic filling during barium enema [50–52]. Glucagon also enhances the reflux of colonic air into the small intestine by relaxing the ileocecal valve; this reflux unfortunately reduces colonic distention. Routine administration of glucagon during CTC is controversial. In a study of 33 patients administered glucagon before CTC versus 27 patients not administered glucagon, glucagon did not significantly improve colonic distention [53].

Scanning Technique

After colonic insufflation, a thin-section abdominopelvic CT is performed from the level of the diaphragm to the level of the perineum. Images are obtained in both the supine and prone positions to (1) differentiate particulate stool from fixed lesions such as polyps or cancers (Fig. 2); (2) distend adequately colonic regions poorly distended in one position because the air is redistributed with a change in patient position; and (3) evaluate adequately colonic regions obscured by residual fluid because fluid is redistributed with a change in patient position. The optimal scanning technique should minimize radiation exposure, minimize scanning time, and maximize image quality.

Radiation exposure

CTC is performed at a 40% to 50% lower radiation dose than conventional abdominopelvic CT. The lower exposure is accomplished by lowering the scan time to 50 to 100 mAs and the scan energy/dose to less than 120 kVp [54]. With the use of multidetector CT scanners, the radiation dose is about half of the radiation dose of a barium enema.

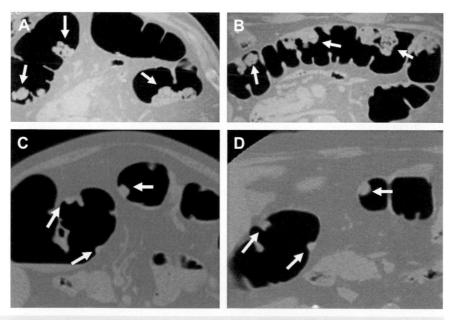

Fig. 2. Usefulness of prone and supine images to distinguish stool from a true polyp based on mobility. (*A* and *B*). Mobile apparent "polyp" (stool). (*A*) The supine 2D axial image shows three polypoid aggregations of stool (*arrows*) lying on the dependent (posterior) wall of the colon. (*B*) The prone 2D axial image shows that these three aggregations of stool (*arrows*) have moved to the now-dependent (anterior) wall of the colon. (*C* and *D*). Immobile true polyp. (*C*) The supine 2D axial image and (*D*) the prone 2D axial image reveal that these three true colonic polyps (*arrows*) remain fixed when the patient turns from supine to prone.

Scanning time

Multidetector CT scanners have the advantage of decreased acquisition time compared with single-detector scanners. For example, the scanning time for a 16-detector CT scanner with 0.75-mm collimation is only 15 seconds, whereas the scanning time for a single-detector scanner with 5-mm collimation is typically 35 to 40 seconds. Multidetector CT machines therefore significantly reduce breath-hold times and essentially eliminate respiratory motion artifacts that otherwise would degrade the image quality.

Image quality

Slice thickness affects polyp conspicuity. Every 1-mm decrease in slice thickness increases polyp detection sensitivity by 5% [55]. Multidetector CT scanners increase the sensitivity for polyp detection compared with single-detector scanners because of the decreased slice thickness. A multidetector CT scan with collimation of 3 mm or less is recommended [56].

Intravenous contrast

Intravenous contrast increases bowel wall conspicuity and improves detection of medium-sized polyps (6–9 mm), especially in a suboptimally prepared colon [57]. Contrast enhancement patterns of polyps, however, are not correlated with histology [58]. Intravenous contrast helps detect synchronous colonic lesions and lymph node involvement in patients who have newly diagnosed colorectal carcinoma, improves the accuracy of preoperative T-and-N staging for colorectal cancer [59], and aids in the detection of local recurrence or distant metastases during colon cancer surveillance [60]. Intravenous contrast is very useful in patients who have had an incomplete conventional colonoscopy because of obstructive colon cancer, and in patients with prior colonic resection for carcinoma because of their frequently inadequate colonic distention. It generally is reserved for these and similar indications.

Disadvantages of intravenous contrast include increased cost, increased invasiveness, occasional contrast reactions, higher radiation dose, and increased interpretation time. Also, intravenous contrast should not be administered simultaneously with oral contrast because the combination enhances both colonic mucosa and colonic lumen and results in a decrease in contrast between the two surfaces.

Interpretation of CT Colonography

After acquiring supine and prone scans, various software packages display images in both 2D and 3D (endoluminal) views.

Primary two-dimensional interpretation

For 2D evaluation, the colon should be able to be viewed in the conventional axial plane or in coronal and sagittal planes [61]. The reader should be able to link supine and prone axial images taken at the same level and place the images side by side. Initially the entire colon is evaluated with lung windows in the axial plane. Images are scrolled from the rectum to cecum to assess the entire colonic mucosal surface on both supine and prone images. Raised areas are evaluated further as needed in the coronal and/or sagittal planes and with soft tissue window settings to determine if the abnormality is a fold, mucosal polyp, lipoma, extrinsic mass, stool, or ileocecal valve (Fig. 3). Soft tissue windows help differentiate mucosal polyps from submucosal lipomas or extracolonic abnormalities and help detect flat colonic lesions.

Primary three-dimensional interpretation

As with the primary 2D method, in the primary 3D interpretation the entire colon is evaluated on both supine and prone images. The colon is evaluated both antegrade and retrograde to visualize regions obscured by colonic folds. The software should permit the reader to fly through the colon either automatically at a variable speed or manually. Primary 3D interpretation is supplemented by 2D views, because polyps, lipomas, and stool cannot be distinguished from each other reliably solely by 3D images.

Two-dimensional versus three-dimensional interpretation

Primary 2D versus 3D evaluation is controversial currently, but most authorities agree that 2D and 3D evaluations are complementary. Most radiologists use 2D for primary evaluation and 3D for problem solving. Reader preference, training, and imaging software often determine the used technique. The computer software should provide a user-friendly means of displaying 2D and 3D views of the same region.

In a study of 42 patients, two different methods were used to evaluate CTC examinations. In method 1, 2D data sets were the primary method of evaluation with 3D display used only if findings were suggestive of an abnormality. In method 2, 2D and 3D fly-through evaluations were performed in all patients. This study revealed that both methods identified the same polyps, but method 1 took less time than method 2 (average of 16 minutes versus average of 40 minutes, respectively) [62]. Pickhardt and colleagues [63] evaluated 1233 asymptomatic patients using primary 3D evaluation, with 2D reserved for

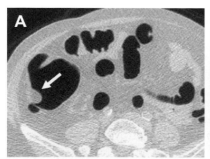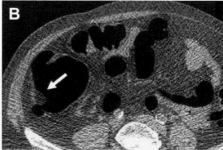

Fig. 3. Usefulness of soft tissue windows. (A) On the 2D axial lung window image, there is an apparent polyp (*arrow*) on the right lateral wall of the ascending colon. (B) On the 2D axial soft tissue window image, the "polyp" (*arrow*) is shown to have fat within it, demonstrating that it is a lipoma.

problem solving, following colon cleansing and fecal tagging with automated subtraction of tagged material. They reported excellent sensitivities for detection of adenomatous polyps: 92% for polyps 10 mm and larger, 93% for polyps 8 mm and larger, and 88% for polyps 6 mm and larger.

Pitfalls of CT Colonography
Pitfalls of two-dimensional and three-dimensional interpretation
Numerous factors can limit the accuracy of CTC:

- Stool/inadequately prepared colon
- Inadequate colonic distention
- Colonic spasm
- Uncooperative patient
- Motion artifacts from respiration
- Old CT machine (single-detector CT scanner)
- Inadequate radiologist training
- Failure to read study using both 2D and 3D imaging
- Flat (nonpolypoid) colonic lesions that are hard to detect by CTC

Technical errors are reduced or avoided by adequate bowel cleansing, adequate colonic distention, and adherence to the CT scanning protocol. Residual fecal material can obscure or mimic a colonic lesion. Several maneuvers can differentiate residual fecal material from true colonic polyps [64]. Fecal material usually does not adhere to the colonic wall and will move to the dependent colon when the patient turns from supine to prone. Rarely, stool adheres to the colonic wall, rendering it difficult to differentiate from a colonic polyp. Adherent stool typically has an irregular shape, contains air, and contains foci of high attenuation (Fig. 4). Occasionally, a pedunculated polyp attached to the bowel wall via a long stalk will seem to migrate when the patient turns.

With colonic underdistention, a narrowed colonic segment can mimic an annular lesion, and a collapsed colonic segment can prevent visualization of a true colonic lesion. Each colonic segment therefore must be adequately distended on at least one of the two (prone or supine) scans.

Pitfalls of two-dimensional interpretation
Perception errors (failure to detect a lesion) may be caused by technical factors (eg, bowel preparation, bowel distention), the primary reading technique (2D versus 3D), or reader skill and experience. Misinterpretation of findings is a major source of error. CTC has numerous potential pitfalls that often can be avoided by careful analysis of the morphology of every potential lesion on multiple views and with several maneuvers (Table 2) [37]. Polyps have rounded or lobulated contours and homogeneous soft tissue attenuation. Submucosal lesions can mimic the smooth and polypoid appearance of mucosal polyps. For instance, lipomas can mimic polyps on 3D and 2D images evaluated with lung windows. The fat within a lipoma is easily recognized, however, on 2D images evaluated with soft tissue windows [65].

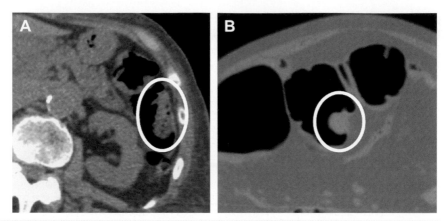

Fig. 4. Characteristics that help differentiate fecal material from polyps on CT colonography. (*A*) Fecal material (*within circle*) typically has an irregular contour, has a heterogeneous density, and usually contains air. (*B*) True polyps (*within circle*) typically have a smooth contour and a homogeneous density.

Bulbous colonic folds may mimic colonic polyps on 2D and 3D images, but sequential review of the suspected abnormality in the axial, coronal, and sagittal images should clarify that the abnormality represents a fold rather than a polyp.

An inverted appendiceal stump may mimic a cecal lesion on 2D and 3D images. When a suspected lesion is demonstrated in the expected region of the appendiceal orifice, an attempt should be made to identify a normal appendix. If the appendix is not identified, it is important to determine whether the patient has had prior inversion-ligation appendectomy [66]. A prominent ileocecal valve can mimic a cecal mass, especially on 3D images (Fig. 5). Therefore, the ileocecal valve should be identified in every study. The normal valve often contains macroscopic fat demonstrated by soft tissue windows. The terminal ileum also can be located and followed to the ileocecal valve on axial or coronal 2D images.

Pitfalls of three-dimensional interpretation
Residual fecal material is a major problem in 3D examination. It can either mask or mimic a colonic polyp or mass. 2D images are a useful adjunct to primary 3D interpretation to differentiate feces from polyps or masses. 2D images can detect air within fecal material and demonstrate fecal material moving to the dependent portion of the colon when the patient turns.

Diverticula can simulate polyps on 3D images, but a complete dense ring surrounds the orifice of a diverticulum, whereas an incomplete ring shadow surrounds the base of a polyp. An inverted diverticulum is difficult to distinguish from a polyp. In this situation, 2D images exhibit pericolonic fat in an inverted diverticulum but exhibit soft tissue density in a true polyp. Stool

Table 2
Differentiation of true mucosal colonic polyps or masses from artifacts or other filling defects

Artifact or Abnormality	Differentiation from a true mucosal polyp
Fecal matter	Stool usually moves to the dependent colon because of gravity when the patient changes position (eg, supine to prone). Polyps do not migrate because they are attached to mucosa. Stool typically has an irregular shape and often contains low-density air or high-density food particles. Polyps usually have a rounded or lobulated contour and are relatively homogeneous in density. Best to avoid stool by using a proper bowel preparation.
Lipomas	Lipomas can mimic polyps when evaluated with lung windows settings but have low attenuation characteristic of fat when evaluated with soft tissue window settings.
Inverted appendiceal stump	When a putative lesion is found near the expected location of the appendiceal orifice, the normal appendix should be identified carefully. If the appendix is not identified, determine whether patient had undergone appendectomy. If the appendix is identified, the putative lesion is likely to be real.
Prominent ileocecal valve	Bulbous valve can mimic a cecal mass on 3D images. Valve typically contains macroscopic fat demonstrated by soft tissue windows. Serially follow images from terminal ileum to the valve on 2D images.
Diverticulum	On 3D images a diverticulum characteristically has a complete, densely dark ring at its orifice because of air, whereas a polyp has an incomplete ring shadow at its base.
Inverted diverticulum	When 2D soft tissue window settings are used, an inverted diverticulum has pericolonic fat, whereas a polyp has the density of soft tissue.
Extrinsic compression	The extrinsic nature of lesion is usually demonstrated by 2D imaging.
Poorly distended colon	A poorly distended colon may mimic an annular colonic lesion (stricture or cancer). Adequate distention of all colonic segments on at least one of the two (prone or supine) views averts this artifact.
Bulbous colonic folds	Serial cinegraphic review should clarify that the finding represents a colonic fold rather than a polyp.

impacted in a diverticulum can project into the colonic lumen and simulate a polyp on the 3D image, but the 2D images typically show dense material admixed with air projecting into the lumen and may show part of the impacted diverticulum projecting outside the lumen (Fig. 6) [67].

The ileocecal valve is a common pitfall on 3D images. It is recognized easily when characteristic in location and in appearance as either a papillary-type domelike protrusion with a mouth at the apex or as a slightly raised fold with a mouth separating the fold margins (labial appearance). When it is round or irregular in shape, however, the valve may mimic a neoplasm. 2D imaging

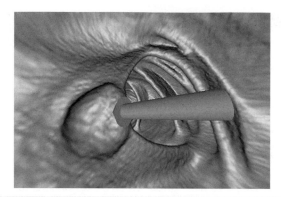

Fig. 5. Ileocecal valve mimicking a polyp. This 3D image at the level of the cecum demonstrates a smooth, round mass (3D *arrow*) that has the appearance of a polyp. This "polyp" was determined to be the ileocecal valve by scrolling through the axial and coronal images and following the path of the terminal ileum into the colon.

often helps in these cases by demonstrating fat within the valve (Fig. 7). Organs or structures adjacent to the colon can produce a mass effect that mimics a colonic polyp or mass on the 3D endoluminal view. In these cases, 2D evaluation should demonstrate the abnormality as extrinsic (Fig. 8).

Air bubbles on the colonic surface can mimic flat lesions on a 3D endoluminal view. The base of a bubble on mucosa may resemble a depressed lesion with a slightly elevated border. An air bubble can be distinguished from a true flat lesion by its characteristic morphology of a smooth, thin, ringlike peripheral elevation; by a lack of colonic wall thickening on soft tissue window views; and by its disappearance upon turning the patient [68].

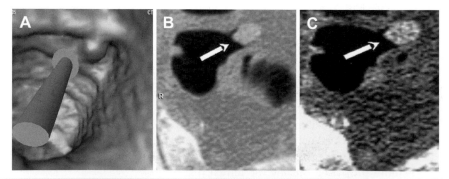

Fig. 6. Impacted, inverted diverticulum mimicking a polyp. (*A*) The 3D image shows an apparent polypoid lesion in the sigmoid colon (3D *arrow*). (*B*) The corresponding 2D axial lung window image shows the same apparent "polyp." (*C*) The corresponding 2D axial soft tissue image shows a dense fecalith within an inverted diverticulum accounting for the suspected polyp (*arrow*).

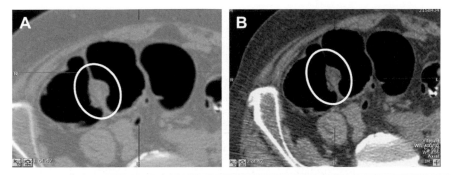

Fig. 7. Utility of soft tissue window images in identifying the ileocecal valve. (A) This 2D supine axial image shows that the ileocecal valve (*within circle*) appears as a polyp on the lung window image. (B) The corresponding 2D axial image in a soft tissue window shows the presence of fat within the circled "polyp," suggesting that it is the ileocecal valve. This finding is confirmed by scrolling through the axial or coronal images to demonstrate that the terminal ileum enters the cecum at the same location.

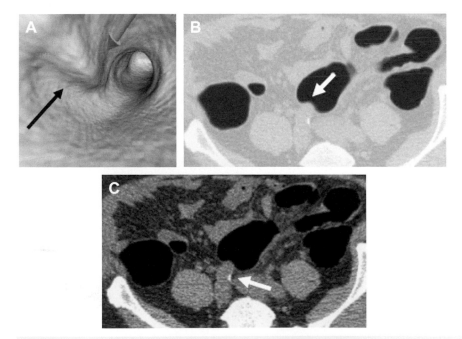

Fig. 8. Extrinsic compression of the colon mimicking a polyp. (A) This 3D image shows an elongated polypoid mass in the sigmoid colon (*arrows*). (B) The 2D axial lung window image also shows a polypoid mass (*arrow*). (C) The 2D axial soft tissue window image reveals that the suspected polyp is caused by extrinsic compression by the adjacent iliac artery (*arrow*).

Accuracy

Sensitivity

In the largest single-center study comparing CTC with conventional colonoscopy, a single-detector CT was used with 3-mm collimation and 1.5-mm reconstructions [69]. Approximately one third of patients were asymptomatic. Two experienced radiologists interpreted the studies by consensus. CTC had a sensitivity of 100% for detection of carcinomas, a sensitivity of 90.2% for polyps 10 mm or larger, and a sensitivity of 80.1% for polyps between 5 and 9.9 mm. In a large multicenter study of 1233 asymptomatic adult patients undergoing CTC and conventional colonoscopy on the same day for colon cancer screening, multidetector CT was performed with a collimation of 1.25 or 2.5 mm and reconstructions of 1 mm [63]. The studies were interpreted by one radiologist using primary 3D interpretation, with 2D for problem solving. Sensitivity was 92% for polyps 10 mm and larger, 93% for polyps 8 mm and larger, and 86% for polyps 6 mm and larger. Other investigators have reported lower sensitivities (Table 3) [42,63,69–75]. Accuracy depends on adequacy of bowel cleansing, colonic distention, imaging technique, interpretation methodology, and reader training/experience. Studies showing a low sensitivity used older CT scanners, inadequate protocols, and suboptimal software, with interpretation by inexperienced radiologists.

Specificity

The specificity of CTC among five different studies ranged from 91% to 97% [42,55,70,72,73].

Flat lesions

Flat or nonpolypoid lesions can be depressed or elevated. When elevated, their height is less than twice the height of adjacent normal mucosa. Initially, flat lesions were believed to affect only native Japanese, but now they are found

Table 3
Sensitivity of CT colonography versus conventional colonoscopy for polyp detection in nine selected comparative studies

Authors, (reference)	No. of patients	Sensitivity for Polyps: No. at CT colonography/No. at conventional colonoscopy (%)		
		< 6 mm in diameter	6–10 mm in diameter	> 10 mm in diameter
Cotton, et al [70]	308	37/265 (14)	18/62 (30)	23/42 (55)
Edwards, et al [71]	184	31/84 (37)	30/43 (70)	9/9 (100)
Johnson, et al [72]	703	–	51/94 (54)	37/59 (63)
Iannaccone, et al [73]	203	27/31 (87)	27/31 (87)	17/17 (100)
Macari, et al [74]	68	9/78 (12)	9/15 (60)	3/3 (100)
Pickhardt, et al [63]	1233	–	104/120 (88)	45/48 (94)
Pineau, et al [42]	205	17/44 (39)	20/25 (80)	18/20 (90)
Rockey, et al [75]	614	–	48/92 (52)	37/63 (59)
Yee, et al [69]	300	65/79 (82)	50/54 (93)	42/49 (86)

with some frequency in the West. In a prospective study of 321 adenomas detected among 1000 symptomatic patients in the United Kingdom, 63% were polypoid, 36% were flat, and 0.6% were depressed [76]. In a prospective study of 344 lesions 6 mm or larger confirmed at conventional colonoscopy among 1233 average-risk patients, 17% of the lesions were flat [77]. Flat lesions are believed to have a higher degree of dysplasia and malignant potential for a given size than polypoid lesions [76,78,79]. An American study contradicted this finding, however [80].

Flat lesions are more difficult to detect than polypoid lesions on both conventional colonoscopy and CTC. On CTC, flat lesions appear as thickened haustral folds, plaque-like mucosal elevations, or nodular elevations (Fig. 9) [68]. These appearances can mimic those of adherent fecal material. Tagging of fecal material can help differentiate flat lesions from adherent stool.

Other colonic findings
CTC may reveal colonic findings other than polyps or cancers. Colonic diverticulosis is diagnosed commonly. CTC is not a first-line test for Crohn's disease or ulcerative colitis because it is less sensitive than conventional colonoscopy in detecting moderate mucosal inflammation and because of the inability to perform colonic biopsies. CTC can, however, demonstrate characteristic abnormalities. Findings include bowel wall thickening, increased mesenteric vascularity, mesenteric lymphadenopathy, and pericolonic fat stranding in uncomplicated Crohn's disease [81] and intestinal fistulae, intra-abdominal abscesses, and colonic strictures in complicated Crohn's disease [81,82]. CTC can identify loss of haustral folds (foreshortening) and pseudopolyps in the colon with chronic ulcerative colitis. CTC can reveal a periappendiceal abscess [83].

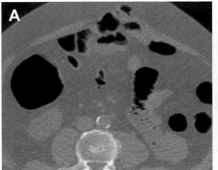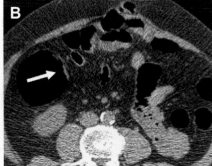

Fig. 9. Use of soft tissue window images for detection of a flat lesion on CT colonography. (A) The 2D axial supine lung window image fails to reveal any evidence of a polyp. (B) The corresponding 2D axial supine soft tissue window image reveals the presence of a flat lesion (*arrow*) along the medial wall of the colon that was inconspicuous on the corresponding lung window image.

Extracolonic findings

CTC evaluates extracolonic abdominopelvic structures. Most extracolonic findings are of little clinical significance and do not merit further investigation, but some are potentially important clinically and require further investigation with additional imaging studies and medical or surgical follow-up [84,85]. Clinically significant extracolonic findings include masses, nodules, aneurysms, metastases, abscesses, contained perforations, and choledocholithiasis (Box 2). In the currently reported review of nine studies, the incidence of significant extracolonic findings ranged from 6.8% to 21.1% (Table 4) [86–94]. The wide discrepancy among studies is caused by (1) variable definitions of clinically significant findings (eg, significance of intra-abdominal lymphadenopathy), (2) patient variability (eg, asymptomatic versus symptomatic patients), (3) CTC variability (eg, multidetector versus single-detector CT machines or use versus nonuse of intravenous contrast), and (4) variations caused by chance in insufficiently powered, small studies. In a meta-analysis of 3488 patients

---

Box 2: Selected reported extracolonic findings at CT colonography

Significant findings

Aortic aneurysm ≥ 5 cm

Liver metastases

Choledocholithiasis

Retroperitoneal perforation

Pelvic mass

Solid renal lesion

Gastric or small intestinal mass

Lung nodule

Ovarian mass

Intra-abdominal abscess

Selected potentially significant findings

Aortic aneurysm < 5 cm

Intra-abdominal lymphadenopathy

Cholelithiasis

Nephrolithiasis

Hepatic cyst

Renal cyst

Gastric or small intestinal polyp

Pelvic fluid

Hydronephrosis

Dilated choledochus

Table 4
Frequency of significant extracolonic findings on CT colonography among selected studies published since 2003

First author (reference)	No. patients with significant extracolonic lesions/total no. of patients (%)
Chin, et al [86]	32/432 (7.4)
Ginnerup Pedersen, et al [87]	9/75 (12.0)
Gluecker, et al [88]	71/681 (10.4)
Hellstrom, et al [89]	26/111 (23.4)
Khan, et al [90]	24/225 (10.7)
Pilch-Kowalczyk, et al [91]	15/71 (21.1)
Rajapaksa, et al [92]	17/250 (6.8)
Spreng, et al [93]	26/102 (25)
Yee, et al [94]	45/500 (9.0)

among 17 studies, extracolonic cancers were detected in 2.7% and aortic aneurysms in 0.9% [85].

The reporting of extracolonic abnormalities is a responsibility that must be handled carefully by the interpreting radiologist [95]. The role of extracolonic findings is controversial. Although detecting important extracolonic findings is beneficial, searching for extracolonic abnormalities has the disadvantages of increased interpretation time, increased costs from further investigation, and potentially increased patient anxiety [96]. Between 69% to 80% of potentially significant findings at CTC prove to be clinically unimportant following thorough evaluation [97]. In a study of 264 patients at increased risk for colon cancer, 11% of patients had highly significant extracolonic findings [98]. Further imaging was required in 7% of patients, including 2.3% who underwent surgery. The cost of the extra examinations prompted by the extracolonic findings in these 7% of patients was small compared with the benefits in the 2.3% group undergoing surgery because of the lesion identification. This study concluded that CTC can help detect clinically important extracolonic disease with negligible additional cost. Similar findings and conclusions were reported in a study of 45 patients who had significant extracolonic findings among 500 patients undergoing CTC [94].

Reader training
Radiologist experience is very important for accurate interpretation. A multicenter study demonstrated that readings by experienced radiologists ($\geq$ 325 CTC studies) were significantly more accurate than readings by inexperienced radiologists (50 CTC studies) [98]. Guidelines for training are lacking, but in 2004 an ad hoc working group of 18 radiologists experienced in CTC recommended training that included hands-on, workstation-based, supervised interpretation of at least 40 examinations with confirmation by conventional colonoscopy [99].

Clinical Applications
Compared with conventional colonoscopy, CTC has advantages and disadvantages (Box 3) [37].

Box 3: Advantages and disadvantages of CTC compared with conventional colonoscopy

Advantages of CTC

Does not require sedation or analgesia

Avoids need for arranging a ride home after the procedure

Generally is performed within 15 minutes

Has a lower risk of colonic perforation than with colonoscopy

Localizes lesions accurately

Detects extracolonic abnormalities

Can replace colonoscopy when colonoscopy is too dangerous

Is less expensive

May be better tolerated by patients

Can identify polyps missed at colonoscopic blind spots (eg, behind a fold)

Can diagnose and stage colon cancer in one examination

Disadvantages of CTC

Involves radiation exposure

Liquid stool is a greater problem because of the ability to aspirate liquids during colonoscopy

Cannot determine polyp histology: detected polyps require colonoscopy for tissue diagnosis

False-positive findings may require a colonoscopy

Many extracolonic findings that require further testing prove to be clinically unimportant

Is not therapeutic: requires subsequent colonoscopic polypectomy for identified polyps

Sensitivity of detecting colonic polyps may be less than that of colonoscopy, particularly for small colonic polyps

Involves patient discomfort because of the insertion of a rectal tube and colonic insufflation without sedation

Common indications for CTC are listed in Box 1. Technical reasons for incomplete colonoscopy include colonic tortuosity, obstructing masses, colonic strictures, and abdominal hernias [40]. Double-contrast barium enemas traditionally had been ordered for the approximately 10% to 15% of conventional colonoscopies that were incomplete [100], but in this situation they typically are poor in quality because of residual colonic fluid from the polyethylene glycol preparation. Residual colonic fluid is not as problematic for CTC, because fluid moves to the dependent colon to expose the submerged mucosa when the patient turns. Patients who have had an incomplete colonoscopy because of obstructing colon cancer should undergo CTC to exclude synchronous polyps or cancers proximal to the obstruction. In a prospective study, CTC performed within 3 hours after conventional colonoscopy in 29 patients who had an obstructing distal cancer demonstrated all the 29 known obstructing cancers and revealed two additional cancers, five polyps 10 mm or larger, and 16 polyps 5 to 9 mm in diameter [101]. In patients who have distal obstructing cancer, intravenous contrast permits simultaneous CT staging of the colon cancer, which avoids the need for another test on another day.

Patients who have symptoms or signs suggesting a colonic lesion may be unable to undergo conventional colonoscopy because of a high risk of anesthesia or colonic bleeding (eg, anticoagulant therapy or thrombocytopenia). CTC is a safe alternative. In a study of 1233 patients who underwent CTC and conventional colonoscopy, 68% of patients preferred CTC, and 24.5% preferred conventional colonoscopy [63]. This preference has been confirmed in other trials [102].

The most important and most controversial question concerns the role of CTC in mass screening of the general population, that is, the applicability of CTC as a routine test in patients at average risk for colon cancer. This application currently has little support from public agencies or insurance carriers. CTC currently is not endorsed by any multidisciplinary organization as a screening test for colon cancer [103]. Medicare insurance pays for CTC for colon cancer screening in Wisconsin but not in any other state [104]. Most private insurance companies do not cover CTC as a screening test [103].

The critical element in this question concerns CTC sensitivity. The sensitivity greatly affects the clinical benefits of CTC and greatly affects clinical comparisons between CTC and conventional colonoscopy. It also should affect the preferences of both informed patients and referring physicians and the guidelines issued by governing bodies. Unfortunately, as mentioned previously, the sensitivity of CTC at detecting polyps is controversial, with widely divergent results.

The answer to this question need not be either all-or-none or immutable. For example, it may be reasonable to refer for CTC a patient at moderate risk for colon cancer who adamantly refuses conventional colonoscopy or who did not tolerate a prior attempt at conventional colonoscopy because of pain or anxiety. As more patient data are accumulated about CTC sensitivity, the role of CTC for mass screening will be clarified further and better understood. Increasing data should clarify ambiguity and reduce controversy. With further progress in computerized software and hardware, development of adjunctive techniques such as digital subtraction of stool, and better training of radiologists in CTC interpretation, test sensitivity may improve sufficiently to render CTC a worthy alternative to conventional colonoscopy for mass screening.

Management of Identified Polyps

At the time of colonoscopy, nearly all identified mucosal polyps are removed by polypectomy [105] to eradicate the polyp and characterize the histology based on microscopic examination of the entire polyp. Polyp histology determines the need for subsequent cancer surgery, the time interval for surveillance colonoscopy, and the patient prognosis. In contrast, polyps cannot be removed during CTC. The need to schedule a subsequent colonoscopy for polypectomy increases medical costs and patient inconvenience substantially. Small colonic polyps are so common that a strategy of prompt colonoscopy for all polyps detected by CTC would be costly. Such a policy would require that the 30% or more of patients who have polyps at CTC undergo colonoscopy [63,106]. This consideration has led to a strategy of selectively performing colonoscopy and polypectomy after CTC based on the size and number of identified polyps. This strategy is controversial because even small polyps entail a small risk of harboring or transforming into malignancy. For example, in a study of 3291 colonoscopies, 10.1% of small adenomas (5–10 mm) had advanced histology (high-grade dysplasia or villous features), and 0.9% harbored cancer, whereas 1.7% of diminutive adenomas (≤4 mm) had advanced histology [107]. In another study of 3536 persons undergoing colonoscopy, 3.4% of small polyps (6–9 mm) had advanced histology [108].

Gastroenterologists and radiologists uniformly agree that polyps 1 cm in diameter or larger detected at CTC require prompt colonoscopy and polypectomy because of both the risk of undiagnosed malignancy in such polyps and the greater than 1% per year risk of malignant transformation within these polyps [13,109]. Gastroenterologists generally agree that colonoscopy and polypectomy are recommended for patients with any polyp 6 mm or larger in size or three polyps of any size. This recommendation has been endorsed by the American College of Gastroenterology [110]. Some radiologists have argued that polyps 9 mm and smaller do not require prompt colonoscopy and polypectomy but could be followed by periodic noninvasive surveillance protocols [108]. In particular, Pickhardt and colleagues [111] have argued strongly that a strategy of reporting diminutive colonic polyps (≤4 mm) for possible colonoscopy and polypectomy is not cost effective.

If logistically possible, patients who have a significant polyp or polyps identified at CTC should be referred directly for colonoscopy and polypectomy on the same day, if oral contrast was not administered. Similarly, patients who have an incomplete colonoscopy should be referred directly for CTC on the same day if the reason for the incomplete colonoscopy was not poor colonic preparation. This patient-friendly strategy avoids another patient visit and another colonic preparation.

The Future of CT Colonography

CTC without colonic cleansing may improve patient acceptance but currently is experimental. Preliminary studies have shown promising results [112]. In a study of 200 patients who received fecal tagging using dilute iodinated contrast material consumed during five low-fat and low-fiber meals without bowel preparation, the sensitivity for detecting polyps 9 mm and larger was 95%, which compares favorably with studies using bowel cleansing [73]. Fecal tagging with subtraction CTC involves electronic cleansing of the colon by subtracting tagged liquid and particulate stool ("digital bowel cleansing") to help the reader detect hidden polyps and avoid false-positive findings. One preliminary study reported a sensitivity of about 78% for detection of polyps, a rate similar to that of CTC with bowel preparation [113]. This study requires confirmation in larger trials.

Computer-aided detection (CAD) using software packages may enhance the ability to detect colorectal lesions [114,115]. Radiologists have used CAD for several years in mammography to detect breast cancer and in chest CT to detect pulmonary nodules. CAD is useful as a secondary but not primary reader for polyp detection because it identifies polyp candidates but cannot differentiate true polyps from structures or abnormalities that mimic polyps, such as fecal material or lipomas. Novel 3D views that appear to slice, open up, and flatten the colonic wall for improved polyp visualization are being developed [116].

In MR colonography, magnetic resonance is combined with colonic distention and administration of contrast into the gastrointestinal tract. In preliminary studies, MR colonography has shown promise in the detection of colonic polyps or colon cancer [117]. It may be superior to CTC for evaluation of inflammatory bowel disease because of the greater contrast within soft tissues. Currently, however, colonoscopy is a more sensitive and specific test than MR colonography for this purpose. MR colonography is superior to CTC for diagnosis of fistulae and sinus tracts associated with Crohn's disease [118]. MR colonography is more expensive than CTC. Unlike CTC, MR colonography involves no exposure to ionizing radiation.

SUMMARY

CTC is becoming more widely available. It can be performed on any multidetector CT with excellent quality if standard protocols are followed. CTC meets criteria for a screening test, because it is safe, relatively inexpensive, and acceptable to patients. It is less time consuming and more convenient for the patient than conventional colonoscopy. The sensitivity of CTC may be comparable to that of conventional colonoscopy when performed under ideal circumstances but has been quite variable in general practice situations.

CTC should not be viewed as a screening method that competes with conventional colonoscopy. Only about half of the patients eligible for colon cancer screening participate in screening programs. If CTC becomes more acceptable for screening, ideally more patients will undergo colon cancer screening, more polyps will be detected, and more conventional colonoscopies will be needed for polypectomy. In this way CTC and conventional colonoscopy can be viewed as complementary. Increased screening should result in a decrease in the incidence and mortality of colon cancer.

References

[1] Jemal A, Siegel R, Ward E, et al. Cancer statistics, 2007. CA Cancer J Clin 2007;57: 43–66.
[2] Mandel JS. Screening of patients at average risk for colon cancer. Med Clin North Am 2005;89:43–59.

[3] Cappell MS. From colonic polyps to colon cancer: pathophysiology, clinical presentation, and diagnosis. Clin Lab Med 2005;25:135–77.

[4] Leslie A, Carey FA, Pratt NR, et al. The colorectal adenoma-carcinoma sequence. Br J Surg 2002;89:845–60.

[5] Winawer S, Fletcher R, Rex D, et al. Colorectal cancer screening and surveillance: clinical guidelines and rationale—update based on new evidence. Gastroenterology 2003;124: 544–60.

[6] Seeff LC, Nadel MR, Klabunde C, et al. Patterns and predictors of colorectal cancer test use in the adult population. Cancer 2004;100:2093–103.

[7] Colorectal cancer test use among persons aged > or = 50 years—United States 2001. MMWR Morb Mortal Wkly Rep 2004;52:193–6.

[8] Harewood GC, Wiersema MJ, Melton LJ III. A prospective, controlled assessment of factors influencing acceptance of screening colonoscopy. Am J Gastroenterol 2002;97: 3186–94.

[9] Morson BC, Dawson IMP. Gastrointestinal pathology. Oxford (UK): Blackwell Scientific; 1972.

[10] Heald RJ, Bussey HJR. Clinical experiences at St. Mark's Hospital with multiple synchronous cancers of the colon and rectum. Dis Colon Rectum 1975;18:6–10.

[11] Day DW, Morson BC. The adenomatous-carcinoma sequence. In: Morson BC, editor. The pathogenesis of colon cancer. Philadelphia: WB Saunders; 1978. p. 58–71.

[12] Cappell MS. The pathophysiology, clinical presentation, and diagnosis of colon cancer and adenomatous polyps. Med Clin North Am 2005;89:1–42.

[13] Stryker SJ, Wolff BG, Culp CE, et al. Natural history of untreated colonic polyps. Gastroenterology 1987;93:1009–13.

[14] Bussey HJR. Familial polyposis coli: family studies, histopathology, differential diagnosis and results of treatment. Baltimore (MD): Johns Hopkins University Press; 1975.

[15] Miyaki M, Knoishi M, Kikuchi-Yanoshita R, et al. Characteristics of somatic mutation of the adenomatous polyposis coli gene in colorectal tumors. Cancer Res 1994;54:3011–20.

[16] Robbins DH, Itzkowitz SH. The molecular and genetic basis of colon cancer. Med Clin North Am 2002;86:1467–95.

[17] Appel MF. Nature and significance of colonic polyps. South Med J 1977;70:1213–4.

[18] Gebbers JO, Laissue JA. Mixed hyperplastic and neoplastic polyp of the colon: an immunohistological study. Virchows Arch A Pathol Anat Histopathol 1986;410:189–94.

[19] Urbanski SJ, Kossakowska AE, Marcon N, et al. Mixed hyperplastic adenomatous polyps: an underdiagnosed entity—report of a case of adenocarcinoma within a mixed hyperplastic adenomatous polyp. Am J Surg Pathol 1984;8:551–6.

[20] Cappell MS, Forde KA. Spatial clustering of multiple hyperplastic, adenomatous, and malignant colonic polyps in individual patients. Dis Colon Rectum 1989;32:641–52.

[21] Rubio CA, Stemme S, Jaramillo E, et al. Hyperplastic polyposis coli syndrome and colorectal carcinoma. Endoscopy 2006;38:266–70.

[22] Young JP, Jenkins MA, Parry S, et al. Serrated pathway colorectal cancer in the population: genetic consideration. Gut 2007;56:1453–9.

[23] Lynch HT, de la Chapelle A. Hereditary colon cancer. N Engl J Med 2003;348:919–32.

[24] Winawer SJ, Zauber AG, Ho MN, et al. Prevention of colorectal cancer by colonoscopic polypectomy. N Engl J Med 1993;329:1977–81.

[25] U.S. Census Bureau. Census 2000 Table PHC-T-9. Population by age, sex, race, and Hispanic or Latino origin for the United States. 2000. Available at: www.census.gov/population/www/cen2000/phc-t9.html. Accessed July 4, 2007.

[26] Imperiale TF, Ransohoff DF, Itzkowitz SH, et al. Fecal DNA versus fecal occult blood for colorectal-cancer screening in an average-risk population. N Engl J Med 2004;351: 2704–14.

[27] Allison JE. Colon cancer screening guidelines 2005: the fecal occult blood test option has become a better FIT. Gastroenterology 2005;125:745–8.

[28] Levin TR. Flexible sigmoidoscopy for colorectal cancer screening: valid approach or short sighted? Gastroenterol Clin North Am 2002;31:1015–29.

[29] Lieberman DA, Weiss DG, Veterans Affairs Cooperative Study Group 380. One-time screening for colorectal cancer with combined fecal occult-blood testing and examination of the distal colon. N Engl J Med 2001;345:555–60.

[30] Petko Z, Ghiassi M, Shuber A, et al. Aberrantly methylated CDKN2A, MGMT, and MLH1 in colon polyps and in fecal DNA from patients with colorectal polyps. Clin Cancer Res 2005;11:1203–9.

[31] Winawer SJ, Stewart ET, Zauber AG, et al. A comparison of colonoscopy and double-contrast barium enema for surveillance after polypectomy: National Polyp Study Work Group. N Engl J Med 2000;342:1766–72.

[32] Cappell MS, Friedel D. The role of sigmoidoscopy and colonoscopy in the diagnosis and management of lower gastrointestinal disorders: technique, indications, and contraindications. Med Clin North Am 2002;86:1217–52.

[33] Fidler JL, Johnson CD, MacCarty RL, et al. Detection of flat lesions in the colon with CT colonography. Abdom Imaging 2002;27:292–300.

[34] Ahlquist DA, Shuber AP. Stool screening for colorectal cancer: evolution from occult blood to molecular markers. Clin Chim Acta 2002;315:157–68.

[35] Vining DJ, Gelfand DW. Non-invasive colonoscopy using helical CT scanning, 3D reconstruction and virtual reality. Presented in the syllabus of the 23rd annual meeting, Society of Gastrointestinal Radiologists. Maui (Hawaii); 1994.

[36] Vining DJ. Virtual colonoscopy: the inside story. In: Dachman A, editor. Atlas of virtual colonoscopy. New York: Springer-Verlag; 2003. p. 3–4.

[37] Lefkovitz Z, Shapiro R, Koch S, et al. The emerging role of virtual colonoscopy. Med Clin North Am 2005;89:111–38.

[38] Chan CC, Ioke TK, Chan JC, et al. Comparison of two oral evacuants (Citromag and Golytely) for bowel preparation before barium enema. Br J Radiol 1997;70:1000–3.

[39] Macari M, Lavelle M, Pedrosa I, et al. Effect of different bowel preparations on residual fluid at CT colonography. Radiology 2001;218:274–7.

[40] Macari M, Bini EJ. CT colonography: where have we been and where are we going? Radiology 2005;237:819–33.

[41] Fletcher JG, Johnson CD, Welch TJ, et al. Optimization of CT colonography technique: prospective trial in 180 patients. Radiology 2000;216:704–11.

[42] Pineau BC, Paskett ED, Chen GJ, et al. Virtual colonoscopy using oral contrast compared with colonoscopy for the detection of patients with colorectal polyps. Gastroenterology 2003;125:304–10.

[43] Lefere PA, Gryspeerdt SS, Dewyspelaere J, et al. Dietary fecal tagging as a cleansing method before CT colonography: initial results—polyp detection and patient acceptance. Radiology 2002;224:393–403.

[44] Lefere P, Gryspeerdt S, Marrannes J, et al. CT colonography after fecal tagging with a reduced cathartic cleansing and a reduced volume of barium. AJR Am J Roentgenol 2005;184:1836–42.

[45] Shinners TJ, Pickhardt PJ, Taylor AJ, et al. Patient-controlled room air insufflation versus automated carbon dioxide delivery for CT colonography. AJR Am J Roentgenol 2006;186:1491–6.

[46] Burling D, Taylor SA, Halligan S, et al. Automated insufflation of carbon dioxide for MDCT colonography: distention and patient experience compared with manual insufflation. AJR Am J Roentgenol 2006;186:96–103.

[47] Burling D, Halligan S, Slater A, et al. Potentially serious adverse events at CT colonography in symptomatic patients: national survey of the United Kingdom. Radiology 2006;239:464–71.

[48] Young BM, Fletcher JG, Earnest F, et al. Colonic perforation at CT colonography in a patient without known colonic disease. AJR Am J Roentgenol 2006;186:119–21.

[49] Sosna J, Blachar A, Barmeir E, et al. Colonic perforation at CT colonography: assessment of risk in a multicenter cohort. Radiology 2006;239:457–63.

[50] Harned RK, Stelling CB, Williams S, et al. Glucagon and barium enema examinations: a controlled clinical trial. AJR Am J Roentgenol 1976;126:981–4.

[51] Bova JG, Jurdi RA, Bennett WF. Antispasmodic drugs to reduce discomfort and colonic spasm during barium enemas: comparison of oral hyoscyamine, IV glucagon, and no drug. AJR Am J Roentgenol 1993;161:965–8.

[52] Meeroff JC, Jorgens J, Isenberg JI. The effect of glucagon on barium enema examinations. Radiology 1975;115:5–7.

[53] Yee J, Hung RK, Akerkar GA, et al. The usefulness of glucagon hydrochloride for colonic distension in CT colonography. AJR Am J Roentgenol 1999;173:169–72.

[54] Barish MA, Rocha TC. Multislice CT colonography: current status and limitations. Radiol Clin North Am 2005;43:1049–62.

[55] Mulhall BP, Veerappan GR, Jackson JF. Meta-analysis: computed tomographic colonography. Ann Intern Med 2005;142:635–50.

[56] Barish MA, Soto JA, Ferrucci JT. Consensus on current clinical practice of CT colonography. AJR Am J Roentgenol 2005;184:786–92.

[57] Morrin MM, Farrell RJ, Kruskal JB, et al. Utility of intravenously administered contrast material at CT colonography. Radiology 2000;217:765–71.

[58] Sosna J, Morrin MM, Kruskal JB, et al. Colorectal neoplasms: role of intravenous contrast-enhanced CT colonography. Radiology 2003;228:152–6.

[59] Filippone A, Ambrosini R, Fuschi M, et al. Preoperative T and N staging of colorectal cancer: accuracy of contrast-enhanced multi-detector row CT colonography—initial experience. Radiology 2004;231:83–90.

[60] Fletcher JG, Johnson CD, Krueger WR, et al. Contrast-enhanced CT colonography in recurrent colorectal carcinoma: feasibility of simultaneous evaluation for metastatic disease, local recurrence, and metachronous neoplasia in colorectal carcinoma. AJR Am J Roentgenol 2002;178:283–90.

[61] Yee J. Screening CT colonography. Radiol Clin North Am 2004;42:757–66.

[62] Macari M, Milano A, Lavelle M, et al. Comparison of time-efficient CT colonography with two- and three-dimensional colonic evaluation for detecting colorectal polyps. AJR Am J Roentgenol 2000;174:1543–9.

[63] Pickhardt PJ, Choi JR, Hwang I, et al. CT colonography to screen for colorectal neoplasia in asymptomatic adults. N Engl J Med 2003;349:2191–200.

[64] Laks S, Macari M, Bini E. Positional change in colon polyps at CT colonography. Radiology 2004;231:761–6.

[65] Pickhardt PJ. Differential diagnosis of polypoid lesions seen at CT colonography (virtual colonoscopy). Radiographics 2004;24:1535–59.

[66] Mang T, Maier A, Plank C, et al. Pitfalls in multi-detector row CT colonography: a systematic approach. Radiographics 2007;27:431–54.

[67] Macari M, Megibow AJ. Pitfalls of using three-dimensional CT colonography with two-dimensional imaging correlation. AJR Am J Roentgenol 2001;176:137–43.

[68] Park SH, Lee SS, Choi EK, et al. Flat colorectal neoplasms: definition, importance, and visualization on CT colonography. AJR Am J Roentgenol 2007;188:953–9.

[69] Yee J, Akerkar GA, Hung RK, et al. Colorectal neoplasia: performance characteristics of CT colonography for detection in 300 patients. Radiology 2001;219:685–92.

[70] Cotton PB, Durkalski VL, Pineau BC, et al. Computed tomographic colonography (CT colonography): a multicenter comparison with standard colonoscopy for detection of colorectal neoplasia. JAMA 2004;291:1713–8.

[71] Edwards JT, Mendelson RM, Fritschi L, et al. Colorectal neoplasia screening with CT colonography in average-risk asymptomatic subjects: community-based study. Radiology 2004;230:459–64.

[72] Johnson CD, Harmsen WS, Wilson LA, et al. Prospective blinded evaluation of computed tomographic colonography for screen detection of colorectal polyps. Gastroenterology 2003;125:311–9.

[73] Iannaccone R, Laghi A, Catalano CR, et al. Computed tomographic colonography without cathartic preparation for the detection of colorectal polyps. Gastroenterology 2004;127: 1300–11.

[74] Macari M, Bini EJ, Jacobs SL, et al. Colorectal polyps and cancers in asymptomatic average-risk patients: evaluation with CT colonography. Radiology 2004;230:629–36.

[75] Rockey DC, Paulson E, Niedzwiecki D, et al. Analysis of air contrast barium enema, computed tomographic colonography, and colonoscopy: prospective comparison. Lancet 2005;365:305–11.

[76] Rembacken BJ, Fujii T, Cairns A, et al. Flat and depressed colonic neoplasms: a prospective study of 1000 colonoscopies in the UK. Lancet 2000;355:1211–4.

[77] Pickhardt PJ, Nugent PA, Choi JR. Flat colorectal lesions in asymptomatic adults: implications for screening with CT colonography. AJR Am J Roentgenol 2004;183:1343–7.

[78] Jaramillo E, Watanabe M, Slezak P, et al. Flat neoplastic lesions of the colon and rectum detected by high-resolution video endoscopy and chromoscopy. Gastrointest Endosc 1995;42:114–22.

[79] Saitoh Y, Wasman I, West AR, et al. Prevalence and distinctive biologic features of flat colorectal adenomas in a North American population. Gastroenterology 2001;120: 1657–65.

[80] O'Brien MJ, Winawer SJ, Zauber AG, et al. Flat adenomas in the National Polyp Study: is there increased risk for high-grade dysplasia initially or during surveillance? Clin Gastroenterol Hepatol 2004;2:905–11.

[81] Andersen K, Vogt C, Blondin D, et al. Multi-detector CT-colonography in inflammatory bowel disease: prospective analysis of CT-findings to high-resolution video colonoscopy. Eur J Radiol 2006;58:140–6.

[82] Ota Y, Matsui T, Ono H, et al. Value of virtual computed tomographic colonography for Crohn's colitis: comparison with endoscopy and barium enema. Abdom Imaging 2003;28:778–83.

[83] Serracino-Inglott F, Atkinson HDE, Jha P, et al. Early experiences with computed axial tomography colonography. Am J Surg 2004;187:511–4.

[84] Hara AK. Extracolonic findings at CT colonography. Semin Ultrasound CT MR 2005;26: 24–7.

[85] Xiong T, Richardson M, Woodroffe R, et al. Incidental lesions found on CT colonography: their nature and frequency. Br J Radiol 2005;78:22–9.

[86] Chin M, Mendelson R, Edwards J, et al. Computed tomographic colonography. Am J Gastroenterol 2005;100:2771–6.

[87] Ginnerup Pedersen B, Rosenkilde M, Christiansen TE, et al. Extracolonic findings at computed tomography colonography are a challenge. Gut 2003;52:1744–7.

[88] Gluecker TM, Johnson CD, Wilson LA, et al. Extracolonic findings at CT colonography: evaluation of prevalence and cost in a screening population. Gastroenterology 2003;124:911–6.

[89] Hellstrom M, Svensson MH, Lasson A. Extracolonic and incidental findings on CT colonography (virtual colonoscopy). AJR Am J Roentgenol 2004;182:631–8.

[90] Khan KY, Xiong T, McCafferty I, et al. Frequency and impact of extracolonic findings detected at computed tomographic colonography in a symptomatic population. Br J Surg 2007;94:355–61.

[91] Pilch-Kowalczyk J, Konopka M, Gibinska J, et al. Extracolonic findings at CT colonography: additional advantage of the method. Med Sci Monit 2004;10(Suppl 3):22–5.

[92] Rajapaksa RC, Macari M, Bini EJ. Prevalence and impact of extracolonic findings in patients undergoing CT colonography. J Clin Gastroenterol 2004;38:767–71.

[93] Spreng A, Netzer P, Mattich J, et al. Importance of extracolonic findings at IV contrast medium-enhanced CT colonography versus those at non-enhanced CT colonography. Eur Radiol 2005;15:2088–95.

[94] Yee J, Kumar NN, Godara S, et al. Extracolonic abnormalities discovered incidentally at CT colonography in a male population. Radiology 2005;236:519–26.

[95] Pickhardt PJ, Taylor AJ. Extracolonic findings identified in asymptomatic adults at screening CT colonography. AJR Am J Roentgenol 2006;186:718–28.

[96] Sosna J, Krukal JB, Bar-Ziv J, et al. Extracolonic findings at CT colonography. Abdom Imaging 2005;30:709–13.

[97] Hara AK, Johnson CD, MacCarty RL, et al. Incidental extracolonic findings at CT colonography. Radiology 2000;215:353–7.

[98] European Society of Gastrointestinal and Abdominal Radiology CT Colonography Study Group Investigators. Effect of directed training on reader performance for CT colonography: multicenter study. Radiology 2007;242:152–61.

[99] Soto JA, Barish MA, Yee J. Reader training in CT colonography: how much is enough? Radiology 2005;237:26–7.

[100] Shah HA, Paszat LF, Saskin R, et al. Factors associated with incomplete colonoscopy: a population-based study. Gastroenterology 2007;132:2297–303.

[101] Fenlon HM, McAneny DB, Nunes DP. Occlusive colon carcinoma: CT colonography in the preoperative evaluation of the proximal colon. Radiology 1999;210:423–8.

[102] Rex DK. Is virtual colonoscopy ready for widespread application? Gastroenterology 2003;125:608–14.

[103] Rex DK, Lieberman D. ACG colorectal cancer prevention action plan: update on CT-colonography. Am J Gastroenterol 2006;101:1410–3.

[104] Pickhardt PJ. Response letter. Ann Intern Med 2005;142:155.

[105] Cappell MS, Friedel D. The role of sigmoidoscopy and colonoscopy in the diagnosis and management of lower gastrointestinal disorders: endoscopic findings, therapy, and complications. Med Clin North Am 2002;86:1253–88.

[106] Rex DK. Pro: patients with polyps smaller than 1 cm on computed tomographic colonography should be offered colonoscopy and polypectomy. Am J Gastroenterol 2005;100:1903–5.

[107] Butterly LF, Chase MP, Pohl H, et al. Prevalence of clinically important histology in small adenomas. Clin Gastroenterol Hepatol 2006;4:343–8.

[108] Kim DH, Pickhardt PJ, Taylor AJ. Characteristics of advanced adenomas detected at CT colonographic screening: implications for appropriate polyp size thresholds for polypectomy versus surveillance. AJR Am J Roentgenol 2007;188:940–4.

[109] Ransohoff DF. Con: immediate colonoscopy is not necessary in patients who have polyps smaller than 1 cm on computed tomographic colonography. Am J Gastroenterol 2005;100:1905–7.

[110] Rex DK. American College of Gastroenterology action plan for colorectal cancer prevention. Am J Gastroenterol 2004;99:574–7.

[111] Pickhardt PJ, Hassan C, Laghi A, et al. Cost-effectiveness of colorectal cancer screening with computed tomography colonography: the impact of not reporting diminutive lesions. Cancer 2007;109:2213–21.

[112] Callstrom MR, Johnson CD, Fletcher JG, et al. CT colonography without cathartic preparation: feasibility study. Radiology 2001;219:693–8.

[113] Zalis ME, Perumpillichira J, Del Ferate C, et al. CT colonography: digital subtraction bowel cleansing with mucosal reconstruction—initial observations. Radiology 2003;226:911–7.

[114] Summers RM, Johnson CD, Pusanik LM, et al. Automated polyp detection at CT colonography: feasibility study in a human population. Radiology 2001;219:51–9.

[115] Taylor SA, Halligan S, Burling D, et al. Computer-assisted reader software versus expert reviewers for polyp detection on CT colonography. AJR Am J Roentgenol 2006;186: 696–702.

[116] Dachman AH, Lefere P, Gryspeerdt S, et al. CT colonography: visualization methods, interpretation, and pitfalls. Radiol Clin North Am 2007;45:347–59.

[117] Ajaj W, Pelster G, Treichel U, et al. Dark lumen magnetic resonance colonography: comparison with conventional colonoscopy for detection of colorectal pathology. Gut 2003;52:1738–43.

[118] MacKalski BA, Bernstein CN. New diagnostic imaging tools for inflammatory bowel disease. Gut 2006;55:733–41.

Gastroenterol Clin N Am 37 (2008) 191–213

GASTROENTEROLOGY CLINICS
OF NORTH AMERICA

Surveillance of Patients at Increased Risk of Colon Cancer: Inflammatory Bowel Disease and Other Conditions

Amulya Konda, MD, Michael C. Duffy, MD*

Division of Gastroenterology, William Beaumont Hospital, 3535 West 13 Mile Road, Royal Oak, MI 48076, USA

C olorectal cancer (CRC) is the second most common cause of cancer-related mortality in the United States. Colonoscopic screening with removal of adenomatous polyps in individuals at average risk is known to decrease the incidence and associated mortality from colon cancer. Certain conditions, notably inflammatory bowel disease (IBD) involving the colon, a family history of polyps or cancer, a personal history of colon cancer or polyps, and other conditions such as acromegaly, ureterosigmoidostomy, and *Streptococcus bovis* bacteremia are associated with an increased risk of colonic neoplasia. This article reviews in detail the CRC risks associated with these conditions and the currently recommended surveillance strategies.

INFLAMMATORY BOWEL DISEASE
Cancer Risk

Patients who have chronic IBD, whether classified as ulcerative colitis or Crohn's colitis, are at greater than average risk of developing CRC [1]. The reported risk varies considerably, however, with older studies generally showing a very high risk (perhaps reflecting referral bias) and recent studies suggesting a much lower risk. A recent meta-analysis of 116 studies found the overall prevalence of CRC in ulcerative colitis to be 3%, with a cumulative risk of CRC of 2% at 10 years, 8% at 20 years, and 18% at 30 years [2]. There also is considerable geographic variation, with higher rates of cancer in the United States and United Kingdom and lower rates in Scandinavia [2]. The mean time from the diagnosis of colitis to the diagnosis of cancer is 17 years, with a mean age at diagnosis of cancer of 51 years for men and 54 for women [3]. Although most studies demonstrate an increased risk of cancer in IBD, this finding is not universal. Indeed, two recent population studies from Denmark and the Mayo Clinic failed to show any increased risk of cancer in patients who had ulcerative colitis compared with a control population [4,5]. Furthermore, the reported

*Corresponding author. E-mail address: mduffymd@comcast.net (M.C. Duffy).

0889-8553/08/$ – see front matter
doi:10.1016/j.gtc.2007.12.013

mortality from the colon cancer is variable. One study suggested that colon cancer accounts for one third of deaths in ulcerative colitis [6], whereas another study found that this cancer accounts for only one sixth of deaths [7].

Crohn's colitis, particularly with extensive colonic involvement, carries a similar risk of developing CRC [8,9]. CRC associated with Crohn's disease and CRC associated with ulcerative colitis seem to share unusual features [10]. Both groups tend to have cancer diagnosed after 8 years of IBD and frequently have multifocal cancer with an aggressive (signet ring or mucinous) histology. The cancers in Crohn's colitis were confined to areas of diseased mucosa. A recent population-based study from Olmsted County, Minnesota showed only a modestly increased risk (standardized incidence ratio, 1.9) for CRC in Crohn's disease but a marked (40-fold) increased risk for small intestinal cancer [5].

Pathogenesis

The precise pathogenesis of CRC in IBD is unclear. The pathogenesis is believed to involve chronic inflammation leading to increased cell proliferation with subsequent development of dysplasia [11,12]. This postulated mechanism is different from the gene deletion sequence that occurs in sporadic, non-IBD carcinomas [13,14]. A detailed discussion of the molecular mechanisms of neoplasia is beyond the scope of this article and has been reviewed elsewhere [15]. The progression to dysplasia and cancer in ulcerative colitis may involve genomic instability with chromosomal breakage caused by shortened telomeres; patients who have IBD may have a mutator phenotype that predisposes them to colon cancer [15]. Colonoscopic surveillance to prevent colon cancer in IBD is based on the concept of stepwise progression from chronic inflammation through low-grade dysplasia (LGD) and high-grade dysplasia to cancer.

Risk Factors

Risk factors for CRC in patients who have IBD are

> Duration of disease
> Extent of colitis
> Primary sclerosing cholangitis
> Family history of CRC
> Inflammatory pseudopolyps
> Degree of histologic inflammation

The duration of disease and extent of colitis are well-established risk factors. Other important clinical risk factors for neoplasia in ulcerative colitis have been identified recently. A recent case-controlled study of 188 patients who had ulcerative colitis–related colon cancer showed that the presence of inflammatory pseudopolyps was an independent risk factor (odds ratio [OR], 2.5), whereas cigarette smoking, the use of aspirin, nonsteroidal anti-inflammatory drugs, or 5-acetyl salicylic acid (5-ASA), and a history of one or two surveillance colonoscopies decreased the risk [16]. More severe histologic inflammation of the colon also has been recognized recently as an important risk factor [17]. The coexistence of primary sclerosing cholangitis (PSC) confers an approximately fivefold increase in

CRC risk [18–21]. A meta-analysis of 11 studies incorporating 16,844 patients who had ulcerative colitis, including 560 who had concomitant PSC, reported an approximately fivefold increase in the CRC risk associated with PSC [22]. The mechanism of this increase in PSC is unknown, but altered bile salt composition in the colonic lumen has been suggested as a mechanism [23]. This increased risk of cancer has led to recommendations that patients who have IBD and PSC undergo more intensive surveillance colonoscopy beginning at the time of diagnosis (see guidelines presented later). In addition, patients who have PSC and IBD have an increased risk of cholangiocarcinoma [18]. Ulcerative colitis associated with ileal inflammation ("backwash ileitis") seems to be a risk factor for colon cancer [24].

The clinical characteristics of cancers associated with IBD are somewhat different from those of sporadic CRC. These cancers occur at a younger age (mean age, 43 years) [2], are more frequently multifocal [25], and exhibit more aggressive histology [26,27]. Despite these unfavorable prognostic factors, a recent case-controlled study of 290 patients who had IBD-related CRC showed that the 5-year survival rates were virtually identical (56% versus 57%) to those of patients who had non–IBD-related CRC [27].

Surveillance Strategies (Secondary Prevention)

Colonoscopy with removal of elevated polypoid precursor lesions (adenomatous polyps) is the most common prevention strategy for sporadic colon cancer. In IBD-related cancers, however, the precursor dysplastic lesion often is flat and may not be readily evident endoscopically. Thus, the primary strategy for preventing CRC in patients who have IBD is surveillance colonoscopy with multiple random biopsies throughout the colon to detect dysplasia, with subsequent proctocolectomy for patients harboring dysplastic lesions in the hopes of preventing progression to cancer or of removing cancer at an earlier, potentially curable, stage.

In a retrospective cohort analysis of 91 screened subjects versus 95 unscreened controls, screening improved overall survival, but the survival benefit was not related to increased cancer-related survival [28]. In contrast, a study of 41 patients who had ulcerative colitis showed that patients undergoing colonoscopic surveillance had cancers diagnosed at an earlier Dukes stage and had an improved 5-year survival (77.2% versus 36.3%) [29]. In a population-based, nested, case-control study of 142 patients who had ulcerative colitis who died from colon cancer, one surveillance colonoscopy was associated with a decreased risk of cancer death (OR, 0.29), and two or more colonoscopies were associated with a further risk reduction [30]. A recent report of a surveillance program involving 600 patients, with up to 40 years of follow-up, reported that the cancer incidence was lower than expected (10.8% at 40 years) and that the 5-year survival rate for those who had cancer was very high (73%) [31]. Indeed, only 2% of the surveillance group died from CRC during the 40-year study period. One half of the cancers, however, were thought to be interval cancers that potentially were missed on the preceding colonoscopy, and this surveillance program did not uniformly prevent advanced cancer.

In a recent Cochrane review, the authors found no direct evidence that colonoscopy prolonged survival in patients who had IBD, although patients in surveillance programs tended to have cancers diagnosed earlier with a correspondingly better prognosis [32]. They could not exclude lead-time bias as a contributing factor for this benefit. On the basis of indirect evidence, however, the authors concluded that surveillance seemed to decrease mortality from CRC and that surveillance was cost effective.

Despite the lack of conclusive evidence of benefit, surveillance colonoscopy with biopsy currently is recommended by the major gastrointestinal societies worldwide, including the American Gastroenterology Association, the American Society for Gastrointestinal Endoscopy, the American College of Gastroenterology, the British Society of Gastroenterology, and the American Society of Colon and Rectal Surgeons. A recent consensus conference of the Crohn's and Colitis Foundation of America also endorsed this recommendation [33].

Dysplasia

Surveillance strategies critically depend on the detection and accurate histologic classification of dysplasia, defined as unequivocal neoplastic transformation of mucosa, and subsequent proctocolectomy to reduce the incidence and mortality from CRC in patients who have IBD. The precise histologic definitions of low-, high-, and indeterminate-grade dysplasia have been reviewed recently and are beyond the scope of this article [34]. Interobserver variability in the diagnosis of dysplasia is common and. may justify outside pathologic review of biopsies initially read as containing dysplasia [35]. Pathologists generally agree when there is no dysplasia or high-grade dysplasia but often disagree in cases of indeterminate- or low-grade dysplasia [36].

High-grade Dysplasia and Dysplasia-associated Lesions or Masses

High-grade dysplasia, when confirmed independently by two experienced pathologists, generally warrants proctocolectomy because of the high (42%–62%) risk of concurrent cancer [31,37]. The finding of any degree of dysplasia in the setting of a grossly visible mass lesion, called a "dysplasia-associated lesion or mass" (DALM), is generally a strong indication for immediate proctocolectomy because up to 50% of these patients have frank cancer at surgery [38,39].

Low-grade Dysplasia

The management of LGD is controversial. Many experts recommend immediate colectomy, but others favor intense colonoscopic surveillance [40]. Patients who have LGD have an approximately 20% risk of harboring concurrent cancer and a 50% risk of progressing to advanced dysplasia with time [31,41]. In a retrospective review of patients who had LGD, one half developed advanced neoplasia (defined as cancer, DALM, or high-grade dysplasia) during a mean follow-up of 32 months [42].

Not all studies show this association between LGD and advanced neoplasia, however. Among 60 patients who had LGD followed for a mean of 10 years, no patient developed cancer, although 11 patients developed DALMs [43]. In a retrospective cohort study of 29 patients who had LGD followed for 10 years, 10% developed high-grade dysplasia or cancer compared with 4% of controls, a difference that was not statistically significant [44].

Rubin and Turner [36] suggest that multifocal LGD is an indication for colectomy but that unifocal LGD can be managed by either colectomy or aggressive colonoscopic surveillance. Other experts suggest that unifocal and multifocal LGD have the same cancer risk and that a policy of increased endoscopic surveillance is unwise because patients may develop advanced (node-positive) CRC despite intensive colonoscopic surveillance [45]. Both unifocal and multifocal LGD were found to progress to high-grade dysplasia or CRC in 50% at 5 years. A recently published meta-analysis of 20 surveillance studies of patients who had LGD found that LGD was associated with a ninefold increased risk of developing cancer and a 12-fold risk of developing high-grade dysplasia or cancer [46]. LGD was associated with concurrent CRC in 22% and subsequent cancer in 7.9%.

Table 1 lists the recommendations for management of dysplasia promulgated by various societies. Proctocolectomy is the preferred management strategy for any patient who has IBD and high-grade dysplasia and for any grade of DALM. The management of LGD remains controversial. Most experts recommend immediate colectomy because of the high risk of concurrent or subsequent cancer [47–49]. Patients choosing intensive colonoscopic surveillance (eg, at 6-month intervals) should be advised of the risk of developing advanced CRC despite this intensive surveillance. Furthermore, reliance on detection of dysplasia alone to predict CRC cannot protect all patients, because 26% of patients who have carcinoma identified at surgery do not harbor concomitant dysplasia [50].

Dysplasia-associated Lesions or Masses Versus Adenoma-like Masses

Patients who have IBD can develop polypoid lesions that resemble sporadic adenomas, which have been called "adenoma-like masses" (ALMs). In two longitudinal studies, patients who had IBD with colonoscopically resected polyps and who had no evidence of dysplasia adjacent to the polyp or elsewhere in the colon did not develop dysplasia or cancer during 4 years of follow-up [51,52]. In a subsequent 7-year follow-up of one of these studies, 58% developed further ALMs, an incidence that was similar to the incidence of sporadic adenomas in the control group of patients who did not have ulcerative colitis, and only one study patient (who had concomitant PSC) developed carcinoma [53]. Thus, pedunculated polyps occurring within areas of colitis or elsewhere in the colon can be managed safely by colonoscopic polypectomy without colectomy, provided biopsies of adjacent mucosa reveal no dysplasia [54,55].

Guidelines for Colonoscopic Surveillance in Irritable Bowel Disease

Table 2 lists the surveillance approaches currently recommended by various national and international societies [36,56–60]. A surveillance program also should include periodic office visits with physical examination and routine

Table 1
Guidelines for management of dysplasia by various professional societies

Condition	ACG	AGA	BSG	ASCRS	CCFA
High-grade dysplasia in flat mucosa	Colectomy	Colectomy if confirmed by two pathologists	Proctocolectomy if confirmed by two pathologists	Proctocolectomy	Proctocolectomy if confirmed by two pathologists
Dysplasia associated lesion or mass (DALM)	Colectomy	Colectomy if confirmed by two pathologists	Proctocolectomy if confirmed by two pathologists	Proctocolectomy	Proctocolectomy
Low-grade dysplasia in flat mucosa	Colectomy may be indicated	Multifocal: colectomy; unifocal low-grade dysplasia: no consensus	Proctocolectomy preferred; colonoscopy every 6 months until two negative examinations if surgery not performed	Proctocolectomy if stricture present	Unifocal or multifocal: proctocolectomy preferred; surveillance every 3 to 6 months if surgery not performed
Indefinite for dysplasia					Repeat colonoscopy in 3 to 6 months

Abbreviations: ACG, American College of Gastroenterology; AGA, American Gastroenterology Association; ASCRS, American Society of Colon and Rectal Surgeons; ASGE, American Society of Gastrointestinal Endoscopy; BSG, British Society of Gastroenterology; CCFA, Crohn's and Colitis Foundation of America.

Table 2
Guidelines for colonoscopic surveillance in irritable bowel disease

	ACG	ASGE	AGA	BSG	ASCRS	CCFA
Time to start surveillance (years)	8–10	8	8	8–10	8	8–10
Interval (years)	1–2	1–2	1–2	Second decade: 3 y; third decade: 2 y; fourth decade: 1 y	1–2	1–2; after two negative examinations, 1–3 y until 20 y, then every 1–2 y
Left-sided disease	Same as for pancolitis	Start after 15 y	Start after 15 y	Start after 15 y	Start after 15 y	> 35 cm: same as for pancolitis; < 35 cm: no special screening
Biopsy protocol	Multiple biopsies every 10 cm	Two to four biopsies every 10 cm	Four biopsies every 10 cm	Two to four biopsies every 10 cm	Four biopsies every 10 cm	> 33 biopsies; four quadrant biopsies every 10 cm with jumbo forceps
PSC	Surveillance at onset	–	–	Surveillance at onset	Surveillance at onset	Surveillance at onset

Abbreviations: ACG, American College of Gastroenterology; AGA, American Gastroenterological Association; ASCRS, American Society of Colon and Rectal Surgeons; ASGE, American Society of Gastrointestinal Endoscopy; BSG, British Society of Gastroenterology; CCFA, Crohn's and Colitis Foundation of America; PSC, Primary sclerosing cholangitis.

laboratory testing. Surveillance colonoscopy should be considered starting after 7 or 8 years of disease. If possible it should be performed when the colitis is in clinical remission to minimize any misinterpretation of inflammatory change as dysplasia. To maximize detection of neoplasia, jumbo biopsy forceps should be used, two to four biopsies should be obtained every 10 cm for a minimum of 33 biopsies, and additional targeted biopsies should be performed for any raised lesions (suspected DALMs) or strictures [61]. Strictures in the setting of ulcerative colitis should be considered neoplastic until proven otherwise, and strictures in Crohn's disease should be biopsied or brushed to exclude malignancy.

Gastroenterologists do not seem to adhere strictly to these guidelines [62,63]. A questionnaire survey of British gastroenterologists showed that all consultants recommended surveillance colonoscopy, but only 4% recommended colectomy for LGD, and, surprisingly, only 53% recommended colectomy for high-grade dysplasia [63]. A questionnaire survey found that 80% of members of the American Gastroenterology Association recommend surveillance colonoscopy beginning at 8 to 10 years of disease, but only half reported performing at least 31 biopsy specimens per colonoscopy, and only 40% recommended immediate colectomy for patients who have LGD [64]. Despite published guidelines, gastroenterologists need further education about performance standards for surveillance colonoscopy. These two surveys also demonstrate a lack of consensus among practicing gastroenterologists regarding management of LGD.

Advanced Endoscopic Techniques

Although standard colonoscopy with 30 or more random biopsies is the reference standard for surveillance, it is imperfect. It requires extra time to obtain and process all the biopsy specimens. The yield of dysplasia per biopsy is low. Hurlstone and colleagues [65] reported only 0.14% of approximately 12,000 nontargeted biopsies showed intraepithelial neoplasia (dysplasia), and Rutter and colleagues [66] found no instances of intraepithelial neoplasia among 2904 biopsies in 100 patients. Several methods to enhance the efficiency of colonoscopic detection of intraepithelial neoplasia in IBD have been developed, including chromoendoscopy, with or without magnification endoscopy, narrow-band imaging, and optical coherence tomography [67].

Chromoendoscopy, the most widely studied technique, involves the topical application of dyes, most commonly indigo carmine or methylene blue, to enhance mucosal detail and to facilitate detection of abnormalities that should undergo targeted biopsy [67–69]. Several studies have shown improved yields for intraepithelial neoplasia in patients who have ulcerative colitis undergoing chromoendoscopy with targeted biopsies compared with conventional colonoscopy with nontargeted biopsies. In a study of 263 patients who had ulcerative colitis randomly assigned to either conventional colonoscopy or chromoendoscopy with methylene blue, the yield for intraepithelial neoplasia was threefold higher in the chromoendoscopy group [70]. In a similar study of 100 patients undergoing back-to-back conventional colonoscopy versus chromoendoscopy with indigo carmine, Rutter and colleagues [66] found no dysplasia by conventional nontargeted biopsies compared with nine dysplastic lesions in the indigo-carmine group and found that chromoendoscopy required many fewer biopsies.

The use of high-magnification colonoscopes in conjunction with chromoendoscopy further enhances the yield for intraepithelial neoplasia and can allow preliminary classification of lesions as neoplastic or non-neoplastic based on chromoendoscopic appearance using a pit-pattern classification [71,72]. In a recent controlled study of 161 patients who had ulcerative colitis randomly assigned to conventional surveillance colonoscopy versus chromoendoscopy with methylenc blue and endomicroscopy, fivefold more neoplastic lesions were found using chromoendoscopy and endomicroscopy than with conventional colonoscopy [73].

Emerging experimental colonoscopic techniques for enhanced neoplasia detection include narrow-band imaging, optical coherence tomography, fluorescence endoscopy, and confocal laser endomicroscopy [67]. More clinical studies of these techniques are needed. Furthermore, most of these techniques require specialized colonoscopes and additional endoscopic training and are more time consuming than conventional colonoscopy; these requirements increase the cost of colonoscopic surveillance.

Primary Prevention Strategies

Patients who have IBD are at increased risk of death from colon cancer because current surveillance strategies are imperfect in detecting early cancer or dysplasia. Pharmacotherapy to decrease this risk is an attractive option. Several drugs have been tried, but direct proof of efficacy for any primary prevention strategy is lacking because of the long required duration of exposure to a potential agent, the relatively low risk of CRC, and the difficult of eliminating confounding factors. The available data come primarily from retrospective observational studies comparing the incidence of cancer in patients using a medication and in those not using this medication.

5-Acetyl Salicylic Acid Compounds

In a nested case-control study of 3112 patients, including 102 cases of colon cancer, sulfasalazine administered for at least 3 months significantly decreased the risk of CRC (relative risk, 0.34) [3]. In a similar case-control study of 102 cases of CRC complicating IBD, regular use of 5-ASA reduced the cancer risk by 75% [74]. In this study, the risk of CRC was reduced dramatically (by 81%) in patients administered more than 1.2 g/d of mesalamine, but simply visiting a doctor more than twice a year had an even greater protective effect (OR, 0.16). Another study of 100 patients who had IBD and CRC also showed significant risk reductions with regular use of 5-ASA [75]. Some studies have not shown this protective effect. A case-controlled retrospective study of 25 cases of IBD and cancer showed no relationship between mesalamine use or dosage and cancer risk [76]. In a similar study of 364 patients who had IBD and cancer, using data extracted from two large insurance claims databases, the use of

5-ASA at any dose or duration for the year preceding the diagnosis of cancer did not reduce the cancer risk [77]. A meta-analysis of nine observational studies, including 334 cases of CRC complicating IBD, showed a decrease in the risk of CRC among patients receiving 5-aminosalicylates (OR, 0.51) [78]. In conclusion, 5-ASA seems to be beneficial in preventing cancer and is useful as a maintenance therapy to prevent flares of colitis with minimal toxicity [79–81].

Ursodeoxycholic Acid

Ursodeoxycholic acid (UDCA) is used commonly to treat PSC. One study of 59 patients who had ulcerative colitis and PSC showed a significantly lower incidence of colonic dysplasia in those administered UDCA (OR, 0.18) [82]. Similar results were seen in a study of 42 patients who had PSC and ulcerative colitis in which patients receiving UDCA had a much lower incidence of developing dysplasia or colon cancer (OR, 0.26) [83]. The use of UDCA in patients who had ulcerative colitis and PSC therefore is reasonable. Whether this apparent benefit extends to patients who have ulcerative colitis but do not have PSC is unknown. The mechanism of this apparent chemoprotective effect also is unknown.

Folic Acid

Low folate levels have been identified as a risk factor for sporadic CRC [84], and patients who have IBD have an increased risk of folic acid deficiency because of decreased intake, decreased intestinal absorption, or the use of concomitant medications such as sulfasalazine that interfere with folic acid metabolism. Studies in patients who have IBD given supplemental folic acid have shown a statistically nonsignificant trend toward a reduced risk of cancer and dysplasia [85,86].

In summary, 5-ASA compounds seem to decrease the risk of dysplasia and cancer in patients who have IBD. In patients who have PSC and ulcerative colitis, UDCA seems to have a beneficial effect. The data on the benefits of folic acid supplementation for cancer prevention in IBD are weak.

OTHER CONDITIONS WITH INCREASED RISK OF CANCER

Personal History of Colon Cancer

The recurrence of colon cancer recurrence after curative resection may result from missed synchronous lesions, new metachronous lesions, or anastomotic recurrence. In a prospective study of patients undergoing colonoscopy either preoperatively or within 6 months postoperatively, synchronous cancers occurred in 5% and adenomatous polyps occurred in 28% of patients [87]. Many of these cancers occurred at a site distant from the original malignancy and would not have been included in the original curative resection. Passman and colleagues [88] similarly reported a 3.3% incidence of synchronous cancers, with most being stage I or II. Metachronous colon cancers occur at a higher frequency in patients who had prior colon cancer than in the general population. In one study, 42 metachronous cancers developed during a total of

15,345 person-years of follow-up for a cumulative incidence of 1.5% at 5 years [89]. More than one half of metachronous lesions were found within 2 years of the original colonic resection, suggesting that some of these apparently metachronous lesions actually are missed synchronous lesions [89,90]. Patients undergoing annual surveillance colonoscopy after curative resection were found to have a 5% risk of anastomotic recurrence and a 2% risk of metachronous cancers after 6 years [91]. Of the metachronous lesions, 80% were found within 2 years of follow-up, and all these were resectable for cure, whereas none in the anastomotic recurrent group underwent curative resection. The benefit of colonoscopy in the first 2 years lies primarily in detecting metachronous cancers rather than anastomotic recurrence [92]. The optimal interval for surveillance colonoscopy after the first year is debated, but several studies have not shown a survival benefit from annual follow-up colonoscopies [93,94].

Rectal cancer has a higher incidence of local recurrence than proximal cancers (20%–30% versus 2%–4%), and surgical excision with neoadjuvant chemoradiation is known to lower recurrence rates significantly (by about 10%) [95]. Frequent proctoscopic evaluations or rectal endoscopic ultrasounds are recommended after low anterior resection for rectal cancer [96]. Current guidelines for surveillance colonoscopy after curative surgery for colon cancer from the American Cancer Society and the United States Multi-Society Task Force on Colorectal Cancer [96] are listed in Table 3.

Personal History of Adenomatous Polyps

Patients who have a history of adenomatous polyps are at increased risk of subsequently developing colonic adenomas and colon cancer [97]. Risk factors for subsequent adenomas include villous histology [98–100], multiplicity of polyps [101,102] and increased polyp size [98,103,104]. Right-sided adenomas may

Table 3
American Cancer Society and the United States Multi-Society Task Force on Colorectal Cancer guidelines for colonoscopy after curative colon cancer resection

Type of malignancy	Initial colonoscopy	Follow-up colonoscopy
Proximal cancer with partial resection	Perioperative colonoscopy (before or within 6 months after surgery)	Follow-up in 1 y. If normal, repeat in 3 y and 5 y subsequently.
Rectal cancer with low anterior resection	Perioperative colonoscopy	Three to 6 monthly proctoscopic evaluations or rectal endoscopic ultrasound for 2–3 y in addition to above follow-up.
Endoscopic removal of malignant polyp		Colonoscopy in 3 to 6 mo.

Data from Rex DK, Kahi CJ, Levin B, et al. Guideline for colonoscopy surveillance after cancer resection: a consensus update by the American Cancer Society and the US Multi-Society task force on colorectal cancer. Gastroenterology 2006;130:1865–71.

carry a higher risk than left-sided adenomas [102,103]. Lesions found on index colonoscopy are categorized as having low risk for subsequent neoplasia (one or two tubular adenomas with LGD) or high risk (more than three adenomas of any size or a single adenoma larger than 1 cm, villous histology, or high-grade dysplasia) [57,97]. The United States Multi-Society Task Force on Colorectal Cancer recommends follow-up colonoscopy at 3 years for patients who have high-risk lesions [57]. If the follow-up colonoscopy demonstrates no polyps, the surveillance interval can be extended to 5 years. If low-risk lesions are detected on the index colonoscopy, follow-up may be delayed from 5 to 10 years [105]. The current recommendations of the United States Multi-Society Task Force on Colorectal Cancer and the American Cancer Society are shown in Table 4.

Family History of Adenomatous Polyps or Cancer

Several studies have documented an increased risk of colorectal neoplasia in patients who have a family history of colon cancer [106] or adenomatous polyps [107]. The risk is increased further when two or more family members are affected or when the neoplasia was diagnosed before the age of 60 years [107]. Two recent meta-analyses have confirmed these findings [108,109]. For persons with a first-degree relative who had colon cancer or two first-degree relatives who had colon cancer, the current American Gastroenterology Association guidelines (Table 5) recommend screening colonoscopy every 5 years beginning at age 40 or 10 years younger than the age at diagnosis of the relative affected with CRC [57]. For individuals with a first-degree relative

Table 4
Recommendations for surveillance after removal of adenomatous polyps

Index colonoscopy findings[a]	Follow-up colonoscopy	Comments
No adenoma or small (< 1-cm) rectal hyperplastic polyps	10 y	Identify hyperplastic polyposis syndrome and follow up earlier for this syndrome
Low risk: one or two small (< 1-cm) tubular adenomas with low-grade dysplasia	5–10 y	Family history, quality of initial colonoscopy, age, and comorbidities of patient may modify decision
High risk: 3–10 adenomas, or any adenoma >1 cm, or villous histology or high-grade dysplasia	3 y	Complete removal of polyp needs to be ascertained. Follow-up is 5 y if low-risk lesions are seen.
> 10 adenomas	< 3 y	Exclude genetic syndromes
Sessile adenoma, piecemeal removal	2–6 mo	Individualized follow-up after first follow-up colonoscopy

[a] Index colonoscopy needs to be complete and of high quality.
Data from Winawer S, Fletcher R, Rex D, et al. Colorectal cancer screening and surveillance: clinical guidelines and rationale-update based on new evidence. Gastroenterology 2003;124:544–60.

Table 5
Guidelines for patients who have a family history of colon cancer or adenomatous polyps

Family history	Initial colonoscopy	Follow-up colonoscopy
Cancer: One first-degree relative diagnosed at age < 60 y or two first-degree relatives of any age	Age 40 y or 10 y younger than the age of relative at cancer diagnosis, whichever is earlier	5-y interval if initial colonoscopy is negative
Cancer: one first-degree relative diagnosed at age > 60 y or two second-degree relatives	Age 40 y or 10 y younger than the age of relative at cancer diagnosis, whichever is earlier	10-y interval if initial colonoscopy is negative
Polyps: first-degree relative diagnosed at age < 60 y	Age 40 y	5-y interval if initial colonoscopy is negative
Polyps: first-degree relative diagnosed at age > 60 y	Age 40 y	10-y interval if initial colonoscopy is negative

Data from Winawer S, Fletcher R, Rex D, et al. Colorectal cancer screening and surveillance: clinical guidelines and rationale-update based on new evidence. Gastroenterology 2003;124:544–60.

who had adenomatous polyps diagnosed before the age of 60 years or two second-degree relatives who had colon cancer, standard average-risk guidelines apply, but screening is recommended beginning at age 40 years.

Serrated adenomas

Hyperplastic polyps (HPP) traditionally were not considered precancerous, but recently some HPPs have been recognized as having adenomatous features and a malignant potential. Originally called "mixed hyperplastic–adenomatous polyps" [110], they now are called "serrated adenomas" (SAs) [111]. They are characterized by architectural distortion including abnormal crypt branching, aberrant dilated crypts, and the presence of mature goblet cells or gastric foveolar cells [112,113].

Recent studies have shown a strong association between SAs and sporadic colon cancer. Makinen and colleagues [114,115] reported SAs adjacent to 5.8% of colon cancers; up to 40% of these colon cancers had microsatellite instability (MSI-H) suggesting that SAs may be precursor lesions to these cancers. Goldstein and colleagues [113] reported 91 patients who had right-sided mismatch repair–deficient (MSI-H) adenocarcinomas who previously had "hyperplastic polyps" removed from the same colonic segment. Retrospective pathologic analysis of these lesions showed them to be SAs based on current histologic criteria. Hawkins and Ward [116] showed that patients who had MSI-H cancers had a higher risk of having synchronous SA or HPP than patients who had microsatellite-stable cancers. SAs with MSI-H cancers also had a higher incidence of loss of enzyme expression of the DNA mismatch repair gene *hMLH1* with increased methylation of hMLH1 promoter, a finding corroborated by Wynter and colleagues [117]. SAs also are associated with a high incidence of *BRAF* mutations, a mutation linked to inhibition of apoptosis [118,119]. Progression of SA to carcinoma based on the sequential acquisition of gene mutations has been proposed [120].

Retrospective analysis has shown that up to 20% of all HPPs are unrecognized SAs [113,121]. SAs are predominantly flat or sessile lesions typically found in the proximal colon (75%–80%) [113,118]. In Goldstein and colleague's [113] retrospective review, the mean interval between the finding of an SA and the development of cancer was 7.3 years, with 90% of cancers developing more than 3 years after the finding of an SA and 55% developing more than 5 years after polypectomy.

Hyperplastic polyposis syndrome is a rare familial syndrome characterized by numerous HPP and SAs throughout the colon [108]. It is associated with an increased risk of proximal cancer and may be associated with MSI [115,122,123]. Suggested criteria for the diagnosis include more than 30 HPP distributed throughout the colon or more than five HPP proximal to the sigmoid with at least two greater than 1 cm, or one or more proximal HPP in an individual with a first-degree relative who has hyperplastic polyposis [124].

The clinical management of patients who have SAs or the hyperplastic polyposis syndrome is not defined. Complete colonoscopic removal of all SAs is recommended, especially right-sided lesions, which may have a greater malignant potential [116,120,125]. In the absence of dysplasia or phenotypic evidence of hyperplastic polyposis, patients who have SAs should undergo colonoscopic surveillance at intervals similar to those for sporadic adenomas [120]. Patients who have dysplasia, especially right-sided, should undergo a follow-up colonoscopy within 1 year, and segmental colectomy may be considered, especially for patients who have hyperplastic polyposis [120].

Acromegaly

Ezzat and colleagues [126] first described an increased risk of colorectal neoplasia in patients who have acromegaly. A recent cohort study noted that patients treated with growth hormone had an increased incidence of and mortality from CRC [127]. As the life expectancy of patients who have acromegaly increases, an increased risk of CRC is being recognized. The relative risk of CRC in acromegalics is increased 7- to 18-fold; the variability may be caused in part by variation in the study population age, different cecal intubation rates at colonoscopy, and the retrospective nature of the studies [128–130]. Patients who have acromegaly also have an increased incidence of adenomatous polyps [128,130]. These polyps may be more frequently right-sided, multiple, and villous in histology [131].

Elevated levels of growth hormone and insulin-like growth factor can potentiate growth of colonic epithelial cells and may play a role in the increased risk of colonic neoplasia in acromegalics [132]. In vitro studies of these cell lines suggest increased high-affinity binding sites for insulin-like growth factor 1. Reduced tumor necrosis factor-α–induced apoptosis of colon cancer cells may play an etiologic role [133].

Given the rarity of acromegaly, no published guidelines exist for colonoscopic screening or surveillance, but one expert has suggested starting screening colonoscopy at age 40 years [130]. Colonoscopy may be more difficult in patients who have acromegaly because of inadequate bowel preparation resulting from slowed colonic transit and difficulty reaching the cecum because of an elongated, tortuous colon [131]. A recent prospective cohort study suggests acromegalics who have prior adenomas and persistently elevated levels of insulin-like growth factor have a high risk of metachronous adenomas [134]. Acromegalics who do not have polyps on the initial colonoscopy seem to have a lower risk of subsequent adenomas [135].

Ureterosigmoidostomy

Ureterosigmoidostomy is used for urinary diversion in the treatment of bladder extrophy, bladder cancer, or trauma. An increased incidence of adenomatous polyps and cancers has been reported at the ureterosigmoid anastomosis, possibly caused by the conversion of urinary nitrates into carcinogenic N-nitroso compounds by colonic bacteria [136,137]. Rectal urine samples in patients undergoing ureterosigmoidostomy have significantly increased urinary nitrite and N-nitroso compounds with decreased nitrates when compared with normal bladder samples [138]. Tumors can be prevented in a rat model by diversion of the fecal stream, suggesting that admixture of fecal and urinary streams may contribute to carcinogenesis [139]. Adenocarcinomas have been reported even after reversal of the ureterosigmoidostomy, however, especially when ureteric stumps have been left in place [140–143]. A recent meta-analysis suggested an incidence of carcinoma ranging from 2% to 15% [144]. Cancers begin to appear as early as 6 to 7 years postoperatively, with a mean duration of 20 to 26 years between the surgery and cancer diagnosis [142,144,145]. The mean age of colon cancer diagnosis is 30 to 35 years in persons treated as children with ureterosigmoidostomy for bladder extrophy [143,146]. Rectal bleeding and obstructive uropathy often are the presenting symptoms of malignancy, and urinary obstruction occurring more than 2 years after ureterosigmoidostomy mandates exclusion of cancer [144,147]. The ureterosigmoidostomy normally has a cherry-red polypoid appearance on colonoscopy. Biopsy rather than snare polypectomy of suspicious lesions is recommended to prevent anastomotic stricture [147]. Surveillance with annual sigmoidoscopies starting 10 years after ureterosigmoidostomy has been suggested by Woodhouse [147], but others suggest annual colonoscopy beginning no later than 6 years after surgery [144]. Sigmoidal resection with excision of the ureteric implants and creation of alternative urinary diversion should be considered in patients unable to undergo surveillance endoscopy [144].

Streptococcus bovis *endocarditis*

An association between *S bovis* infections and colorectal neoplasia is well recognized [148,149]. The incidence of fecal carriage of *S bovis* is increased in patients who have colonic neoplasia [150,151]. *S bovis* was recovered from the feces of 56% of patients who had colon cancer as compared with only 10% of controls [152]. A recent prospective, controlled study, however, found a similar rate of fecal carriage of *S bovis* among patients and matched controls, perhaps reflecting the application of more stringent bacteriologic techniques to isolate *S bovis* [153]. *S bovis* septicemia, with or without endocarditis, is associated with a high risk of colon cancer (27%) and adenomatous polyps (44%) as well as noncolonic tumors [152]. Another study showed an 11% risk of colon cancer in patients who have *S bovis* septicemia [154]. *S bovis* bacteremia may precede the diagnosis of colonic neoplasia by several years [155]. The reason for this association is unclear, but colonic neoplasia may promote bacterial invasion and septicemia [156]. *S bovis* itself may be carcinogenic in a rat model [157]. Patients who have *S bovis* bacteremia require extensive endoscopic evaluation for gastrointestinal neoplasia. If initial endoscopic examinations are negative, these patients may need more frequent surveillance than average-risk patients.

SUMMARY

Patients who have IBD have an increased risk of colonic cancer compared with the general population, but the increased risk is much less than previously thought. Colonoscopy with nontargeted surveillance biopsies to detect dysplasia and colectomy when dysplasia is identified is the standard strategy to prevent colon cancer. Chromoendoscopy and other advanced endoscopic techniques will play an increasing role in targeting surveillance biopsies in the future. The significance of LGD remains controversial, but most authorities recommend colectomy for any degree of dysplasia. PSC confers a much higher risk of colon cancer, and such patients deserve more intensive screening. 5-ASA compounds seem to have a role in preventing colon cancer. UDCA seems to prevent colon cancer in patients who have ulcerative colitis and PSC, but it is unknown whether this protective effect extends to patients who have ulcerative colitis alone.

Patients who have a personal history of resected CRC are at increased risk for synchronous and metachronous cancer and require increased colonoscopic surveillance. Patients who have a family history of colon cancer or adenomatous polyps occurring before age 60 years and patients who have a history of advanced adenomas also are at increased risk for CRC and require more intensive colonoscopic surveillance.

SAs also carry an increased risk of CRC and should be removed completely with follow-up colonoscopic surveillance intervals similar to those for sporadic adenomas.

Patients who have acromegaly are at increased risk for CRC, and achieving adequate colonoscopy may be difficult because of their frequently elongated colons and their difficulty in achieving an adequately clean bowel.

Patients who have undergone ureterosigmoidostomy have an increased risk of CRC at the anastomosis. Rectal bleeding or urinary obstruction is a frequent sign of this cancer.

S bovis bacteremia is associated with an increased risk of concurrent or subsequent gastrointestinal neoplasia.

References

[1] Bernstein CN, Blanchard JF, Kliewer E, et al. Cancer risk in patients with inflammatory bowel disease: a population-based study. Cancer 2001;91:854–62.
[2] Eaden JA, Abrams KR, Mayberry JF. The risk of colorectal cancer in ulcerative colitis: a meta-analysis. Gut 2001;48:526–35.

[3] Pinczowski D, Ekbom A, Baron J, et al. Risk factors for colorectal cancer in patients with ulcerative colitis: a case-control study. Gastroenterology 1994;107:117–20.

[4] Winther KV, Jess T, Langholz E, et al. Long term risk of cancer in ulcerative colitis: a population-based cohort study from Copenhagen county. Clin Gastroenterol Hepatol 2004;2: 1088–95.

[5] Jess T, Loftus EV, Valeyos FS, et al. Risk of intestinal cancer in inflammatory bowel disease: a population-based study from Olmsted County, Minnesota. Gastroenterology 2006;130: 1039–46.

[6] Eaden JA, Mayberry JF. Colorectal cancer complicating ulcerative colitis: a review. Am J Gastroenterol 2000;95:2710–9.

[7] Gyde S, Rrior P, Dew NJ, et al. Mortality in ulcerative colitis. Gastroenterology 1982;83: 36–43.

[8] Friedman S, Rubin PH, Bodian C, et al. Screening and surveillance colonoscopy in chronic Crohn's colitis. Gastroenterology 2001;120:820–6.

[9] Gillen CD, Walmsley RS, Prior P, et al. Ulcerative colitis and Crohn's disease: a comparison of the colorectal cancer risk in extensive colitis. Gut 1994;35:1590–2.

[10] Choi PM, Zelig MP. Similarity of colorectal cancer in Crohn's disease and ulcerative colitis: implications for carcinogenesis and prevention. Gut 1994;35:950–4.

[11] Clevers H. At the crossroads of inflammation and cancer. Cell 2004;118:671–4.

[12] Itzkowitz SH, Xio X. Inflammation and cancer IV: colorectal cancer in inflammatory bowel disease: the role of inflammation. Am J Physiol Gastrointest Liver Physiol 2004;287: G7–17.

[13] Vogelstein B, Fearon ER, Hamilton SR, et al. Genetic alterations during colorectal-tumor development. N Engl J Med 1988;19:525–32.

[14] Fearon ER, Vogelstein B. A genetic model for colorectal tumorignesis. Cell 1990;61: 759–67.

[15] Brentnall TA. Molecular underpinnings of cancer in ulcerative colitis. Curr Opin Gastroenterol 2003;19:64–8.

[16] Valeyos FS, Loftus EV, Jess T, et al. Predictive and protective factors associated with colorectal cancer in ulcerative colitis: a case-control study. Gastroenterology 2006;130: 1941–9.

[17] Rutter M, Saunders B, Wilkinson K, et al. Severity of inflammation is a risk factor for colorectal neoplasia in ulcerative colitis. Gastroenterology 2004;126:451–9.

[18] Broome U, Lofberg R, Veress B, et al. Primary sclerosing cholangitis and ulcerative colitis: evidence for increased neoplastic potential. Hepatology 1995;22:1404–8.

[19] Broome U, Bergquist A. Primary sclerosing cholangitis, inflammatory bowel disease and colon cancer. Semin Liver Dis 2006;26:31–41.

[20] Brentnall TA, Haggitt RC, Rabinovitch PS, et al. Risk and natural history of colonic neoplasia in patients with primary sclerosing cholangitis and ulcerative colitis. Gastroenterology 1996;110:331–8.

[21] Kornfeld D, Eckom A, Ihre T. Is there an excess risk for colorectal cancer in patients with ulcerative colitis and primary sclerosing cholangitis? A population based study. Gut 1997;41:522–5.

[22] Soetikno RM, Lin OS, Heidenreich PA, et al. Increased risk of colorectal neoplasia in patients with primary sclerosing cholangitis and ulcerative colitis: a meta-analysis. Gastrointest Endosc 2002;56:48–54.

[23] Naggengast F, Grubben M, van Munster I. Role of bile acids in colorectal carcinogenesis. Eur J Cancer 1995;31:1067–70.

[24] Hueschen UA, Hinz U, Allemeyer EH, et al. Backwash ileitis is strongly associated with colorectal carcinoma in ulcerative colitis. Gastroenterology 2001;120:841–7.

[25] Greenstein AJ, Slater G, Heimann TM, et al. A comparison of multiple synchronous colorectal cancer in ulcerative colitis, familial polyposis coli and de novo cancer. Ann Surg 1986;203:123–8.

[26] Harpaz N, Tlbot IC. Colorectal cancer in idiopathic inflammatory bowel disease. Semin Diagn Pathol 1996;13:339–57.

[27] Delauoit T, Limburg PJ, Goldberg RM, et al. Colorectal cancer prognosis among patients with inflammatory bowel disease. Clin Gastroenterol Hepatol 2006;4:335–42.

[28] Lashner BA, Kane SV, Hanauer SB. Colon cancer surveillance in chronic ulcerative colitis: historical cohort study. Am J Gastroenterol 1990;85:1083–7.

[29] Choi PM, Nugent FW, Schoetz DJ, et al. Colonoscopic surveillance reduces mortality from colorectal cancer in ulcerative colitis. Gastroenterology 1993;105:418–24.

[30] Karlen P, Kornfeld D, Brostrom O, et al. Is colonoscopic surveillance reducing colorectal cancer mortality in ulcerative colitis? A population based case control study. Gut 1998;42:711–4.

[31] Rutter MD, Saunders BP, Wilkinson KW, et al. Thirty-year analysis of a colonoscopic surveillance program for neoplasia in ulcerative colitis. Gastroenterology 2006;130:1030–8.

[32] Collins PD, Mpofu C, Watson AJ, et al. Strategies for detecting colon cancer and/or dysplasia in patients with inflammatory bowel disease. Cochrane Database Syst Rev 2006;4(2):CD000279.

[33] Itzkowitz SH, Present DH. Consensus conference: colorectal cancer screening and surveillance in inflammatory bowel disease. Inflamm Bowel Dis 2005;11:314–21.

[34] Odze RD. Pathology of dysplasia and cancer in inflammatory bowel disease. Gastroenterol Clin North Am 2006;35:533–52.

[35] Dixon MF, Brown LJ, Gilmour HM, et al. Observer variation in the assessment of dysplasia in ulcerative colitis. Histopathology 1988;13:385–97.

[36] Rubin DT, Turner JR. Surveillance of dysplasia in inflammatory bowel disease: the gastroenterologist-pathologist partnership. Clin Gastroenterol Hepatol 2006;4:1309–13.

[37] Bernstein CN, Shanahan F, Weinstein WM. Are we telling patients the truth about surveillance colonoscopy in ulcerative colitis? Lancet 1994;353:71–4.

[38] Torres C, Antonioli D, Odze RD. Polypoid dysplasia and adenomas in inflammatory bowel disease. A clinical, endoscopic and pathological study of 89 polyps in 59 patients. Am J Surg Pathol 1998;22:275–84.

[39] Ridell RH, Goldman H, Ransohoff DF, et al. Dysplasia in inflammatory bowel disease: standardized classification with provisional clinical applications. Hum Pathol 1983;14:931–68.

[40] Bernstein CN. The color of dysplasia in ulcerative colitis. Gastroenterology 2003;124:1135–49.

[41] Ullman T, Croog V, Harpaz N, et al. Progression of flat low-grade dysplasia to advanced neoplasia in patients with ulcerative colitis. Gastroenterology 2003;125:1311–9.

[42] Ullman TA, Loftus EV, Kakar S, et al. The fate of low grade dysplasia in ulcerative colitis. Am J Gastroenterol 2002;97:922–7.

[43] Befrits R, Ljung T, Jaramillo E, et al. Low-grade dysplasia in extensive, long-standing inflammatory bowel disease: a follow up study. Dis Colon Rectum 2002;45:615–20.

[44] Lim CH, Dixon MF, Vail A, et al. Ten year follow up of ulcerative colitis patients with and without low grade dysplasia. Gut 2003;52:1127–32.

[45] Ullman TA. Low-grade colorectal dysplasia and the need for colectomy. Gastroenterology & Hepatology 2006;2:868–70.

[46] Thomas T, Abrams KA, Robinson RJ, et al. Meta-analysis: cancer risk of low-grade dysplasia in chronic ulcerative colitis. Aliment Pharmacol Ther 2007;25:657–68.

[47] D'Haens G. Dysplasia and cancer in ulcerative colitis: too many questions, too few answers. Digestion 2006;73:9–10.

[48] Bernstein CN. Natural history and management of flat and polypoid dysplasia in inflammatory bowel disease. Gastroenterol Clin North Am 2006;35:573–9.

[49] Itzkowitz SH, Harpaz N. Diagnosis and management of dysplasia in patients with inflammatory bowel diseases. Gastroenterology 2004;126:1634–48.

[50] Taylor BA, Pemberton JH, Carpenter HA, et al. Dysplasia in chronic ulcerative colitis: implications for colonoscopic surveillance. Dis Colon Rectum 1992;35:950–6.

[51] Rubin PH, Friedman S, Harpaz N, et al. Colonoscopic polypectomy in chronic colitis: conservative management after endoscopic resection of dysplastic polyps. Gastroenterology 1999;117:1295–300.

[52] Engelsgjerd M, Farraye FA, Odze RD. Polypectomy may be adequate treatment for adenoma-like dysplastic lesions in chronic ulcerative colitis. Gastroenterology 1999;117: 1288–94.

[53] Odze RD, Farraye FA, Hecht JL, et al. Long-term follow-up after polypectomy treatment for adenoma-like dysplastic lesions in ulcerative colitis. Clin Gastroenterol Hepatol 2004;2: 534–41.

[54] Bernstein CN. ALMs versus DALMs in ulcerative colitis: polypectomy or colectomy? Gastroenterology 1999;117:1488–91.

[55] Marion JF. Polypectomy versus proctocolectomy for adenoma patients with long-standing ulcerative colitis. Inflamm Bowel Dis 2006;12:914–5.

[56] American Society for Gastrointestinal Endoscopy. The role of colonoscopy in the management of patients with inflammatory bowel disease. Gastrointest Endosc 1998;48:689–90.

[57] Winawer S, Fletcher R, Rex D, et al. Colorectal cancer screening and surveillance: clinical guidelines and rationale-update based on new evidence. Gastroenterology 2003;124: 544–60.

[58] Eaden JA, Mayberry JF. Guidelines for screening and surveillance of asymptomatic colorectal cancer in patients with inflammatory bowel disease. Gut 2002;51(Suppl V): v10–2.

[59] Cohen JL, Strong SA, Hyman NH, et al. Practice parameters for the surgical treatment of ulcerative colitis. Dis Colon Rectum 2005;48:1997–2009.

[60] Kornbluth A, Sachar DB. Ulcerative colitis practice guidelines in adults (update): American College of Gastroenterology, Practice Parameters Committee. Am J Gastroenterol 2004;99:1371–85.

[61] Connell WR, Lennard-Jones JE, William CB, et al. Factors affecting the outcome of endoscopic surveillance for cancer in ulcerative colitis. Gastroenterology 1994;107:934–44.

[62] Bernstein CN, Weinstein WM. Physician's perceptions of dysplasia and approaches to surveillance colonoscopy in UC. Am J Gastroenterol 1995;90:2106–14.

[63] Eaden JA, Ward BA, Mayberry JF. How gastroenterologists screen for colonic cancer in ulcerative colitis: an analysis of performance. Gastrointest Endosc 2000;51:123–8.

[64] Rodriguez SA, Collins JM, Knigge KL, et al. Surveillance and management of dysplasia in ulcerative colitis. Gastrointest Endosc 2007;65:432–9.

[65] Hurlstone DP, Sanders DS, Lobo AJ, et al. Indigo carmine-assisted high-magnification chromoscopic endoscopy for the detection and characterization of intraepithelial neoplasia in UC: a prospective evaluation. Endoscopy 2005;37:1186–92.

[66] Rutter MD, Saunders BP, Schofield G, et al. Pancolonic indigo carmine dye spraying for detection of dysplasia in ulcerative colitis. Gut 2004;53:256–60.

[67] Kiesslich R, Neurath MF. Chromoendoscopy and other novel techniques. Gastroenterol Clin North Am 2006;35:605–19.

[68] Thorlacius H, Toth E. Role of chromoendoscopy in colon cancer surveillance in inflammatory bowel disease. Inflamm Bowel Dis 2007;13:911–7.

[69] Rutter M, Bernstein C, Matsumoto T, et al. Endoscopic appearance of dysplasia in ulcerative colitis and the role of staining. Endoscopy 2004;36:1109–14.

[70] Kiesslich R, Fritsch J, Holtmann M, et al. Methylene blue-aided chromoendoscopy and colon cancer in ulcerative colitis. Gastroenterology 2003;124:880–8.

[71] Hurlstone DP, Sanders DS, McAlindon ME, et al. High-magnification chromoscopic colonoscopy in ulcerative colitis: a valid tool for in vivo optical biopsy and assessment of disease extent. Endoscopy 2006;38:1213–7.

[72] Kato S, Fu KI, Sano Y, et al. Magnifying colonoscopy as a non-biopsy technique for differential diagnosis of non-neoplastic and neoplastic lesions. World J Gastroenterol 2006;12: 1416–20.

[73] Kiesslich R, Goetz M, Lammersdorf K, et al. Chromoscopy-guided endomicroscopy increases the diagnostic yield of intraepithelial neoplasia in ulcerative colitis. Gastroenterology 2007;132:874–82.

[74] Eaden J, Abrams K, Ekbom A, et al. Colorectal cancer prevention in ulcerative colitis: a case-control study. Aliment Pharmacol Ther 2000;14:145–53.

[75] van Staa TP, Card T, Logan RF, et al. 5-aminosalicylate use and colorectal cancer risk in inflammatory bowel disease: a large epidemiological study. Gut 2005;54:1573–8.

[76] Bernstein CN, Blanchard JF, Metge C, et al. Does the use of 5-aminosalicylates in inflammatory bowel disease prevent the development of colorectal cancer? Am J Gastroenterol 2003;98:2784–8.

[77] Terdiman JP, Steibuch M, Blumentals WA, et al. 5-aminosalicylic acid therapy and the risk of colorectal cancer among patients with inflammatory bowel disease. Inflamm Bowel Dis 2007;13:367–71.

[78] Valeyos FS, Terdiman JP, Walsh JM. Effect of 5-aminosalicylate use on colorectal cancer and dysplasia risk: a systematic review and metaanalysis of observational studies. Am J Gastroenterol 2005;100:1345–53.

[79] Bernstein CN, Eaden J, Steinhart AH, et al. Cancer prevention in inflammatory bowel disease and the chemoprophylactic potential of 5-aminosalicylic acid. Inflamm Bowel Dis 2002;8:356–61.

[80] Eaden J. Review article: the data supporting a role for salicylates in chemoprevention of colorectal cancer in patients with inflammatory bowel disease. Aliment Pharmacol Ther 2003;18(Suppl 2):15–21.

[81] Rubin DT, Lashner BA. Will a 5-ASA a day keep the cancer (and dysplasia) away? Am J Gastroenterol 2005;100:1354–6.

[82] Tung BY, Edmond MJ, Haggitt RC, et al. Ursodiol use is associated with lower prevalence of colonic neoplasia in patients with ulcerative colitis and primary sclerosing cholangitis. Ann Intern Med 2001;134:89–95.

[83] Pardi DS, Loftus EV, Kremers WK, et al. Ursodeoxycholic acid as a chemopreventive agent in patients with ulcerative colitis and primary sclerosing cholangitis. Gastroenterology 2003;124:889–93.

[84] Giovannucci E, Stampfer MJ, Colditz GA, et al. Folate, methionine and alcohol intake and risk of colorectal adenoma. J Natl Cancer Inst 1993;85:875–84.

[85] Lashner BA, Heidenreich PA, Su GL, et al. Effect of folate supplementation on the incidence of dysplasia and cancer in chronic ulcerative colitis. Gastroenterology 1989;97:255–9.

[86] Lashner BA, Provencher KS, Seidner DL, et al. The effect of folic acid supplementation on the risk for cancer or dysplasia in ulcerative colitis. Gastroenterology 1997;112:29–32.

[87] Langevin JM, Nivatvongs S. The true incidence of synchronous cancer of the large bowel: a prospective study. Am J Surg 1984;147:330–3.

[88] Passman MA, Pommier RF, Vetto JT. Synchronous colon primaries have the same prognosis as solitary colon cancers. Dis Colon Rectum 1996;39:329–34.

[89] Green RJ, Metlay JP, Propert K, et al. Surveillance for second primary colorectal cancer after neo-adjuvant chemotherapy: an analysis of intergroup 0089. Ann Intern Med 2002;136:261–9.

[90] Barillari P, Ramacciato G, Manetti G, et al. Effectiveness of early detection of intraluminal recurrences on prognosis and survival of patients treated for cure. Dis Colon Rectum 1996;38:388–93.

[91] Juhl G, Larsin GM, Mullins R, et al. Six-year results of annual colonoscopy after resection of colorectal cancer. World J Surg 1990;14:255–60.

[92] Jeffery GM, Hickey BE, Hider P. Follow-up strategies for patients treated for non-metastatic colorectal cancer. Cochrane database Sys Rev 2002:CD002200.

[93] Schoemaker D, Black R, Giles L, et al. Yearly colonoscopy, liver CT and chest radiography do not influence 5-year survival of colorectal cancer patients. Gastroenterology 1998; 114:7–14.

[94] Renehan AG, Egger M, Saunders MP, et al. Impact on the survival of intensive followup after curative resection for colorectal cancer: systematic review and meta-analysis of randomized trials. Br Med J 2002;324:813.

[95] Kapiteijn E, Marijnen CA, Nagtegaal ID, et al. Dutch colorectal cancer group. Preoperative radiotherapy combined with total mesorectal excision for resectable rectal cancer. N Engl J Med 2001;345:638–46.

[96] Rex DK, Kahi CJ, Levin B, et al. Guideline for colonoscopy surveillance after cancer resection: a consensus update by the American Cancer Society and the US Multi-Society task force on colorectal cancer. Gastroenterology 2006;130:1865–71.

[97] Atkin WS, Morson BC, Cuzick J. Long-term risk of colorectal cancer after excision of rectosigmoid adenomas. N Engl J Med 1992;326:658–62.

[98] Yang G, Zheng W, Sun QR, et al. Pathologic features of initial adenomas as predictors for metachronous adenomas of the rectum. J Natl Cancer Inst 1998;90:1661–5.

[99] Loeve F, Van Ballegooijen M, Boer R, et al. Colorectal cancer risk in adenoma patients. A nation wide study. Int J Cancer 2004;111:147–51.

[100] Lieberman DA, Weiss DG. Five year surveillance of patients with adenomas or colorectal cancer at screening colonoscopy. results from the VA Co-operative Study #380 [abstract]. Gastroenterology 2004;126:A22.

[101] Robertson DJ, Greenberg ER, Beach M, et al. Colorectal cancer in patients under close colonoscopic surveillance. Gastroenterology 2005;129:34–41.

[102] Bonithon-Kopp C, Piard F, Fenger C, et al. Colorectal adenomas characteristics as predictors of recurrence. Dis Colon Rectum 2004;47:323–33.

[103] Martinez ME, Sampliner R, Marshall JR, et al. Adenoma characteristics as risk factors for recurrence of advanced adenomas. Gastroenterology 2001;120:1077–83.

[104] Noshirwani K, Van Stolk RU, Rybicki LA, et al. Adenoma size and number are predictive of adenoma recurrence: implications for surveillance colonoscopy. Gastrointest Endosc 2000;51:433–7.

[105] Winawer SJ, Zauber AG, Fletcher RH, et al. Guidelines for colonoscopy surveillance after polypectomy: a consensus update by the US Multi-Society Task Force on colorectal cancer and the American Cancer Society. CA Cancer J Clin 2006;56:143–59.

[106] Fuchs CS, Giovannucci EL, Colditz GA, et al. A prospective study of family history and risk of colorectal cancer. N Engl J Med 1994;331:1669–74.

[107] Winawer SJ, Zauber AG, Gerdes H, et al. Risk of colorectal cancer in families of patients with adenomatous polyps. N Engl J Med 1996;334:82–7.

[108] Johns LE, Houlston RS. A systematic review and meta-analysis of familial colorectal cancer risk. Am J Gastroenterol 2001;96:2992–3003.

[109] Butterworth AS, Higgins JP, Pharoah P. Relative and absolute risk of colorectal cancer for individuals with a family history: a meta-analysis. Eur J Cancer 2006;42:216–27.

[110] Urbanski SJ, Kossakowska AE, Marcon N, et al. Mixed hyperplastic adenomatous polyps: an underdiagnosed entity; report of a case of adenocarcinoma arising within mixed hyperplastic polyp. Am J Surg Pathol 1984;8:551–6.

[111] Longacre TA, Fenoglio-Preiser CM. Mixed hyperplastic adenomatous polyps/serrated adenomas. A distinct form of colorectal neoplasia. Am J Surg Pathol 1990;14:524–37.

[112] Torlakovic E, Snover DC. Serrated adenomatous polyposis in humans. Gastroenterology 1996;110:748–55.

[113] Goldstein NS, Bhanot P, Odish E, et al. Hyperplastic-like colon polyps that preceded microsatellite-unstable adenocarcinomas. Am J Clin Pathol 2003;119:778–96.

[114] Mäkinen MJ, George SM, Jernvall P, et al. Colorectal carcinoma associated with serrated adenoma–prevalence, histological features, and prognosis. J Pathol 2001; 193:286–94.

[115] Jass JR. Serrated route to colorectal cancer: back street or super highway? J Pathol 2001;193:283–5.

[116] Hawkins NJ, Ward RL. Sporadic colorectal cancers with microsatellite instability and their possible origin hyperplastic polyps and serrated adenomas. J Natl Cancer Inst 2001;93: 1307–13.

[117] Wynter CVA, Walsh MD, Higuchi T, et al. Methylation patterns define two types of hyperplastic polyp associated with colorectal cancer. Gut 2004;53:573–80.

[118] Spring KJ, Zhao ZZ, Karamatic R, et al. High prevalence of sessile serrated adenomas with BRAF mutations: a prospective study of patients undergoing colonoscopy. Gastroenterology 2006;131:1400–7.

[119] Kambara T, Simms LA, Whitehall VLJ, et al. BRAF mutation and CpG island methylation: an alternative pathway to colorectal cancer. Gut 2004;53:1137–44.

[120] Snover DC, Jass JR, Preiser CF, et al. Serrated polyps of the large intestine. A morphologic and molecular review of an evolving concept. Am J Clin Pathol 2005;124:380–91.

[121] Torlakovic E, Skovland E, Snover DC, et al. Morphological reappraisal of serrated colorectal polyps. Am J Surg Pathol 2003;27:65–81.

[122] Rashid A, Houlihan PS, Booker S, et al. Phenotypic and molecular characteristics of hyperplastic polyposis. Gastroenterology 2000;119:323–32.

[123] Leggett BA, Devereaux B, Biden K, et al. Hyperplastic polyposis: association with colorectal cancer. Am J Surg Pathol 2001;25:65–81.

[124] Renaut AJ, Douglas PR, Newstead GL. Hyperplastic polyposis of the colon and rectum. Colorectal Dis 2002;4:213–5.

[125] Higuchi T, Jass JR. My approach to serrated polyps of the colorectum. J Clin Pathol 2004;57:682–6.

[126] Ezzat S, Strom C, Melmed S. Colon polyps in acromegaly. Ann Intern Med 1991;114: 754–5.

[127] Swerdlow A, Higgins C, Adlard P, et al. Risk of cancer in patients treated with human pituitary growth hormone in the UK, 1959–85: a cohort study. Lancet 2002;360:273–7.

[128] Jenkins PJ, Fairclough OD, Richards T, et al. Acromegaly, colon polyps and carcinoma. Clin Endocrinol 1997;47:17–22.

[129] Ladas SD, Thalassinos NC, Ioannides G, et al. Does acromegaly really predispose to an increased prevalence of gastrointestinal tumors? Clin Endocrinol 1994;41:597–601.

[130] Terzolo M, Reimondo G, Gasperi M, et al. Colonoscopic screening and follow-up in patients with acromegaly: a multicenter study in Italy. J Clin Endocrinol Metab 2005;90: 84–90.

[131] Renehan AG, Bhaskar P, Painter JE, et al. The prevalence and characteristics of colorectal neoplasia in acromegaly. J Clin Endocrinol Metab 2000;85:3417–24.

[132] Cats A, Dullaart RP, Kleibeuker JH, et al. Increased epithelial cell proliferation in the colon of patients with acromegaly. Cancer Res 1996;56:523–6.

[133] Remacle-Bonnet MM, Garrouste FL, Heller S, et al. Insulin-like growth factor-I protects colon cancer cells from death factor-induced apoptosis by potentiating tumor necrosis factor α-induced mitogen-activated protein kinase and nuclear factor κB signaling pathways. Cancer Res 2000;60:2007–17.

[134] Jenkins PJ, Frajese V, Jones AM, et al. Insulin-like growth factor I and the development of colorectal neoplasia in acromegaly. J Clin Endocrinol Metab 2000;85:3218–21.

[135] Bogazzi F, Cosci C, Sardella C, et al. Identification of acromegalic patients at risk of developing colonic adenomas. J Clin Endocrinol Metab 2006;91:1351–6.

[136] Hammer E. Cancer du colon sigmoide dix ans après implantation aux ureters d'une versie extrophies. J Urol 1929;28:260–4.

[137] Stewart M, Macrae FA, Williams CB. Neoplasia and ureterosigmoidostomy: a colonoscopic survey. Br J Surg 1982;69:414–6.

[138] Tricker AR, Kalble T, Preussmann R. Increased urinary nitrosoamine excretion in patients with urinary diversions. Carcinogenesis 1989;10:2379–82.

[139] Crissey MM, Steele GD, Gittes RF. Rat model for carcinogenesis in ureterosigmoidostomy. Science 1980;207:1079–80.

[140] Parsons CD, Thomas M, Garrett R. Colonic adenocarcinoma: a delayed complication of ureterosigmoidostomy. J Urol 1977;118:31–4.

[141] Sooriyaarachchi G, Johnson RO, Carbone P. Neoplasms of the large bowel following ureterosigmoidostomy. Arch Surg 1977;112:1174–7.

[142] Strachan JR, Woodhouse CR. Malignancy following ureterosigmoidostomy in patients with extrophy. Br J Surg 1991;78:1216–8.

[143] Schipper H, Decter A. Carcinoma of the colon arising at ureteral implant sites despite early external diversion. Cancer 1981;47:2062–5.

[144] Azimuddin K, Rosen L, Khubchandani IT, et al. Neoplasia after ureterosigmoidostomy. Dis Colon Rectum 1999;42:1632–8.

[145] Urdaneta H, Duffell D, Creevey CD. Development of primary carcinoma of the colon following ureterosigmoidostomy. Ann Surg 1982;164:503–13.

[146] Brekkan E, Colleen S, Myrvoid H. Colonic neoplasia: a late complication of ureterosigmoidostomy. Scand J Urol Nephrol 1972;6:197–202.

[147] Woodhouse CRJ. Guidelines for monitoring of patients with ureterosigmoidostomy. Gut 2002;51(Suppl V):v15–6.

[148] Keush GT. Opportunistic infections in colon carcinoma. Am J Clin Nutr 1974;27:1481–5.

[149] McCoy WC, Mason JM. Enterococcal endocarditis associated with carcinoma of the sigmoid: report of a case. J Med Assoc State Ala 1951;21:162–6.

[150] Burns CA, McCaughey R, Lauter CB. The association of Streptococcus bovis fecal carriage and colon neoplasia: possible relationship with polyps and their premalignant potential. Am J Gastroenterol 1985;80:42–6.

[151] Leport C, Bure A, Leport J, et al. Incidence of colonic lesions in Streptococcus bovis and enterococcal endocarditis. Lancet 1987;1:748.

[152] Klein RS, Recco RA, Catalano MT, et al. Association of Streptococcus bovis with carcinoma of the colon. N Engl J Med 1977;287:800–2.

[153] Potter MA, Cunliffe NA, Smith M, et al. A prospective controlled study of the association of Streptococcus bovis with colorectal carcinoma. J Clin Pathol 1998;51:473–4.

[154] Murray HW, Roberts RB. Streptococcus bacteremia and underlying gastrointestinal disease. Arch Intern Med 1978;138:1097–9.

[155] Honberg OZ, Gutschick E. Streptococcus bovis bacteremia and its association with alimentary-tract neoplasm. Lancet 1987;1(8525):163–4.

[156] Wanke CA, Bistrian B. Recombinant human tumor necrosis factor and recombinant murine interleukin-1 alter the binding of *Escherichia coli* to intestine, mucine glycoprotein, and the HT29-C1 intestinal cell line. Nutrition 1997;13:959–64.

[157] Ellmericch S, Schöller M, Duranton B, et al. Promotion of intestinal carcinogenesis by Streptococcus bovis. Carcinogenesis 2000;21:753–6.

Gastroenterol Clin N Am 37 (2008) 215–227

GASTROENTEROLOGY CLINICS
OF NORTH AMERICA

SEVIER
UNDERS

Endoscopic Ultrasound in the Diagnosis, Staging and Management of Colorectal Tumors

Manoop S. Bhutani, MD, FASGE, FACG, FACP

Department of Gastroenterology, Hepatology and Nutrition, Unit 436, UT MD Anderson Cancer Center, Faculty Center Room 10.2028, 1515 Holcombe Boulevard, Houston, TX 77030-4009, USA

Endoscopic ultrasound (EUS) has evolved as a useful technique for imaging and intervention in the colon and rectum. Instruments, manufactured by various companies, for imaging the colorectal area include radial (cross-sectional) and linear (longitudinal) flexible endoscopic ultrasound echoendoscopes, rigid endorectal probes, and high-frequency catheter miniprobes that can be passed through the biopsy channel of conventional endoscopes. Interventional EUS procedures require use of the linear array echoendoscopes to permit visualization of a needle along its length. This article reviews the clinical applications of EUS for imaging and intervention in colorectal cancer, with an emphasis on the most recent clinical studies.

ARTIFACTS IN COLORECTAL ENDOSCOPIC ULTRASOUND

Artifacts in colorectal EUS include pseudomasses created by beam thickness during imaging of rectal folds and mirror image reflection at an intraluminal fluid level [1]. Simulation of malignant infiltration may occur because of beam thickness, attenuation, or refraction. The understanding of the physical properties of ultrasound, with recognition of these artifacts, is important to avoid EUS misinterpretation.

ENDOSCOPIC ULTRASOUND IN RECTAL CANCER

EUS is a highly useful technique for preoperative local staging of rectal cancer to help determine the type of surgery required and whether preoperative neoadjuvant chemoradiation is needed. Savides and Master [2] concisely summarized the indications for EUS in rectal cancer based on therapeutic impact,

E-mail address: manoop.bhutani@mdanderson.org

0889-8553/08/$ – see front matter
doi:10.1016/j.gtc.2007.12.001

stratified according to cancer stage. Indications for EUS in rectal cancer include:

- To determine the suitability for endoscopic mucosal resection or transanal excision (if the lesion is T1 by EUS) for a large polyp or small rectal cancer
- To determine whether preoperative chemotherapy and radiation are necessary for a large, rectal cancer (T2: radical resection, T3-4 or N1: preoperative chemoradiation followed by radical resection)
- Surveillance after surgery for rectal cancer

Glancy and colleagues [3] analyzed the accuracy of EUS for selection for local excision by transanal endoscopic microsurgery (TEM) in 156 patients who had rectal neoplasia (Fig. 1). EUS (uT stage) was compared with the postoperative histopathological stage of the resected specimens (pT stage). Of the 62 patients undergoing TEM, three were overstaged, and none were understaged by EUS (95% overall accuracy). Among the other 94 patients undergoing an alternative procedure, the accuracy of EUS at predicting advanced disease was 89%, and the overall accuracy was 92%. The accuracy of EUS for assessing local depth of invasion of rectal carcinoma (T stage) ranges from 80% to 95% (Fig. 2) [2,4,5]. This accuracy compares favorably with the accuracy of CT of 65% to 75% and the accuracy of MRI of 75% to 85% [6–10]. Concerning T stage, the major limitation of EUS is overstaging of T2 tumors [11]; peritumorous inflammation cannot be distinguished from malignant tissue by ultrasound. On the other hand, the inability to detect microscopic malignant infiltration can lead to understaging. Stenotic rectal cancers sometimes are staged suboptimally by EUS because of an inability of the echoendoscope to traverse the stenosis [11,12], but stenotic tumors usually are advanced lesions.

The accuracy of EUS for lymph node staging is less than that for T staging, because the echo features of benign/inflammatory and malignant lymph nodes overlap. It ranges from 70% to 75%. This accuracy compares favorably with that for CT (55% to 65%) and with that for MRI (60% to 65%) [4]. Round, echo-poor or hypoechoic lymph nodes that are more than 5 mm in diameter

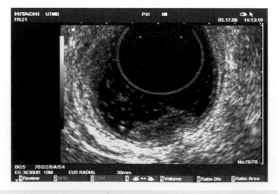

Fig. 1. Endoscopic ultrasound image of a T1 rectal cancer, with an intact muscularis propria.

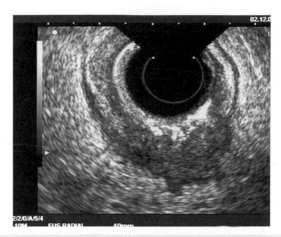

Fig. 2. Endoscopic ultrasound image of a T3 rectal cancer with penetration through the muscularis propria into the peri-rectal fat.

are considered suspicious for metastases in rectal cancer (Fig. 3) [2,13]. EUS-guided fine needle aspiration (FNA) (Fig. 4) can improve the accuracy of lymph node staging, but this can be done only for lymph nodes not immediately adjacent to the primary tumor, because traversing of the EUS FNA needle through the primary tumor will lead to spurious false-positive results.

Numerous studies have compared EUS with MRI and other imaging modalities. A recent study compared the ability of EUS versus either body coil MRI or phased-array coil MRI to locally stage rectal carcinoma before surgery in 49 patients [12]. The EUS and MRI findings were compared with the histologic findings on the surgical specimen. For local T staging, the accuracy of EUS was 70%; the accuracy of body coil MRI was 43%, and the accuracy of phased-array coil MRI was 71%. For N stage, the accuracy of EUS, body

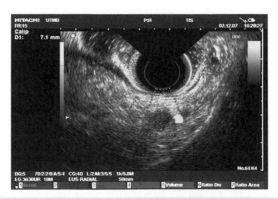

Fig. 3. Endoscopic ultrasound image of a 7 mm round, hypoechoic, peri-rectal lymph node in a patient with T3 rectal cancer.

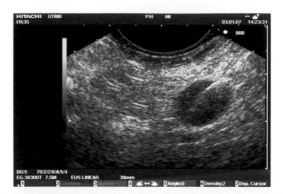

Fig. 4. Endoscopic ultrasound-guided FNA of a peri-rectal lymph node. Note the needle tip within the lymph node.

coil MRI, and phased-array coil MRI was 63%, 64%, and 76%, respectively. For T staging, EUS had the best sensitivity (80%), but the same specificity (67%) as phased-array coil MRI. For N stage, phased-array coil MRI had the best sensitivity (63%), but the same specificity (80%) as the other methods. In this study, EUS and phased-array coil MRI provided similar results for assessing T stage. No method provided satisfactory assessments of local N stage, although phased-array coil MRI was marginally better in assessing this important parameter.

THREE DIMENSIONAL ENDOSCOPIC ULTRASOUND

Conventional two-dimensional (2D) EUS provides limited spatial information. Three-dimensional (3D) EUS image reconstruction may improve the accuracy of EUS and decrease errors in staging. Kim and colleagues [14] studied both 3D and 2D EUS for staging rectal cancer in 33 patients. Accuracy of 3D EUS was 90.9% for pT2 and 84.8% for pT3, whereas that of conventional EUS was 84.8% and 75.8%, respectively. Lymph node metastasis was predicted accurately by 3D EUS in 28 patients (84.8%), but was predicted accurately in only 22 patients (66.7%) by 2D EUS.

Kim and colleagues [15] recently reported a study comparing the efficacy of 3D EUS with that of 2D EUS and CT for staging of rectal cancer. Eighty-six rectal cancer patients were evaluated before surgery by 2D EUS, 3D EUS, and CT. EUS imaging was performed with rigid rectal probes. The accuracy of T staging was 78% for 3D EUS, 69% for 2D EUS, and 57% for CT, while the accuracy of detecting lymph node metastases was 65%, 56%, and 53%, respectively. Examiner errors were the most frequent cause of misinterpretation, occurring in 47% of 2D EUS examinations and 65% of 3D EUS examinations. By eliminating examiner errors, the accuracy rates of T staging and lymph node evaluation could be improved to 88% and 76%, respectively, for 2D EUS, and could be improved to 91% and 90%, respectively, for 3D EUS. Poorly differentiated or mucinous rectal tumors with adverse prognostic factors were closely associated with infiltration grade detected by 3D EUS in this study [15]. The 3D reconstruction of rectal tumors revealed conical protrusions along the deep margins with the number of cones closely correlating with infiltration grade, advanced local T stage, and presence of lymph node metastases.

Giovannini and colleagues [16] recently reported the staging of rectal cancer in 35 patients using a new software program for 3D EUS that can be used with electronic radial or linear rectal probes. No differences were evident with 3D EUS versus 2D EUS for superficial tumors (T1 and T2N0). In 6 of 15 patients classified as having T3N0 lesions, however, 3D EUS revealed malignant lymph nodes, a finding that was confirmed surgically in five of the six cases. Three-dimensional EUS also correctly assessed the degree of infiltration of the meso-rectum, demonstrating complete invasion of the mesorectum in eight cases. These findings were confirmed by surgery in all the cases. Two-dimensional EUS was accurate for T and N staging in 25 of 35 rectal tumors (71.4%), whereas 3D EUS was accurate in 31 of 35 cases (88.6%). The authors con-cluded that 3D EUS provided more precise staging of lesions and better defini-tion of the mesorectal margins in patients who had rectal cancer; this difference impacted on the therapeutic decisions.

INTEROBSERVER VARIABILITY

Burtin and colleagues [17] studied interobserver variability in EUS at two cen-ters for rectal cancer staging in 37 patients. Six months later, the video taped examinations were reviewed by four independent observers who assessed the stage of the tumor, from uT1 to uT4, and lymph node invasion. Interob-server agreement was estimated using the kappa coefficient (k) and the intra-class correlation coefficient (ICC). Agreement was fair for uT1 tumors (k = .40), but poor for uT2 tumors (k = .20). Agreement was good (k = .58; CI, .51 to .65) for uT3 tumors. There was significant interobserver corre-lation for the extent of rectal fat invasion (ICC = .65). The agreement was also good (k = .54, CI, .47 to .61) for metastatic lymph nodes. Roubein and col-leagues [18] also studied interobserver variability in the interpretation of EUS for staging rectal carcinoma in 26 patients prospectively evaluated by three endoscopists. One performed sigmoidoscopy; the second (primary endo-sonographer) performed an EUS staging examination with full knowledge of the patient history and the sigmoidoscopic appearance of the lesion, and the third endoscopist (secondary endosonographer) performed EUS blinded to this information. The two endosonographers agreed about the T stage in 88% of patients, with the following kappa coefficients: T1 (k = 0.00); T2 (k = −.04); T3 (k = −.05); T4 (k = .00). N stage agreed in 73% of patients (k = .42).

CLINICAL IMPACT AND COST EFFECTIVENESS OF ENDOSCOPIC ULTRASOUND IN RECTAL CANCER

Harewood and colleagues [4,19–22] have analyzed the clinical impact of EUS in rectal cancer thoroughly. In a study of cost effectiveness [21], evaluation with abdominal CT plus EUS was found to be the most cost-effective approach

($24,468/y), compared with abdominal CT plus pelvic MRI ($24,870), or CT alone ($26,076). In another study [22], EUS staging of rectal cancer in 31% of cases changed the surgeon's original treatment plan based on CT alone. T staging accuracy was 71% for CT and 91% for EUS ($P = .02$). N staging accuracy was 76% for CT, 82% for EUS, and 76% for EUS with FNA ($P =$ not significant [NS]). Preoperative EUS resulted in more frequent use of preoperative neoadjuvant therapy than if staging was performed by CT alone. The addition of FNA of lymph nodes changed the management of only one patient. The authors concluded that FNA seems to offer the greatest potential impact on management in patients who have early T stage disease, and its use should be confined to these patients. In another study, 73 patients who had nonmetastatic rectal cancer undergoing EUS (study group) were compared with 68 patients not undergoing EUS (control group). In patients who had advanced T or N stage cancer, preoperative adjuvant therapy was administered to 58.5% of patients in the EUS group versus 14.9% of patients in the non-EUS group. EUS staging of rectal cancer appeared to facilitate appropriate institution of preoperative neoadjuvant therapy in patients who had advanced disease, and was associated with a recurrence-free survival advantage in patients. EUS also can impact on rectal cancer therapy by classifying T3 tumors into early versus advanced [20]. In a study of 42 patients with T3 rectal tumors who had surgical resection without preoperative neoadjuvant therapy, including 14 minimally invasive T3 and 28 advanced T3 by preoperative EUS, the tumor recurrence rate was 14.3% for minimally invasive T3 tumors and 39.3% for advanced T3 tumors ($P = .02$, log-rank test) [20]. Identification of advanced T3 disease by EUS provides important prognostic information that may help improve selection of patients for neoadjuvant therapy.

Harewood [4] analyzed all published articles about EUS accuracy in staging rectal cancer between 1985 and 2003 in the English literature for accuracy of EUS, year of publication, number of subjects studied, journal impact factor, and type of journal. EUS T staging accuracy was reported in 40 studies, while EUS N staging accuracy was reported in 27 studies. The experience of 4118 subjects was reported with an overall mean T staging accuracy of 85.2% (median 87.5%) and N-staging accuracy of 75.0% (median 76.0%). Both T staging and N staging accuracy declined over time, with the lowest accuracy reported most recently. The author concluded that the accuracy of EUS in staging rectal cancer may be overestimated in the literature because of a publication bias; an inflated estimate of the accuracy of EUS may lead to unrealistic expectations of this technology.

Even though Harewood and colleagues [22] concluded in 2002 that EUS FNA had a negligible role in the initial management of rectal cancer, a recent study from the same institution by Levy and colleagues [23] seeks to expand the role of EUS FNA in the staging of rectal cancer. The presence of malignant iliac lymph nodes (ILN), designated M1 stage in rectal cancer, alters patient management in terms of surgical candidacy, extent of resection, and/or radiotherapy field. Rectal EUS studies traditionally have not included evaluation of lymph nodes in the iliac area, even though this area is accessible to flexible EUS probes, in contrast to rigid EUS instruments that cannot be advanced in the colon to the level of the iliac lymph nodes. In this prospective study, 457 rectal cancer patients underwent T, N, and M staging by EUS. Suspicious nonperitumoral LNs were sampled by FNA. EUS identified suspicious iliac lymph nodes (ILNs) in 32 of 457 rectal cancer patients (7.0%), of which 15 of 32 (47%) were found to be malignant ILNs by EUS-FNA. In contrast, CT identified iliac lymph nodes in only 7 of 15 (47%) patients who had confirmed malignant ILNs. Discovery of malignant ILNs by EUS-FNA resulted in expansion of the radiation field and extended lymphadenectomy in four patients, and expansion of the radiation field and nonoperative palliative therapy in 11 patients. The authors concluded that rectal cancer patients who undergo EUS should have routine evaluation of ILN status. If these results concerning the impact of iliac lymph node imaging and FNA are confirmed by other centers, then flexible echoendoscopes with FNA capability may provide a definite advantage over rigid rectal probes.

RESTAGING RECTAL CANCER AFTER CHEMORADIATION

Accuracy of EUS for staging rectal cancer after radiation therapy is decreased because of postradiation edema, inflammation, necrosis, and fibrosis [2,24,25]. Vanagunas and colleagues [26] studied the accuracy of EUS in staging rectal cancer performed before and after concurrent 5-fluorouracil and radiotherapy in 82 patients who had recently diagnosed, locally advanced rectal cancer. All patients underwent subsequent surgical resection and complete pathologic staging. After chemoradiation, 16 patients (20%) had no residual disease at pathologic staging (T0N0). The overall accuracy of EUS post-chemoradiation for pathologic T-stage was only 48%. Fourteen percent were understaged, and 38% were overstaged. EUS accuracy for N-stage was 77%. The T-category was staged correctly before surgery in 23 of the 56 responders (41%) and in 16 of the 24 nonresponders (67%). EUS was unable to accurately distinguish postradiation changes from residual tumor. Another recent study [25] compared the accuracy of EUS staging for rectal cancer before (group 1) and following chemoradiation (group 2). The accuracy of the T staging for group 1 was 86% (57/66). Inaccurate staging mainly arose from overstaging of EUS T2 tumors. In group 2, following chemoradiation, the EUS staging predicted postchemoradiation T0N0 stage correctly in only 50% of cases. Inaccurate staging mainly arose from overstaging of EUS T3 tumors. Restaging with EUS after chemoradiation should be performed cautiously, with an understanding of its limitations and pitfalls by the ultrasonographers, oncologists, and surgeons in using the EUS information for therapeutic decisions.

Romagnuolo and colleagues [27] used a novel brachytherapy (BT) protocol for downstaging and achieving high tumor sterilization rates in rectal cancer and showed that the sensitivity, specificity, and positive and negative predictive values of post-BT EUS in predicting residual tumor were 82%, 29%, 64% and

50%, respectively. Post-BT EUS accurately predicted the -stage in eight (44%) patients. Most errors arose from overstaging. The authors concluded that EUS appears to be sensitive in predicting the presence or absence of residual tumor in rectal adenocarcinoma after preoperative BT, but the low predictive value in this setting limits its current utility.

ENDOSCOPIC ULTRASOUND FOR DETECTION OF RECURRENT RECTAL CANCER

The risk of recurrence of rectal cancer is greatest during the first 2 years after surgery. Detection of local recurrence in a resectable stage provides an opportunity for repeat surgery with curative intent or other treatment with improved survival. Several studies have shown EUS is very accurate in detecting recurrent rectal cancer around the anastomotic site, with EUS/FNA being able to provide tissue confirmation [28–32]. Lohnert and colleagues [28] prospectively analyzed the role of endorectal and endovaginal ultrasound to detect asymptomatic resectable local recurrence in 338 patients. Local recurrence was detected in 116 patients (34.3%), which was suggested by EUS and proven by EUS-guided needle biopsy in all cases of ambiguous pararectal structures that could not be verified by endoscopic biopsy. In a study by Rotondano and colleagues [29], 62 patients were followed prospectively after surgery for rectal cancer by endorectal ultrasound, serial serum carcinoembryonic antigen (CEA) levels, digital rectal examination, colonoscopy, and pelvic CT. Local recurrence occurred in 11 patients; in all 11 cases the recurrence was suggested by EUS. In two of these patients (18%), recurrent disease was identified only by EUS. Hunerbein and colleagues [30] prospectively investigated the role of EUS with biopsy in the postoperative follow-up of rectal cancer in 312 patients. Local recurrence was found in 36 patients. Intraluminal recurrence was diagnosed by proctoscopy in 12 patients. Transrectal EUS-guided biopsy showed pelvic recurrence in 22 of 68 patients who had perirectal masses. There was a strong agreement between EUS-guided transrectal biopsy results and the final diagnosis (k = .84), with a sensitivity of 91% and a specificity of 93%. In comparison, clinical examination (k = .27), CT (k = .47), or EUS imaging alone (k = .42) demonstrated only moderate levels of agreement with the histopathologic diagnosis.

Despite many studies showing the value of EUS in detecting local recurrence in rectosigmoid cancer, the optimal interval for repeating EUS after surgery is unclear. A recent joint update of guidelines by the American Cancer Society and the US Multi-Society Task Force on Colorectal Cancer [33] addresses colonoscopy and EUS surveillance of rectal cancer. This update recognizes that patients undergoing low anterior resection of rectal cancer generally have higher rates of local cancer recurrence than patients who have colon cancer. Although effectiveness is unproven, the joint update states that performance of EUS or flexible sigmoidoscopy at 3- to 6-month intervals for the first 2 years after resection can be considered to detect surgically curable recurrence of rectal cancer.

ENDOSCOPIC ULTRASOUND AND RECTAL LINITIS PLASTICA

Linitis plastica is a diffuse infiltrating carcinoma that classically occurs in the stomach. Linitis plastica, however, rarely can occur as a primary neoplasm or can occur as a metastatic lesion in the rectum because of a primary lesion elsewhere, such as the stomach, breast, or prostate. The diagnosis is difficult to establish, because the clinical and endoscopic findings may be nonspecific, and endoscopic biopsies may be nondiagnostic in up to 50% of cases [34–37]. Dumontier and colleagues [36] analyzed 22 video-recorded EUS examinations performed in 11 patients who had histologically-proven rectal linitis plastica. Response to conservative treatment was evaluated in three patients who had secondary rectal linitis plastica. In every case, EUS showed circumferential thickening of the rectal wall (mean 13 mm), with thickening mainly of the submucosa and muscularis propria. In nine cases, EUS demonstrated signs of locoregional involvement, including perirectal fat infiltration in six cases, ascites in five cases, and lymph nodes in three cases, that were not detected by CT. In follow-up evaluation, EUS showed no response to treatment in two patients who had rectal linitis secondary to a gastric primary. In the remaining patient who had rectal linitis secondary to breast carcinoma, EUS showed improvement only after the chemotherapy was intensified. EUS shows typical, diagnostic features of rectal linitis plastica. Limited data suggest that EUS can be used to evaluate the response of this disease to treatment.

ENDOSCOPIC ULTRASOUND FOR LARGE ADENOMAS FOR MINIMIZING BLEEDING

Polkowski and colleagues [38] performed EUS before endoscopic polypectomy of 42 large (at least 20 mm) nonpedunculated adenomatous polyps in the rectosigmoid area to evaluate the vessels in the polyp and in the underlying rectal wall. In eight polyps (20.5%, group 1), EUS revealed vessels measuring 2 to 4 mm, while in 31 polyps (79.5%, group 2), no vessels were detected. The postpolypectomy bleeding incidence (per polyp treated) was 12.5% in group 1 and 12.9% in group 2 ($P > .05$). The absence of vessels on EUS did not exclude the possibility of bleeding. The detection of vessels on EUS did not increase the risk for bleeding, but the authors felt that the sample size was too small to draw definite conclusions.

EMERGING CONCEPTS IN ENDOSCOPIC ULTRASOUND FOR COLORECTAL CANCER: MOLECULAR MARKERS

Recent evidence suggests that micrometastases can be present in lymph nodes that cannot be detected by standard pathologic methods. Pellise and colleagues [39] evaluated hypermethylation gene promoter analysis on samples obtained by EUS-FNA from 42 suspicious lymph nodes in 27 consecutive patients with esophageal, gastric, rectal, and nonsmall cell lung cancer (rectal cancer in seven patients). Hypermethylation analysis was performed on the MGMT, p16(INK4a), and p14(ARF) gene promoter CpG islands by methylation-specific polymerase chain reaction (PCR). Accuracy of conventional cytology, methylation analysis, and their combination was compared with respect to the definitive diagnosis. Sensitivity, specificity, and overall accuracy were 76%, 100%, and 88%, respectively, for conventional cytology, and were 81%, 67%, and 74%, respectively, for methylation analysis. Combination of both techniques increased sensitivity (90%), but decreased specificity (67%) with respect to conventional cytology. More work is needed on this technique before recommending routine clinical application.

ENDOSCOPIC ULTRASOUND-GUIDED DRAINAGE OF PERIRECTAL ABSCESSES

Perirectal abscesses may occur in the postoperative period after low anterior resection for rectal cancer. EUS-guided drainage may be an option for treating perirectal pelvic abscesses [40,41]. Attwell and colleagues [40] reported one case of EUS-guided drainage of a perirectal abscess as an adjunct to surgical therapy. Giovannini and colleagues [41] reported the clinical efficacy of EUS-guided transrectal aspiration and drainage by plastic prosthesis of deep pelvic abscesses, using a therapeutic echoendoscope in 12 patients, with no major complications. A transrectal stent was deployed successfully in nine of the patients. Complete drainage without relapse was achieved in eight of the nine patients with a stent at a mean follow-up of 10.6 months. The stent was removed by endoscopic means after 3 to 6 months. The remaining patient subsequently needed surgical drainage. In the other three patients, aspiration was performed, but a stent could not be deployed for drainage. Two of these three patients developed a recurrence of the abscess that required surgical treatment. Hopefully, larger studies on this technique will be available in the future. Recently, Varadarajulu and Drelichman [42] reported a prospective case series of EUS-guided transrectal catheter placement for drainage of pelvic abscesses in high-risk surgical patients who were not amenable for drainage by ultrasound or CT-guidance because of the lack of an adequate window. After accessing the abscess cavity with a 19-gauge needle, a .035 in guide wire was passed into the abscess cavity. The tract was dilated using dilating catheters and over-the-wire balloon dilators, and a 10-Fr trans-rectal single pig-tail catheter, used for percutaneous biliary drainage by interventional radiologists, was deployed. The catheter was flushed periodically with normal saline and discontinued after a follow-up CT demonstrated abscess resolution. Of six patients referred for EUS, two were excluded, including one who had a large rectocele and one who had a multiloculated fluid collection with immature walls. The remaining four patients underwent EUS-guided drainage. The procedure was technically successful in all patients, without complications. Three patients experienced immediate symptomatic relief. The mean duration for abscess resolution was 6 days. These studies in a limited number of patients show that EUS-guided drainage of deep pelvic abscesses can be considered in carefully selected patients as an adjunctive or alternative treatment to surgery.

SUMMARY

In conclusion, EUS is a very useful technique for staging rectal carcinoma. Technological improvements, such as 3D EUS, may improve EUS performance further. EUS is useful for assessing recurrence of rectal carcinoma, and this technique has become part of postoperative surveillance guidelines. Emerging concepts include assessment of molecular markers of EUS-guided FNA material and development of techniques for EUS-guided therapy. Assessment for residual cancer after chemoradiation is currently problematic, and more work is needed to improve the accuracy of EUS in this situation.

References

[1] Hulsmans FJ, Castelijns JA, Reeders JW, et al. Review of artifacts associated with transrectal ultrasound: understanding, recognition, and prevention of misinterpretation. J Clin Ultrasound 1995;23(8):483–94.

[2] Savides TJ, Master SS. EUS in rectal cancer. Gastrointest Endosc 2002;56(4 Suppl):S12–8.

[3] Glancy DG, Pullyblank AM, Thomas MG. The role of colonoscopic endoanal ultrasound scanning (EUS) in selecting patients suitable for resection by transanal endoscopic microsurgery (TEM). Colorectal Dis 2005;7(2):148–50.

[4] Harewood GC. Assessment of publication bias in the reporting of EUS performance in staging rectal cancer. Am J Gastroenterol 2005;100(4):808–16.

[5] Bhutani MS, Nadella P. Utility of an upper echoendoscope for endoscopic ultrasonography of malignant and benign conditions of the sigmoid/left colon and the rectum. Am J Gastroenterol 2001;96(12):3318–22.

[6] Meyenberger C, Huch Boni RA, Bertschinger P, et al. Endoscopic ultrasound and endorectal magnetic resonance imaging: a prospective, comparative study for preoperative staging and follow-up of rectal cancer. Endoscopy 1995;27(7):469–79.

[7] Guinet C, Buy JN, Ghossain MA, et al. Comparison of magnetic resonance imaging and computed tomography in the preoperative staging of rectal cancer. Arch Surg 1990; 125(3):385–8.

[8] Rifkin MD, Ehrlich SM, Marks G. Staging of rectal carcinoma: prospective comparison of endorectal US and CT. Radiology 1989;170(2):319–22.

[9] Kwok H, Bissett IP, Hill GL. Preoperative staging of rectal cancer. Int J Colorectal Dis 2000;15(1):9–20.

[10] Thaler W, Watzka S, Martin F, et al. Preoperative staging of rectal cancer by endoluminal ultrasound vs. magnetic resonance imaging. Preliminary results of a prospective, comparative study. Dis Colon Rectum 1994;37(12):1189–93.

[11] Hawes RH. New staging techniques. Endoscopic ultrasound. Cancer 1993;71(12 Suppl): 4207–13.

[12] Bianchi PP, Ceriani C, Rottoli M, et al. Endoscopic ultrasonography and magnetic resonance in preoperative staging of rectal cancer: comparison with histologic findings. J Gastrointest Surg 2005;9(9):1222–7 [discussion: 1227–8].

[13] Schwartz DA, Harewood GC, Wiersema MJ. EUS for rectal disease. Gastrointest Endosc 2002;56(1):100–9.

[14] Kim JC, Cho YK, Kim SY, et al. Comparative study of three-dimensional and conventional endorectal ultrasonography used in rectal cancer staging. Surg Endosc 2002;16(9): 1280–5.

[15] Kim JC, Kim HC, Yu CS, et al. Efficacy of 3-dimensional endorectal ultrasonography compared with conventional ultrasonography and computed tomography in preoperative rectal cancer staging. Am J Surg 2006;192(1):89–97.

[16] Giovannini M, Bories E, Pesenti C, et al. Three-dimensional endorectal ultrasound using a new freehand software program: results in 35 patients with rectal cancer. Endoscopy 2006;38(4):339–43.

[17] Burtin P, Rabot AF, Heresbach D, et al. Interobserver agreement in the staging of rectal cancer using endoscopic ultrasonography. Endoscopy 1997;29(7):620–5.

[18] Roubein LD, Lynch P, Glober G, et al. Interobserver variability in endoscopic ultrasonography: a prospective evaluation. Gastrointest Endosc 1996;44(5):573–7.

[19] Harewood GC. Assessment of clinical impact of endoscopic ultrasound on rectal cancer. Am J Gastroenterol 2004;99(4):623–7.

[20] Harewood GC, Kumar KS, Clain JE, et al. Clinical implications of quantification of mesorectal tumor invasion by endoscopic ultrasound: all T3 rectal cancers are not equal. J Gastroenterol Hepatol 2004;19(7):750–5.

[21] Harewood GC, Wiersema MJ. Cost-effectiveness of endoscopic ultrasonography in the evaluation of proximal rectal cancer. Am J Gastroenterol 2002;97(4):874–82.

[22] Harewood GC, Wiersema MJ, Nelson H, et al. A prospective, blinded assessment of the impact of preoperative staging on the management of rectal cancer. Gastroenterology 2002;123(1):24–32.

[23] Levy MJ, Alberts SR, Clain JE, et al. Endoscopic ultrasound guided fine needle aspiration (EUS FNA) detection of malignant iliac lymph nodes in rectal cancer [abstract]. Gastrointest Endosc 2006;63(65):AB97.

[24] Rau B, Hunerbein M, Barth C, et al. Accuracy of endorectal ultrasound after preoperative radiochemotherapy in locally advanced rectal cancer. Surg Endosc 1999;13(10):980–4.

[25] Napoleon B, Pujol B, Berger F, et al. Accuracy of endosonography in the staging of rectal cancer treated by radiotherapy. Br J Surg 1991;78(7):785–8.

[26] Vanagunas A, Lin DE, Stryker SJ. Accuracy of endoscopic ultrasound for restaging rectal cancer following neoadjuvant chemoradiation therapy. Am J Gastroenterol 2004;99(1):109–12.

[27] Romagnuolo J, Parent J, Vuong T, et al. Predicting residual rectal adenocarcinoma in the surgical specimen after preoperative brachytherapy with endoscopic ultrasound. Can J Gastroenterol 2004;18(7):435–40.

[28] Lohnert MS, Doniec JM, Henne-Bruns D. Effectiveness of endoluminal sonography in the identification of occult local rectal cancer recurrences. Dis Colon Rectum 2000;43(4):483–91.

[29] Rotondano G, Esposito P, Pellecchia L, et al. Early detection of locally recurrent rectal cancer by endosonography. Br J Radiol 1997;70(834):567–71.

[30] Hunerbein M, Totkas S, Moesta KT, et al. The role of transrectal ultrasound-guided biopsy in the postoperative follow-up of patients with rectal cancer. Surgery 2001;129(2):164–9.

[31] Woodward T, Menke D. Diagnosis of recurrent rectal carcinoma by EUS-guided fine-needle aspiration. Gastrointest Endosc 2000;51(2):223–5.

[32] Sasaki Y, Niwa Y, Hirooka Y, et al. The use of endoscopic ultrasound-guided fine-needle aspiration for investigation of submucosal and extrinsic masses of the colon and rectum. Endoscopy 2005;37(2):154–60.

[33] Rex DK, Kahi CJ, Levin B, et al. Guidelines for colonoscopy surveillance after cancer resection: a consensus update by the American Cancer Society and the US Multi-Society Task Force on Colorectal Cancer. Gastroenterology 2006;130(6):1865–71.

[34] Wiersema MJ, Wiersema LM, Kochman ML. Primary linitis plastica of the colon. Gastrointest Endosc 1993;39(5):716–8.

[35] Papp JP Jr, Levine EJ, Thomas FB. Primary linitis plastica carcinoma of the colon and rectum. Am J Gastroenterol 1995;90(1):141–5.

[36] Dumontier I, Roseau G, Palazzo L, et al. Endoscopic ultrasonography in rectal linitis plastica. Gastrointest Endosc 1997;46(6):532–6.

[37] Bhutani MS. EUS and EUS-guided fine-needle aspiration for the diagnosis of rectal linitis plastica secondary to prostate carcinoma. Gastrointest Endosc 1999;50(1):117–9.

[38] Polkowski M, Regula J, Wronska E, et al. Endoscopic ultrasonography for prediction of post-polypectomy bleeding in patients with large nonpedunculated rectosigmoid adenomas. Endoscopy 2003;35(4):343–7.

[39] Pellise M, Castells A, Gines A, et al. Detection of lymph node micrometastases by gene promoter hypermethylation in samples obtained by endosonography-guided fine-needle aspiration biopsy. Clin Cancer Res 2004;10(13):4444–9.

[40] Attwell AR, McIntyre RC, Antillon MR, et al. EUS-guided drainage of a diverticular abscess as an adjunct to surgical therapy. Gastrointest Endosc 2003;58(4):612–6.

[41] Giovannini M, Bories E, Moutardier V, et al. Drainage of deep pelvic abscesses using therapeutic echo endoscopy. Endoscopy 2003;35(6):511–4.

[42] Varadarajulu S, Drelichman ER. EUS-guided drainage of pelvic abscess. Gastrointest Endosc 2007;65(5):AB106.

Gastroenterol Clin N Am 37 (2008) 229–251

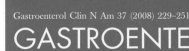

GASTROENTEROLOGY CLINICS
OF NORTH AMERICA

Colonoscopic Polypectomy

Kevin A. Tolliver, MD, Douglas K. Rex, MD*

Division of Gastroenterology, Department of Medicine, Indiana University School of Medicine,
Indiana University Hospital #4100, 550 North University Boulevard,
UH 4100, Indianapolis, IN 46202, USA

C olonoscopic polypectomy is the most effective visceral cancer prevention tool in clinical medicine. Two cohort studies have shown that polypectomy prevents colorectal cancer [1,2]. The National Polyp Study estimated that polypectomy prevented 76% to 90% of incident colorectal cancers (CRC), by comparing the rates of incident cancers after a clearing colonoscopy with the expected rates based on reference populations [1]. Another cohort of patients who had adenoma was calculated to incur an 80% reduction in incident CRC using similar methodology [2]. A randomized controlled trial comparing flexible sigmoidoscopy, with colonoscopy and polypectomy for any detected polyp, versus no screening reported an 80% reduction in CRC incidence in the screened group [3]. Colonoscopy is clearly imperfect in protecting against CRC, however [4]. Two studies have suggested that 27% to 31% of incident cancers after colonoscopy result from ineffective polypectomy [5,6]. All colonoscopists must therefore be highly proficient in polypectomy. Polypectomy has risks, however. The removal of any colon polyp should balance the likelihood that the polyp will turn into cancer with the risks associated with the technique used for its removal.

OPTICAL ENHANCEMENT TECHNIQUES

Colonoscopic technology has undergone numerous recent innovations that enhance its diagnostic capabilities. Optical enhancement could potentially improve the exposure of colonic mucosa, the detection of flat lesions, and the determination of histology in real time (Box 1). Because the focus of this article is polypectomy, we do not review techniques for improved detection, but focus on the assessment of polyps in real time before polypectomy because these technologies may assist in determining whether polypectomy is necessary.

Generally, all adenomas, or potential adenomas, should be removed during colonoscopy, as should hyperplastic polyps in the proximal colon, particularly larger hyperplastic polyps [7,8]. Larger Peutz-Jeghers polyps and juvenile polyps should also be removed because of a risk for adenomatous

*Corresponding author. E-mail address: drex@iupui.edu (D.K. Rex).

0889-8553/08/$ – see front matter
doi:10.1016/j.gtc.2007.12.009

Box 1: Optical enhancement technologies for colonoscopy

See behind folds better
- Wide-angle colonoscopy
- Cap-fitted colonoscopy
- Third-Eye Retroscope

See flat lesions better
- Pancolonic chromoendoscopy
- Narrow band imaging
- High definition
- Autofluorescence

Interpret histology in real time
- Chromoendoscopy with high magnification
- Narrow band imaging
- Confocal laser microscopy
- Autofluorescence

transformation. Small distal colon hyperplastic polyps are the most commonly seen lesions for which there is no clear benefit from removal. Similarly, mucosal polyps and lymphoid hyperplasia, along with inflammatory polyps and true filiform pseudopolyps in inflammatory bowel disease, need not be removed during colonoscopy.

Clues about polyp histology are observed with white light. Diminutive, pale, sessile lesions in the distal colon, sometimes with visible blood vessels running across the surface, or that flatten with insufflation, are typically hyperplastic [8]. Large proximal colonic polyps that are covered with mucus, in which folds or wrinkles develop during manipulation with the electrocautery snare, are typically hyperplastic polyps or serrated adenomas that should be removed (Fig. 1) [8]. Ruddy, pedunculated polyps are most often adenomas, although juvenile polyps and Peutz-Jeghers polyps can have the same appearance. Mucosal prolapse in the sigmoid colon also can be confused with a pedunculated adenoma. Polyps with exudate on the surface are typically inflammatory, although juvenile polyps may have exudate, and some larger pedunculated adenomas have a superficial exudate. Superficial ulceration of an otherwise obvious sessile adenoma indicates the presence of cancer or high-grade dysplasia. Endoscopic resection should typically not be pursued unless the polyp appears benign or can be fully lifted with submucosal injection.

White-light clues to histology are insufficient to accurately determine whether resection is necessary. A reliable way of determining histology is by pit pattern analysis, first described by Professor Kudo and colleagues [9] in Japan. Polyps with type I and II pits are hyperplastic (Fig. 2), whereas types III through VI

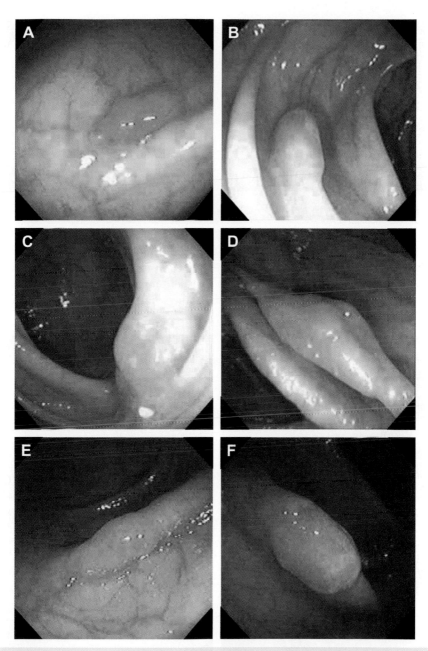

Fig. 1. (A–F) Proximal colon hyperplastic polyps. These lesions may be precursors of serrated adenomas and should be removed. These lesions may be subtle endoscopically. The miss rate for these lesions is unknown. Typical features include pale color, sessile shape, indistinct edges, and a mucus covering. During snare manipulation, the polyps often wrinkle, a phenomenon not seen with adenomas.

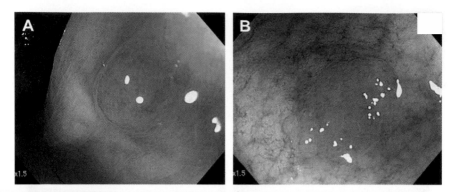

Fig. 2. (*A*, *B*) Small hyperplastic polyps in the distal colon seen in narrow band imaging.

are neoplastic (Fig. 3). The critical differentiation is between hyperplastic and adenomatous polyps. Most adenomas have type IIIL or IV pits. The great majority of studies of pit pattern have used high magnification colonoscopes, which are seldom available in the United States. High magnification is typically combined

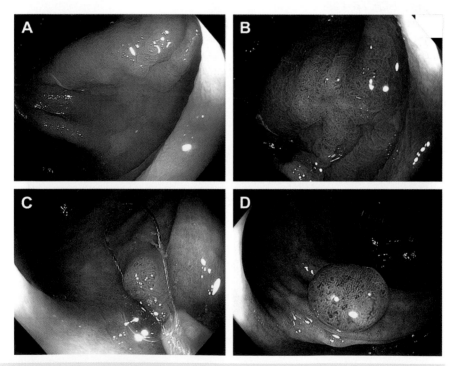

Fig. 3. (*A*) A 1-cm flat right colon adenoma in white light. (*B*) The same lesion in narrow band imaging showing 3 L pits. (*C*) A small flat adenoma with 3 L pits. (*D*) A sessile adenoma with 3 L pits.

with chromoendoscopy or narrow band imaging (NBI) to clearly define the pit pattern [10,11]. NBI also permits display of microcapillaries on the polyp surface, which can reliably differentiate adenomas. In NBI, adenomas appear browner than hyperplastic polyps because of their large numbers of microcapillaries and their tufted vascular pattern (Fig. 4) [11]. The accuracy of NBI using standard and high-definition colonoscopes without optical zoom functions, as currently available in the United States, has not been defined.

Other techniques that are not widely available but can allow accurate real-time histologic evaluation of colon polyps include autofluorescence and confocal laser microscopy. Autofluorescence is rarely used in the United States. It is based on the observation that autofluorescence patterns of dysplastic tissue, including adenomas, are different than those of normal tissue or hyperplastic polyps [12]. Confocal laser microscopy is now available in commercial colonoscopes. It has been highly accurate in skilled hands in determining the real-time histology of colonic polyps [13]. The level of training required for confocal laser microscopy and its practicality for routine use remain to be determined.

SMALL POLYP REMOVAL

Despite the frequency of polypectomy, there are few data on the techniques of polypectomy to most effectively remove polyps and minimize complications. The most serious complication of polypectomy is perforation, and most colonoscopic perforations are polypectomy-related [14]. Nearly all polypectomy-related perforations seem to result from electrocautery, but electrocautery is unnecessary to remove many small (<1 cm) polyps [15,16]. Most polypectomy complications result from removal of small polyps [14] because these polyps are so numerous (80% ≤5 mm in size and 90% ≤9 mm in size). The best approach to polypectomy in small polyps is therefore important.

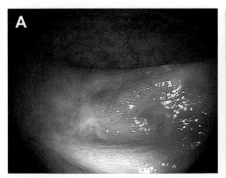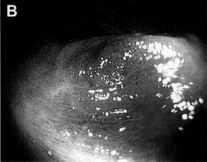

Fig. 4. (A, B): White light (*left*) and narrow band (*right*) images of a small flat adenoma. The fine brown lines visible on the surface of the polyp are abnormal microcapillaries. They impart a dark brown color to the polyp relative to normal mucosa (seen also in Fig. 3 B–D).

Given the paucity of data from randomized controlled trials and the absence of formal recommendations regarding polypectomy techniques, it is not surprising that polypectomy techniques across the United States are inconsistent. In a survey of American College of Gastroenterology (ACG) members (Table 1) [17], forceps methods were most often used to remove polyps 1 to 3 mm in size, including cold forceps in 50% of cases. For the 4- to 6-mm size range, no method was found to be predominant (see Table 1). For polyps 7 to 9 mm in size, the most commonly used modality was hot snaring, but a small number of physicians used hot forceps. An American Society of Gastrointestinal Endoscopy (ASGE) position statement recommends that hot forceps should be used only for polyps 5 mm or smaller [18]. Both hot and cold forceps techniques for larger polyps are associated with ineffective (incomplete) polypectomy [19,20].

Forceps have the advantage of being easier to place on very small flat polyps as compared with snares. Cold forceps are appropriate for 1- to 3-mm polyps, particularly if they engulf the polyp in one piece. Jumbo or large-capacity forceps are useful to engulf slightly larger polyps. Cold forceps are devoid of complication risks and can be safely used to resect diminutive polyps in patients who are therapeutically anticoagulated. The primary disadvantage of forceps techniques, whether hot or cold, is the possibility of leaving residual polyp behind [19,20]. This risk almost certainly increases with increasing polyp size. With cold forceps this results from the requirement for a piecemeal technique, which may leave residual polyp and may obscure the exact margins of the polyp as the endoscopic field of view becomes bloodied after repeated biopsy.

The correct sequential technique for hot forceps is to grasp the tip of the polyp, tent or lift it, deflate the lumen, and apply electrocautery. Electrocautery spreads into the polyp and destroys it while preserving the portion in the forceps for pathologic examination. Although hot forceps are easy to apply, the electrocautery burn sometimes develops asymmetrically, resulting in coagulation of normal tissue. In addition, it is impossible to determine whether the central portion of the polyp has been destroyed. In two series of hot-forceps polypectomies, residual polyp was subsequently identified at the site in 16%

Table 1
Methods of polypectomy for different size polyps

Method	Number (%) of physicians reporting this method stratified according to polyp size		
	1–3 mm polyp	4–6 mm polyp	7–9 mm polyp
Cold forceps	95 (50.3)	35 (18.5)	4 (2.1)
Hot forceps	63 (33.3)	40 (21.2)	8 (4.2)
Hot snare	9 (4.8)	59 (31.2)	151 (79.9)
Cold snare	9 (4.8)	28 (14.8)	11 (5.8)
Combined methods	13 (6.9)	27 (14.4)	15 (7.8)

Adapted from Singh N, Harrison M, Rex DK. A survey of colonoscopic polypectomy practices among clinical gastroenterologists. Gastrointest Endosc 2004;60:414–8; with permission.

to 28% of cases [19,20]. There has been anecdotal evidence suggesting a higher incidence of postpolypectomy bleeding with hot forceps [21], but there is no controlled evidence yet to support or refute this notion. We no longer use hot forceps under any circumstances; however, it is apparent from the afore-mentioned survey [17] that their use remains within the standard of medical care. Hot forceps polypectomy has limited effectiveness [19,20], and its use should be restricted to polyps 5 mm or smaller.

Both hot and cold snaring are more effective than forceps techniques to completely remove polyps [20]. It is unknown whether a large study would demonstrate that hot snaring is slightly more effective than cold snaring in completely removing small polyps. One obvious benefit of cold snaring, however, is elimination of cautery-related complications [15]. The development of diminutive snares has made snaring 1- to 5-mm polyps relatively simple in most cases.

Polyp shape and size are important considerations in deciding whether cold- versus hot-snare polypectomy is appropriate. Cold snaring has been shown to be safe and effective for polyps up to 7 mm in size [15]. During cold-snare polypectomy, the authors' practice is to attempt to ensnare a 1- to 2-mm rim of normal tissue around the polyp edge (Fig. 5). This technique is inadvisable when

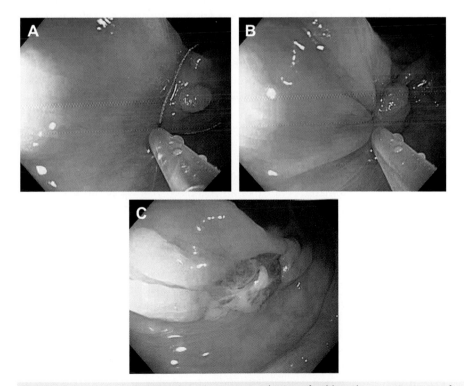

Fig. 5. Cold-snaring technique. The polyp is grasped (A), preferably with a 1- to 2-mm rim of normal tissue (B), and guillotined (C).

using snare electrocautery, because it increases the size of the cautery burn. We typically do not tent during cold-snare removal because this may cause the polyp to pop out of the endoscopic field of view immediately after transection. If the polyp is not tented, it almost invariably remains on or near the site after transection for easy retrieval [22]. We typically use cold snaring on pedunculated polyps up to 4 to 5 mm in size, and on bulky or dome-shaped sessile polyps up to about the same size. We use cold snaring for flat polyps up to 7 to 10 mm in size, occasionally using a piecemeal cold snaring technique. For hot-snare polypectomy of polyps less than 1 cm, tenting the lesion and deflating the lumen are advised to protect the muscularis propria from cautery injury.

There is currently no standard of care with regard to the type of current used for polypectomy. The survey of ACG members on polypectomy revealed that 46% of respondents used pure low-power coagulation, 46% used blended current, and 3% used cutting current [17]. Low-power coagulation is associated with a lower risk for immediate bleeding but a higher risk for delayed bleeding [23,24]. Contrariwise, cutting or blended current is more likely to be associated with immediate bleeding than delayed bleeding. Because the endoscopist may control immediate bleeding during the procedure, blended or cutting current seems advantageous. Both types of current are presently considered acceptable, however.

LARGE PEDUNCULATED POLYPS

Large pedunculated adenomas are most common in the sigmoid colon. Pedunculated mucosal prolapse in the sigmoid is sometimes confused with an adenoma, but can be distinguished by the punctate (rather than uniform) erythema on the surface of the prolapsing tissue, the gradual transition from erythema to normal-colored mucosa and the normal pit pattern of the mucosa [22]. Lipomas can also be confused with adenomas if they exhibit erythema on their surface from prolapse. Of note, lipomas should not be removed endoscopically, unless symptomatic, because of an increased risk for perforation.

The authors' practice is to remove large pedunculated polyps without pretreatment to reduce the risk for bleeding. Most endoscopists who use cutting or blended current prefer pretreatment to prevent immediate bleeding. A commonly recommended approach is to consider pretreatment for patients who have polyps with a stalk thicker than 1 cm, because such stalks can contain a substantial artery [22]. Pretreatment by injection of the stalk with epinephrine in saline has proved to prevent immediate, but not delayed, bleeding in randomized controlled trials [25–27]. It is unclear whether this effect is from local tamponade or the vasoconstrictive effects of epinephrine. In the previously cited survey of ACG members, preinjection with epinephrine was the most commonly used method to prevent bleeding from large pedunculated polyps [17]. In two randomized, controlled trials, detachable snares were found to be effective in the prevention of bleeding in pedunculated polyps 1 cm or larger [25,28]. The risk for bleeding from pedunculated polyps is low, however [29], and some endoscopists reserve the use of detachable snares for patients who are considered high risk, such as those who must resume anticoagulation shortly after polypectomy. Detachable snares have been associated with complications, including pedicle transection from overtightening and inadequate tightening [30,31]. If used for polyps with a short stalk, a detachable snare may slip off, resulting in massive bleeding [31,32].

When removing pedunculated polyps, the electrocautery snare should be placed between one third to one half the distance from the base of the polyp head to the colonic wall to leave residual stalk after resection that can be grabbed if immediate bleeding occurs. Removing some stalk with the polyp increases the likelihood that if cancer is found in the polyp head, the resection line will be free of cancer. Very large snares are useful for very large pedunculated polyps. Polyps in the sigmoid colon are often best approached by opening the snare with the colonoscope tip proximal to the polyp and then withdrawing the colonoscope. If the polyp is in an awkward position, repositioning the patient may make the polyp more accessible. It is sometimes impossible to remove a large pedunculated polyp en bloc, so piecemeal removal must instead be performed. This approach is acceptable, but the portion of the polyp nearest the stalk or colonic wall should be separately submitted to pathology because this section is most important with regard to whether cancer is present.

Immediate postpolypectomy bleeding is managed in several ways. First, traditional management includes regrasping the stalk and holding it for 10 to 15 minutes. It is inadvisable to retransect the stalk with electrocautery, because this might leave no residual stalk to grasp if bleeding continues. Injection of epinephrine or application of multipolar electrocautery may be used to manage bleeding from a polypectomy stalk. Detachable snares can be used after hemostasis has been achieved, but it is impractical to place a detachable snare on the polypectomy stalk after transection in the presence of brisk bleeding. Clips have been clearly effective in arresting immediate postpolypectomy hemorrhage and delayed bleeding when applied to visible vessels in either sessile or pedunculated polyps [33,34]. Clips were ineffective in preventing postpolypectomy hemorrhage after endoscopic polypectomy in a randomized controlled trial that included primarily small polyps at low risk for bleeding [35]. Further study is needed regarding whether prophylactic clipping is effective when a high risk for postpolypectomy bleeding is present. In an uncontrolled series, prophylactic clipping was associated with no subsequent hemorrhage when polypectomy with electrocautery was used to resect polyps 1 cm or smaller [36].

LARGE SESSILE POLYPS

Large sessile polyps are the most difficult polyps to remove endoscopically. In one American study, many large sessile polyps that might have been endoscopically removed were sent for surgical resection [37]. Obstacles to endoscopic removal include the higher risk for bleeding or perforation associated with large sessile polyps and the substantial time required for their removal.

Reimbursement is insufficient for the work and resources required [38]. The mean cost of surgical resection, however, is more than fivefold greater than the cost of endoscopic polypectomy [37].

Whether or not a sessile polyp is amenable to endoscopic removal depends on the size of the polyp and its location within the colon. Sessile lesions in the sigmoid that occupy more than 30% of the circumference are difficult to remove endoscopically because snares may be difficult to fully deploy in the sigmoid, and snares may not effectively close on the polyp because of the tight turning radius of the sigmoid colon. Contrariwise, sessile polyps in the rectum, transverse colon, or ascending colon that occupy 50% to 60% of the circumference can be resected endoscopically. In the cecum, broad lesions can be technically difficult to resect if they extend across multiple sacculations formed by the cecal strap folds or are more than 4 to 5 cm in size (Fig. 6). Furthermore, polyps that extend into the ileocecal valve orifice or through the ileocecal valve into the ileum (Fig. 7), or polyps that overlie the appendiceal orifice in a patient who has not had prior appendectomy, should generally be sent for surgical resection (Fig. 8). Endoscopic removal of polyps that extend over two haustral folds may be completed if the interhaustral valley is not deep or if the valley can be elevated by submucosal fluid injection.

Contraindications to endoscopic resection of sessile polyps include polyps with an ulcerated surface because they have a high probability of containing cancer or high-grade dysplasia. Such polyps are generally biopsied with cold forceps, and endoscopic removal is subsequently attempted if the biopsies fail to reveal frank cancer. Also, in the setting of the nonlifting sign (if there has been no prior attempt at endoscopic removal using snare electrocautery) endoscopic resection should not be performed because this sign indicates the

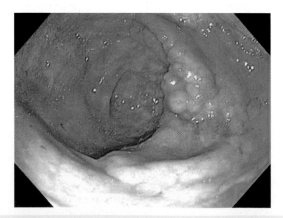

Fig. 6. Large sessile cecal polyp that the senior author (DKR) declined to attempt endoscopic resection based on its large size and flat portions. The polyp extends over the fold seen in the center and extends on the right beyond the edge of the photograph.

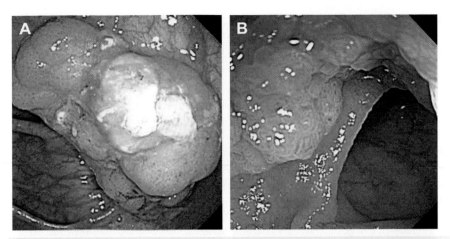

Fig. 7. Large polyp on ileocecal valve (A) that extends into the terminal ileum (B). Patients who have such polyps are best referred for surgical resection.

presence of cancer extending into the muscularis propria, or at least into the deep submucosa.

Because of their size, most sessile polyps greater than 2 cm are removed piecemeal (Fig. 9). Submucosal saline injection is prudent in most cases but not mandatory. It is used to minimize the chance of injury to the muscularis

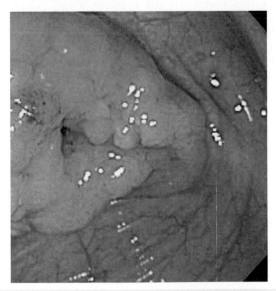

Fig. 8. Polyp engulfing the appendiceal orifice. The depression in the center of the polyp is the location of the appendiceal orifice.

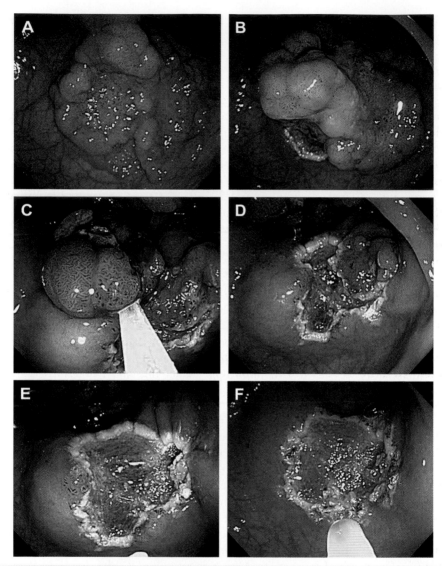

Fig. 9. Piecemeal resection of a large sessile polyp. Large sessile rectal polyp (A), after initial injection and piecemeal resection (B), during resection of another piece of the polyp (C), just before removing the last large piece (D), after last large piece removed (E), and after resection of small pieces and treatment with argon plasma coagulator (F).

propria (which has been demonstrated in animal studies but not in humans) and to facilitate polyp resection [39]. There is no controlled evidence regarding whether submucosal injection reduces the risk for perforation. Furthermore, there are no data to suggest that submucosal injection decreases the chance of postpolypectomy hemorrhage, although the inclusion of epinephrine does reduce the risk for immediate bleeding [25–27].

Most experts in the United States inject saline; 50% dextrose remains in the tissue about twice as long as saline but has a sclerosing effect [40]. Hydroxypropyl methylcellulose (artificial tears) is viscous and must be diluted to 1% to 1.5% and injected through a 23-gauge needle. It persists about 15 times as long as saline [40]. Methylene blue can be added to the injection to help visually delineate the injected mound and to demarcate the edges of the polyp.

In many instances injection should begin through the polyp. The only contraindication to injection through the polyp is surface ulceration. If the injection is started just before the needle penetrates the polyp, then as the needle advances, the submucosal space expands. This is the simplest method to locate the submucosal space. The volume that can or should be injected is unspecified; rather an amount should be injected that facilitates the resection. Usually the injection causes the submucosal mound to spread just beyond the polyp margin.

The resection is typically started with a large snare, removing large pieces if possible [22]. Small, flat areas of residual polyp are often best approached with a diminutive snare or special snares, such as barbed or spiral snares, designed to remove flat pieces. Polyp access can become the rate-limiting factor during polypectomy. Polyps located on the proximal side of sharp bends or folds may be more accessible by retroflexion (Fig. 10). Retroflexion can be achieved in the left colon with a thin upper endoscope using maximal tip deflection, and is facilitated in the proximal colon by use of a pediatric colonoscope.

Large sessile polyps may have to be injected several times if the injection fluid diffuses out of the submucosal space. Injection of very large polyps in sections may facilitate resection by rendering a flat portion of the polyp polypoid followed by resection of that portion, and then reinjection and resection of another portion. This piecemeal injection simplifies resection of each polyp portion, whereas injection of the entire polyp at the outset can transform a flat polyp into a still flat polyp on top of a broad flat injection mound. During snaring, suctioning can help get the polyp to fall into the snare. Any flat portions that cannot be snared may be ablated with the argon plasma coagulator (APC). The depth of injury with APC is more related to the duration of the pulse than the power setting [39]. Lower power settings are used in the proximal compared with the distal colon.

Tattooing is an effective method to mark polypectomy sites for endoscopic follow-up or surgical localization. Large polyps outside the cecum or rectum should be tattooed so that the polypectomy scar can be reliably identified during subsequent examinations. The best material for this purpose is carbon black, available commercially as "SPOT." If tattooing is purely for endoscopic identification, tattooing to the endoscopic right and left of the polypectomy site is sufficient (Fig. 11). If surgical identification is needed, tattooing in three or four quadrants is required.

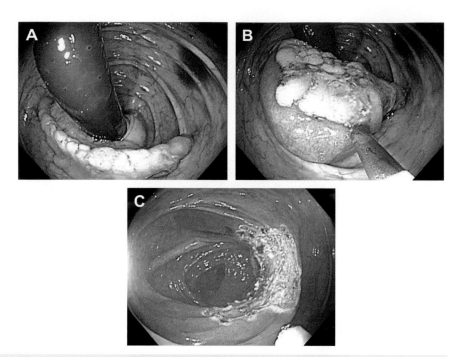

Fig. 10. (A) Large right colon polyp. Note large portion of the polyp made visible by retroflexion. (B) Large-volume injection on the proximal edge rolls this edge into the lumen. (C) Forward view of same polyp after complete resection, argon plasma coagulator treatment, and tattooing. Note the proximal edge of the defect is still visible because of prior injection.

For piecemeal polypectomy, suctioning small pieces through the endoscope into a trap is the most efficient means of retrieval. If a single large fragment cannot be suctioned, this piece can be grasped with a snare and brought into a position 3 to 4 cm beyond the colonoscope tip to permit visualization of the colon during colonoscopic withdrawal. Multiple large fragments can be removed using a Roth retrieval basket. The main disadvantage of this basket is that if additional polyps are detected during withdrawal, they cannot be resected before withdrawing the colonoscope, emptying the basket, and then reinserting the colonoscope.

FOLLOW-UP OF POLYPS

Current guidelines recommend that patients who have 1 or 2 tubular adenomas less than 1 cm with low-grade dysplasia undergo repeat colonoscopy in 5 to 10 years [41]. These recommendations assume that the bowel preparation was adequate and that the examination was completed to the cecum. Patients who have 3 to 10 adenomas or have a single adenoma 1 cm or larger or with high-grade dysplasia or containing villous elements should undergo surveillance colonoscopy in

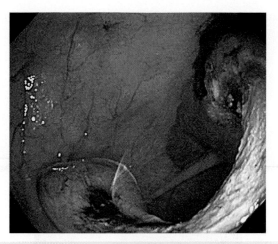

Fig. 11. Endoscopic tattoos placed on either side of a polypectomy defect.

3 years. Patients who have numerous adenomas should undergo surveillance sooner than 3 years to ensure complete clearing of the colon [41].

Patients who undergo piecemeal resection of large sessile adenomas should have an initial follow-up colonoscopy in 3 to 6 months, followed by an additional colonoscopy 1 year later. In the event that the large polyp was located in the rectosigmoid, the follow-up examinations can be done by flexible sigmoidoscopy. The authors biopsy the polypectomy site at the 3- to 6-month evaluation because biopsies showing only normal tissue or scar are highly predictive that subsequent examination at 1 year will continue to show no residual polyp, whereas dysplasia in the flat mucosa at the site of the polypectomy scar at 3 to 6 months predicts the development of a recurrent adenomatous polyp in the resection site [42]. An alternative approach to evaluate the polypectomy scar at the 3- or 6-month interval is chromoendoscopy, with or without high-magnification endoscopy. If polyp is identified at the polypectomy site at the 3- to 6-month follow-up it is snare resected, if possible, or obliterated using the argon plasma coagulator (Fig. 12). An additional examination is then required in 3 to 6 months.

Recurrence rates of adenomas at the prior polypectomy site of large sessile polyps removed in piecemeal fashion have varied from 14% to 55%. This variability likely represents the aggressiveness with which the polyp was initially removed, especially the extent of ablation of flat areas during the initial polypectomy [43]. After resection of adenomas, if subsequent colonoscopy reveals only small hyperplastic polyps or is normal then repeat colonoscopy is recommended every 5 years. For patients who have only had small tubular adenomas on prior examinations, extending the surveillance interval to 10 years is feasible [41]. The occurrence of only small hyperplastic polyps in the distal colon is considered normal and the screening interval can remain at 10 years. Patients who have hyperplastic polyps in the proximal colon are considered to be at

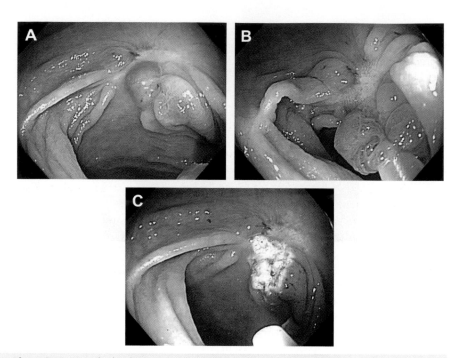

Fig. 12. (A) Residual polyp in a tattooed polypectomy site. (B) Snare cautery resection of the polyp. (C) After APC therapy of edge of the snare defect.

increased risk for CRC, but optimal surveillance intervals have not been defined [41]. Anecdotally, we typically repeat colonoscopy in 5 years when patients have several small proximal hyperplastic polyps. If large proximal hyperplastic polyps are found, we repeat colonoscopy in 1 to 3 years, depending on their number and size. Various definitions have been proposed for the hyperplastic polyposis syndrome [44]. The definition requires prospective validation. The genetic basis for the syndrome remains unknown [44], but an increased risk for CRC and a shorter follow-up interval are needed.

MANAGEMENT OF ANTICOAGULATION AND ANTIPLATELET AGENTS DURING POLYPECTOMY

Given the current high prevalence of cardiovascular disease and its associated therapy, endoscopists must be familiar with the appropriate management of anticoagulation and antiplatelet agents during polypectomy. The ASGE recommends that aspirin need not be stopped before polypectomy [45]. If aspirin causes an increase in the absolute risk for bleeding after polypectomy, the effect is small [46,47]. Despite this, endoscopists often discontinue aspirin and other nonsteroidal anti-inflammatory drugs (NSAIDs) for 1 to 2 weeks after resection of large polyps. The main indication for clopidogrel is coronary artery stent placement. The decision whether to discontinue this medication must be weighed against the risks associated with stoppage, including coronary stent occlusion. Currently, for high-risk procedures, including polypectomy, it is recommended that clopidogrel should be stopped 7 to 10 days before the procedure [45]. Management of clopidogrel is an individualized decision that may need to be made in conjunction with the patient's cardiologist.

Management of warfarin in the peripolypectomy period depends on the indication for anticoagulation and the specific procedure to be performed. Endoscopic procedures have been stratified by the ASGE into high- and low-risk categories, depending on the risk for bleeding [48]. High risk entails a 1% to 6% chance of bleeding; polypectomy and laser ablation are in this category. Box 2 shows the risk of various conditions for thromboembolism and the risks of various endoscopic procedures for bleeding.

For patients undergoing polypectomy at low risk for thromboembolism (see Box 2), anticoagulation is withheld 3 to 5 days before the procedure. For patients at high risk for thromboembolism, one approach is to perform diagnostic colonoscopy with the patient still anticoagulated. Polypectomy of very small polyps using cold-forceps biopsy can be performed in patients who are therapeutically anticoagulated. We extend this rule to cold snaring of polyps up to 4 to 5 mm in size. Polyps up to 1 cm in size have been resected in

---

Box 2: Low- and high-risk conditions for thromboembolism and low- and high-risk colonoscopic procedures for bleeding

Low-risk conditions for thromboembolism

Paroxysmal atrial fibrillation

Mechanical valves in the aortic position

Deep venous thrombosis

High-risk conditions for thromboembolism

Atrial fibrillation plus mitral valve disease

Mechanical valves in the mitral position

Valve disease with a history of thromboembolism

Low-risk procedures for bleeding

Colonoscopy with cold-forceps biopsy examination

High-risk procedures for bleeding

Colonoscopy with polypectomy

Colonoscopy with laser treatment

Colonoscopy with dilation

Adapted from Eisen GM, Baron TH, Dominitz JA, et al. Guideline on the management of anticoagulation and antiplatelet therapy for endoscopic procedures. Gastrointest Endosc 2002;55(7):775–9; with permission.

anticoagulated patients followed by placement of one or two hemostatic clips without subsequent bleeding [36]. This approach has not been tested in larger polyps. If larger polyps must be resected or if the patient prefers to not undergo an initial colonoscopy on anticoagulation, then anticoagulation should be transiently discontinued. Warfarin is held 3 to 5 days before the procedure and the INR allowed to trend toward normal. As the INR reaches the lower limits of the therapeutic range, heparin or low molecular weight heparin (LMWH) is administered as a bridge. One advantage of LMWH is that it can be administered on an outpatient basis, which reduces costs and is more convenient to the patient [48]. The efficacy of this approach in preventing thromboembolism is not established, however.

Intravenous heparin is stopped 4 to 6 hours before colonoscopy or if LMWH is used it is stopped 8 to 12 hours before the procedure. Colonoscopy and polypectomy are then performed. During the procedure potential alternatives to simple snare polypectomy are the use of hemoclips to close the polypectomy site after snaring or ablation of the polyp using laser ablation or argon plasma coagulation. Neither method is proved to reduce the risk for hemorrhage, however. Anticoagulation following the procedure is usually started within 4 to 6 hours, but the starting time should be individualized and determined in conjunction with the cardiologist or cardiac surgeon. We typically resume warfarin on the evening of the procedure but delay heparin or LMWH for a day or two after resection of a large polyp, which is usually acceptable to the cardiac specialist.

MANAGEMENT OF COMPLICATIONS

Complications after colonoscopic polypectomy include perforation, postpolypectomy syndrome, and postpolypectomy hemorrhage. Prompt identification and appropriate management minimize the morbidity and mortality of these complications. Perforation is the most feared complication. It is the most likely to result in medical–legal action against the endoscopist. The reported incidence of perforation has varied, ranging from 1 per 100 polypectomies to 1 per several thousand colonoscopies [14,49,50]. The classic symptoms and signs of perforation include abdominal pain, fever, leukocytosis, and peritoneal findings on physical examination. The diagnosis is made by demonstrating free air in the peritoneal cavity or retroperitoneal space. About 5% of perforations are fatal, usually the result of sepsis and multiorgan failure.

Perforation after polypectomy is invariably the result of thermal injury to the colonic wall from electrocautery. Perforation can occur immediately or be delayed for several hours or days. The delay is believed to be because of transmural thermal injury of the colonic wall, which becomes necrotic and then frankly perforates. The risk for postpolypectomy perforation increases with the size of the resected polyp and is more prevalent with sessile polyps than pedunculated polyps. It is also more likely in the proximal colon, especially the cecum, because the colonic wall is thin at this location. Removal of rectal polyps with electrocautery is less likely to lead to perforation because the rectal wall is thicker and the distal rectum is retroperitoneal. The risk for perforation is decreased by using cold techniques when feasible.

Initial management of perforation includes making the patient nil per os, treating with antibiotics, and prompt surgical consultation. Large perforations (polypectomy perforations are seldom large) or those diagnosed in the first few hours after colonoscopy should undergo surgical repair. If the patient exhibits signs of sepsis or progressing peritoneal signs, prompt surgery is necessary. Patients who present to the emergency room with complaints of abdominal pain after polypectomy should always be examined by an expert, have vital signs and leukocyte count measured, and undergo urgent radiographic imaging. A high index of suspicion for colonic perforation should prompt the physician to obtain a CT scan, even if the plain abdominal radiographs are within normal limits. If there is no evidence of intraperitoneal free air or retroperitoneal air on CT scan, the patient can be considered to have the postpolypectomy syndrome. This syndrome results from a transmural burn through the colonic wall without actual perforation. It represents the second most common complication (behind hemorrhage) and occurs after 0.5% to 1% of polypectomies [29,51,52]. Risk factors include large (>2 cm) sessile polyps and proximal colonic polyp location [53]. Inadvertent snaring of normal mucosa adjacent to the polyp is also a risk factor [54].

Postpolypectomy syndrome presents similarly to colonic perforation, with fever, abdominal pain, and leukocytosis, but does not cause free air. The presentation occurs soon after polypectomy, usually within 12 hours, but can be delayed for several days. Management includes nil per os, antibiotics, and close clinical observation. Having a surgeon follow the patient is appropriate. The chance of evolution to frank perforation is low in properly managed patients [54]. Measures to minimize the risk for postpolypectomy syndrome are the same as those to prevent perforation.

Hemorrhage is the most common complication of colonoscopic polypectomy [55]. It can occur immediately or be delayed [29,56]. Two studies found that immediate bleeding is more common with cutting or blended current and delayed bleeding is more common with coagulation current [23,56]. Risk factors for hemorrhage include large polyp size and location in the proximal colon [56,57]. Immediate bleeding after cold forceps or cold snare removal of small polyps is nearly always capillary in nature and clinically insignificant.

Immediate hemorrhage may be treated with injection of epinephrine followed by multipolar cautery or clipping. We prefer not to use clipping when the polyp is or may not yet be fully resected, because the clip may interfere with completion of resection if it is placed too close to the residual polyp. The endoscopist can almost invariably achieve hemostasis [57,58]. Those patients who suffer delayed hemorrhage should be instructed to return promptly to the emergency room. Delayed bleeding classically presents as passage of large-volume bloody bowel movements. It can occur up to 21 days after polypectomy, although it most commonly occurs within the first week. Up to two thirds of patients have stopped passing bloody bowel movements when they present [55], but they should be hospitalized for observation if they are elderly, have comorbidities, live far away from the treating hospital, or if endoscopic reexamination is not pursued. Patients who continue to pass bloody bowel movements usually have ongoing arterial hemorrhage from the polypectomy site. We promptly perform colonoscopy without bowel purging [55]. Blood acts as a cathartic and the likely site of bleeding is usually already known,

---

Box 3: Pearls and pitfalls in colonoscopic polypectomy

- Gastroenterologists should be experts in bowel preparation and quality colonoscopic withdrawal technique. To remove polyps, one first has to find them.

- Electrocautery causes virtually all polypectomy-related perforations and most delayed bleeding. Small polyps can be removed effectively with cold technique, including cold forceps for 1- to 3-mm polyps and cold snaring for 3- to 10-mm polyps, depending on the shape. Careful consideration should be given to whether electrocautery is necessary for the removal of small polyps because most small polyps will not harm the patient.

- Aspirin and NSAIDs are NOT clearly established risk factors for postpolypectomy bleeding.

- The use of pure low-power coagulation current is associated with an increased risk for delayed bleeding, whereas blended and cutting current are associated with increased risk for immediate bleeding.

- Detachable snares are effective in preventing both immediate and delayed bleeding from pedunculated polyps.

- Inclusion of epinephrine in the submucosal injection fluid has been shown to prevent immediate bleeding from pedunculated and sessile polyps.

- Clipping has not yet been proved to prevent bleeding after polypectomy.

- During cold snaring it is acceptable to include a strip of one to a few millimeters of normal mucosa around the polyp.

- The ASGE recommends that hot forceps not be used for polyps larger than 5 mm. Contrary to the belief of some, hot forceps do not ensure obliteration of polyps and have been shown to leave residual polyp in 16% to 28% of cases.

- The depth of injury from argon plasma coagulation is related primarily to the duration of the pulse and secondarily to the power. Low power and brief pulses are needed in the cecum and ascending colon.

- Pure carbon black is the best tattoo for polyps because it avoids the risk for immunologic reactions seen with India ink.

- Patients who have severe abdominal pain after polypectomy should be assumed to have colonic perforation. Their evaluation should include abdominopelvic CT scan.

- Guidelines for appropriate postpolypectomy surveillance intervals are available from the United States Multi-Society Task Force and the American Cancer Society. Patients who undergo large sessile polyp resection in piecemeal fashion undergo the closest follow-up, typically 3 to 6 months after the initial resection.

unless multiple large polyps have been resected. The endoscope is passed to the area of prior polypectomy and hemostasis is achieved by either injection of epinephrine followed by the application of multipolar cautery [54,55,59] or by application of hemoclips [60].

SUMMARY

Box 3 lists selected "pearls and pitfalls" in colonoscopic polypectomy. In general, risks associated with the technique of polyp removal should match the likelihood that the polyp will become or already is malignant (eg, low-risk technique for low risk for malignant potential). Cold techniques are preferred for most diminutive polyps. Polypectomy techniques must be effective and minimize complications. Complications can occur even with proper technique, however. Aggressive evaluation and treatment of complications helps ensure the best possible outcome.

References

[1] Winawer SJ, Zauber AG, Ho MN, et al. Prevention of colorectal cancer by colonoscopic polypectomy. The National Poly Study Workgroup. N Engl J Med 1993;329:1977–81.

[2] Citarda F, Tomaselli G, Capocaccia R, et al. Efficacy in standard clinical practice of colonoscopic polypectomy in reducing colorectal cancer incidence. Gut 2001;48:812–5

[3] Thiis-Evensen E, Hoff GS, Sauar J, et al. Population-based surveillance by colonoscopy: effect on the incidence of colorectal cancer. Telemark Polyp Study I. Scand J Gastroenterol 1999;34:414–20.

[4] Rex DK. Maximizing detection of adenomas and cancers during colonoscopy. Am J Gastroenterol 2006;101:2866–77.

[5] Pabby A, Schoen RE, Weisfeld JL, et al. Analysis of colorectal cancer occurrence during surveillance colonoscopy in the dietary Polyp Prevention Trial. Gastrointest Endosc 2005;61: 385–91.

[6] Farrar WD, Sawhney MS, Nelson DB, et al. Colorectal cancers found after a complete colonoscopy. Clin Gastroenterol Hepatol 2006;4:1259–64.

[7] Spring KJ, Zhao ZZ, Karamatic R, et al. High prevalence of sessile serrated adenomas with BRAF mutations: a prospective study of patients undergoing colonoscopy. Gastroenterology 2006;131:1400–7.

[8] Rex DK, Ulbright TM. Step section histology of proximal colon polyps that appear hyperplastic by endoscopy. Am J Gastroenterol 2002;97:1530–4.

[9] Kudo S, Hirota S, Nakajima T, et al. Colorectal tumours and pit pattern. J Clin Pathol 1994;47:880–5.

[10] Helbig C, Rex DK. Chromoendoscopy and its alternatives for colonoscopy: useful in the United States? Rev Gastroenterol Disord 2006;6:209–20.

[11] Sano Y, Horimatsu T, Fu KI, et al. Magnified observation of microvascular architecture using narrow band imaging (NBI) for the differential diagnosis between non-neoplastic and neoplastic colorectal lesion. A prospective study. Gastrointest Endosc 2006;63:AB102.

[12] Zanati S, Marcon NE, Cirocco M, et al. Onco-life fluorescence imaging during colonoscopy assists in the differentation of adenomatous and hyperplastic polyps and improves detection rate of dysplastic lesions in the colon. Gastroenterology 2005;128:A27–8.

[13] Kiesslich R, Burg J, Vieth M, et al. Confocal laser endoscopy for diagnosing intraepithelial neoplasias and colorectal cancer in vivo. Gastroenterology 2004;127:706–13.

[14] Levin TR, Zhao W, Conell C, et al. Complications of colonoscopy in an integrated health care delivery system. Ann Intern Med 2006;145:880–6.

[15] Tappero G, Gaia E, De Giuli P, et al. Cold snare excision of small colorectal polyps. Gastrointest Endosc 1992;38:310–3.

[16] Deenadayalu VP, Rex DK. Colon polyp retrieval after cold snaring. Gastrointest Endosc 2005;62:253–6.

[17] Singh N, Harrison M, Rex DK. A survey of colonoscopic polypectomy practices among clinical gastroenterologists. Gastrointest Endosc 2004;60:414–8.

[18] ASGE Technology Assessment Report. Hot biopsy forceps. Gastrointest Endosc 1992;38: 753–6.

[19] Peluso F, Goldner R. Follow-up of hot biopsy forceps treatment of diminutive colon polyps. Gastrointest Endosc 1991;37:604–6.

[20] Ellis K, Shiel M, Marquis S, et al. Efficacy of hot biopsy forceps, cold micro-snare and micro-snare with cautery techniques in the removal of diminutive colonic polyps. Gastrointest Endosc 1997;45:AB107.

[21] Weston AP, Campbell DR. Diminutive colonic polyps—histopathologically, spatial distribution, concomitant significant lesions and treatment complications. Am J Gastroenterol 1995;90:24–8.

[22] Rex DK. Colonoscopic polypectomy. Rev Gastroenterol Disord 2005;5(3):115–25.

[23] Van Gossum A, Cozzoli A, Adler M, et al. Colonoscopic snare polypectomy: analysis of 1485 resections comparing two types of current. Gastrointest Endosc 1992;38(4):472–5.

[24] Parra-Blanco A, Kaminaga N, Kojima T, et al. Colonoscopic polypectomy with cutting current: is it safe? Gastrointest Endosc 2000;51:676–81.

[25] DiGiorgio P, De Luca L, Calcagno G, et al. Detachable snare versus epinephrine injection in the prevention of postpolypectomy bleeding: a randomized and controlled trial. Endoscopy 2004;36:860–3.

[26] Hsieh V-H, Lin H-J, Tseng G-Y, et al. Is submucosal injection necessary before polypectomy? A prospective, comparative study. Hepatogastroenterology 2001;48:1379–82.

[27] Dobrowolski S, Dobosz M, Babicki A, et al. Prophylactic submucosal saline-adrenaline injection in colonoscopic polypectomy: prospective randomized study. Surg Endosc 2004;18(6):990–3.

[28] Iishi H, Tatsuta M, Narahara H, et al. Endoscopic resection of large pedunculated colorectal polyps using a detachable snare. Gastrointest Endosc 2004;44:594–7.

[29] Waye JD, Lewis BS, Yessayan S. Colonoscopy: a prospective report of complications. J Clin Gastroenterol 1992;15(4):347–51.

[30] Brandimarte G, Tursi A. Endoscopic snare excision of large pedunculated colorectal polyps: a new, safe, and effective technique. Endoscopy 2001;33(10):854–7.

[31] Matsushita M, Hajiro K, Takakuwa H, et al. Ineffective use of a detachable snare for colonoscopic polypectomy of large polyps. Gastrointest Endosc 1998;47(6):496–9.

[32] Soetikno RM, Friedland S, Lewit V, et al. Lift and ligate: a new technique to treat a bleeding polypectomy stump. Gastrointest Endosc 2000;52(5):681–3.

[33] Church JM. Experience in the endoscopic management of large colonic polyps. ANZ J Surg 2003;73(12):988–95.

[34] Cipolletta L, Bianco MA, Rotondano G, et al. Endoclip-associated resection of large pedunculated colon polyps. Gastrointest Endosc 1999;50(3):405–6 [see comment].

[35] Shioji K, Suzuki Y, Kobayashi M, et al. Prophylactic clip application does not decrease delayed bleeding after colonoscopic polypectomy. Gastrointest Endosc 2003;57(6):691–4 [see comment].

[36] Friedland S, Soetikno R. Colonoscopy with polypectomy in anticoagulated patients. Gastrointest Endosc 2006;64(1):98–100.

[37] Onken JE, Friedman JY, Subramanian S, et al. Treatment patterns and costs associated with sessile colorectal polyps. Am J Gastroenterol 2002;97:2896–901.

[38] Overhiser AJ, Rex DK. Work and resources needed for endoscopic resection of large sessile colorectal polyps. Clin Gastroenterol Hepatol 2007;5:1076–9.

[39] Norton ID, Wang L, Levine SA, et al. Efficacy of colonic submucosal saline solution injection for the reduction of iatrogenic thermal injury. Gastrointest Endosc 2002;56:95–9.

[40] Conio M, Rajan E, Sorbi D, et al. Comparative performance in the porcine esophagus of different solutions used for submucosal injection. Gastrointest Endosc 2002;56:513–6.

[41] Winawer SJ, Zauber AG, Fletcher RH, et al. Guidelines for colonoscopy surveillance after polypectomy: a consensus update by the US Multi-Society Task Force on Colorectal Cancer and the American Cancer Society. Gastroenterology 2006;130:1872–85.

[42] Rusche M, Chadalawada V, Bratcher LL, et al. Negative scar biopsy after large polypectomy at 3 months predictive of cure. Am J Gastroenterol 2005;100:S393.

[43] Brooker JC, Saunders BP, Shah SG, et al. Treatment with argon plasma coagulation reduces the recurrence after piecemeal resection of large colonic polyps: a randomized trial and recommendations. Gastrointest Endosc 2002;55:371–5.

[44] Chow E, Lipton L, Lynch E, et al. Hyperplastic polyposis syndrome: phenotypic presentations and the role of MBD4 and MYH. Gastroenterology 2006;131(1):30–9.

[45] Zuckerman MJ, Hirota WK, Adler DG, et al. ASGE guideline: the management of low-molecular-weight heparin and nonaspirin antiplatelet agents for endoscopic procedures. Gastrointest Endosc 2005;61(2):189–94.

[46] Hui AJ, Wong RM, Ching JY, et al. Risk of colonoscopic polypectomy bleeding with anticoagulants and antiplatelet agents: analysis of 1657 cases. Gastrointest Endosc 2004;59(1): 44–8.

[47] Yousfi M, Gostout CJ, Baron TH, et al. Postpolypectomy lower gastrointestinal bleeding: potential role of aspirin. Am J Gastroenterol 2004;99(9):1785–9.

[48] ASGE. Guideline on the management of anticoagulation and antiplatelet therapy for endoscopic procedures. Gastrointest Endosc 2002;55(7):775–9.

[49] Smith LE. Fiberoptic colonoscopy: complications of colonoscopy and polypectomy. Dis Colon Rectum 1976;19(5):407–12.

[50] Fatima H, Rex DK. Minimizing endoscopic complications: colonoscopic polypectomy. Gastrointest Endosc Clin N Am 2007;17:145–56.

[51] Waye JD, Kahn O, Auerbach ME. Complications of colonoscopy and flexible sigmoidoscopy. Gastrointest Endosc Clin N Am 1996;6(2):343–77.

[52] Nivatvongs S. Complications in colonoscopic polypectomy: lessons to learn from an experience with 1576 polyps. Am Surg 1988;54(2):61–3.

[53] Christie JP, Marrazzo J III. "Mini-perforation" of the colon—not all postpolypectomy perforations require laparotomy. Dis Colon Rectum 1991;34(2):132–5.

[54] Conio M, Repici A, Demarquay JF, et al. EMR of large sessile colorectal polyps. Gastrointest Endosc 2004;60(2):234–41.

[55] Rex DK, Lewis BS, Waye JD. Colonoscopy and endoscopic therapy for delayed postpolypectomy hemorrhage. Gastrointest Endosc 1992;38(2):127–9.

[56] Sorbi D, Norton I, Conio M, et al. Postpolypectomy lower GI bleeding: descriptive analysis. Gastrointest Endosc 2000;51(6):690–6.

[57] Binmoeller KF, Bohnacker S, Seifert H, et al. Endoscopic snare excision of "giant" colorectal polyps. Gastrointest Endosc 1996;43(3):183–8 [see comment].

[58] Doniec JM, Lohnert MS, Schniewind B, et al. Endoscopic removal of large colorectal polyps: prevention of unnecessary surgery. Dis Colon Rectum 2003;46(3):340–8.

[59] Alberti-Flor JJ, Hernandez ME, Ferrer JP. Combined injection and thermal therapy in the management of early post-polypectomy bleeding. Am J Gastroenterol 1992;87(11): 1681–2.

[60] Letard JC, Kaffy F, Rousseau D, et al. Post-polypectomy colonic arterial hemorrhage can be treated by hemoclipping. Gastroenterol Clin Biol 2001;25(3):323–4 [in French].

Gastroenterol Clin N Am 37 (2008) 253–267

GASTROENTEROLOGY CLINICS
OF NORTH AMERICA

Surgical Therapy for Colorectal Adenocarcinoma

Neal Wilkinson, MD, Carol E.H. Scott-Conner, MD, PhD*

Department of Surgery, University of Iowa Carver College of Medicine, 200 Hawkins Drive, Iowa City, IA 52240, USA

Colon and rectal adenocarcinoma was projected to afflict 153,800 Americans in 2007 and was estimated to cause more than 52,000 deaths [1]. Colorectal cancer (CRC) remains the second leading cause of cancer mortality among men, and the third leading cause among women. Worldwide, CRC is the fourth most common cancer with approximately 1 million new cases annually. North America, Europe, Australia, and New Zealand are high-risk regions [2]. Unfortunately, advanced disease at diagnosis is still all too common. Locally advanced rectal cancer, node-positive colon cancer, and metastatic disease still compose a significant proportion of colon and rectal cancer [1]. Surgery is the mainstay of treatment, providing definitive management and potential cure in early cases, and effective palliation in advanced cases. Chemotherapy and, sometimes, radiotherapy are essential components of effective treatment. This article briefly reviews the general principles of surgical management and describes recent developments.

GENERAL PRINCIPLES OF SURGICAL TREATMENT

CRC is generally diagnosed by colonoscopy or contrast radiography. An increasing percentage of cases are first detected by abdominal CT. Surgical planning is influenced by the cancer location, the clinical stage, and other factors, such as comorbid conditions, patient frailty, and prior surgery. Preoperative colonoscopy provides a secure histologic diagnosis and determines whether the remainder of the colon is clean of polyps or synchronous cancers. A preoperative CT scan provides additional staging information and assesses whether adjacent vital structures, such as the ureters (for low pelvic lesions) or the duodenum (for right transverse colon lesions), are involved. The local extent of rectal carcinoma is best assessed by endorectal ultrasound, as described in an accompanying article by Bhutani, elsewhere in this issue. Neither histologic grade nor molecular markers currently influence the contemplated surgery, but these factors may become important in subsequent therapy.

*Corresponding author. E-mail address: carol-scott-conner@uiowa.edu (C.E.H. Scott-Conner).

0889-8553/08/$ – see front matter
doi:10.1016/j.gtc.2007.12.012

Similarly, serum carcinoembryonic antigen levels do not influence preoperative decision making, but may assist in postsurgical monitoring.

Resection is based on standard anatomic regions according to the regional lymphatic drainage and blood supply (Figs. 1 and 2). An adequate lymphadenectomy should remove all draining lymphatics at risk for metastatic involvement. Numerous large clinical trials have demonstrated that surgery alone results in a 5- or 10-year survival of 50% to 60% for stage III cancer [3,4]. The Cancer Staging Handbook of the American Joint Committee on Cancer recommends that at least 12 lymph nodes draining the primary cancer should be excised and examined to ensure proper staging and provide adequate surgical clearance [5]. For cancers above the peritoneal reflection, the length of colon resected is generally determined by the mesenteric vascular segmental

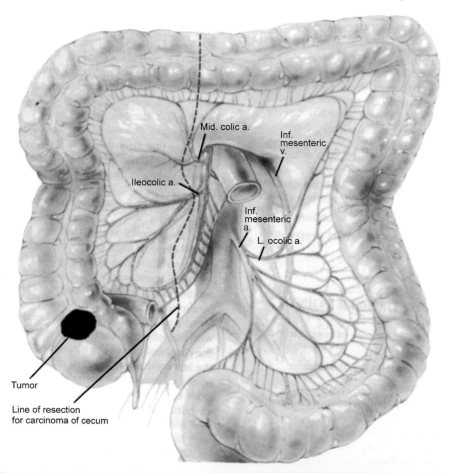

Fig. 1. Extent of resection (*dashed line*) for right hemicolectomy for carcinoma of the cecum. From Scott-Conner CEH, editor. Chassin's operative strategy in colon and rectal surgery. New York: Springer Verlag; 2006; with kind permission of Springer Science and Business Media.)

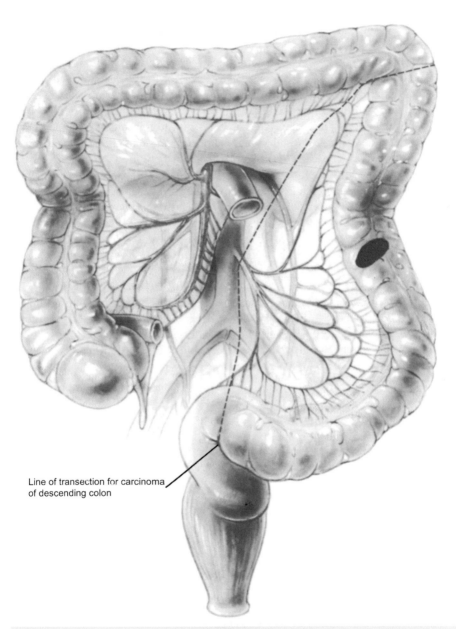

Line of transection for carcinoma
of descending colon

Fig. 2. Extent of resection (*dashed line*) for left hemicolectomy for carcinoma of the descending colon. (*From* Scott-Conner CEH, editor. Chassin's operative strategy in colon and rectal surgery. New York: Springer Verlag; 2006; with kind permission of Springer Science and Business Media.)

anatomy and the surgical margins are usually ample. Frozen sections are rarely required.

Below the peritoneal reflection, the desire for wide surgical margins must be balanced against sphincter preservation. The most difficult margin to control may, in fact, not be the longitudinal margin (ie, distance from the cancer to the sphincters) but the radial margin using the total mesorectal excision (TME) technique. This technique has been thoroughly analyzed, and is now considered standard for rectal cancer. The role of staging and neoadjuvant therapy for rectal cancer is discussed later.

Approximately 5% of patients who undergo colon cancer surgery have synchronous lesions. The management depends on the relative location of the synchronous lesions, family history, patient age, and other factors. Most surgeons prefer an extended resection encompassing both lesions with a single anastomosis, rather than two discontinuous segmental resections with two anastomoses. Subtotal colectomy may be required to accomplish this goal.

High-risk situations, such as chronic ulcerative colitis with severe dysplasia or familial adenomatous polyposis, are best managed by prophylactic surgery (restorative proctocolectomy) before carcinoma develops. When frank carcinoma is encountered in these situations, treatment of the existing malignancy takes precedence over prevention of a subsequent cancer, and a slightly more conservative resection, such as a subtotal colectomy, rather than restorative proctocolectomy or even proctocolectomy with ileostomy, may be elected to minimize complications.

In preparation for elective colon resection, the patient undergoes careful assessment of risk, including cardiac, pulmonary, and hematologic evaluation. Mechanical bowel cleansing is obtained by a combination of cathartics and enemas, or by antegrade lavage. If a CRC is nearly obstructing, the bowel preparation may require modification. Mechanical bowel preparation is supplemented by preoperative administration of antibiotics. Surgery is usually performed under general anesthesia. Epidural catheters are placed for postoperative pain control.

RIGHT AND LEFT HEMICOLECTOMY

As an example of open colon resection, consider elective right hemicolectomy, performed for cancer of the cecum or ascending colon. The lateral peritoneal attachment is incised, and the colon is mobilized medially, to expose the right kidney, ureter, and duodenum. The peritoneum is incised over the base of the mesenteric vessels—in this case, the ileocolic artery and vein. Typically the colon is divided just proximal to the main trunk of the middle colic artery, to preserve a robust blood supply to the transverse colon, and the entire cecum and a few centimeters of terminal ileum are included in the resection. These points of division are identified and windows are made in the mesenteric surface of the bowel (Fig. 3). The bowel is divided with a stapling device. The mesentery is divided between clamps and the resected specimen is removed. Gastrointestinal

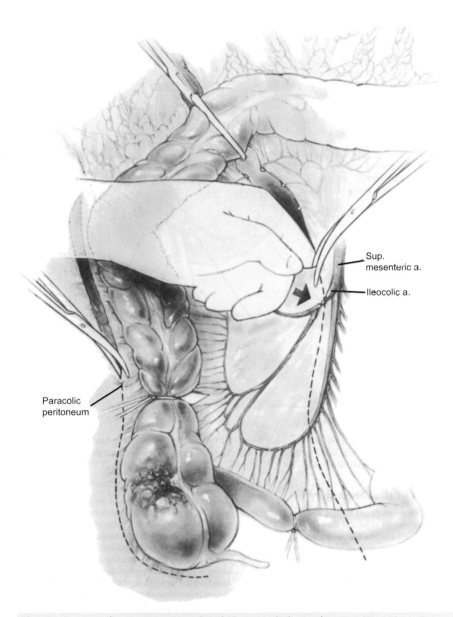

Sup.
mesenteric a.

Ileocolic a.

Paracolic
peritoneum

Fig. 3. Division of mesentery (*arrowhead*) during right hemicolectomy. (*From* Scott-Conner CEH, editor. Chassin's operative strategy in colon and rectal surgery. New York: Springer Verlag; 2006; with kind permission of Springer Science and Business Media.)

continuity is established by a stapled (Fig. 4) or hand-sewn (Fig. 5) anastomosis. The abdomen is closed without external drains.

When the lesion is in the left colon, particularly when below the peritoneal reflection, technical modifications allow restoration of intestinal continuity in

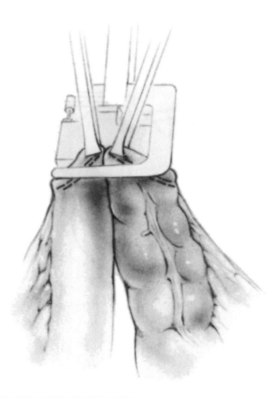

Fig. 4. Completion of stapled anastomosis for right hemicolectomy. (*From* Scott-Conner CEH, editor. Chassin's operative strategy in colon and rectal surgery. New York: Springer Verlag; 2006; with kind permission of Springer Science and Business Media.)

the deep and narrow confines of the pelvis. The most common method is transanal insertion of a circular stapling device (Fig. 6).

Unexpected findings at surgery can require surgical modifications. Despite preoperative workup, peritoneal implants or small hepatic metastases may be identified by careful palpation at surgery. Generally the surgeon proceeds with resection of the primary cancer as planned, and performs a biopsy to document the extent of metastatic disease. When a single isolated metastasis is identified, it may be excised. Controversy surrounds the issue of whether to resect a single hepatic metastasis. Surgeons often individualize this decision based on the size and ease of removal of the lesion. Often, a staged curative surgery is performed for isolated hepatic metastasis. Proper documentation of the presence or absence of peritoneal disease strongly impacts on the surgical decision. Standard therapeutic lymphadenectomy should be performed if future surgical management of metastatic disease is to be entertained. Aggressive debulking is generally not performed during the primary procedure. It may be elected later as part of comprehensive multimodality therapy.

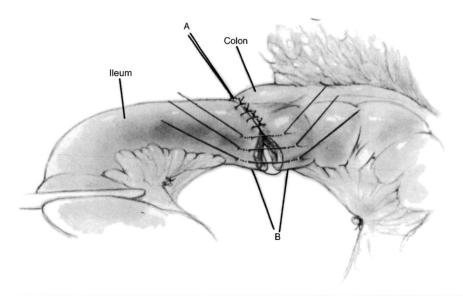

Fig. 5. Completion of suture anastomosis for right hemicolectomy. (*From* Scott-Conner CEH, editor. Chassin's operative strategy in colon and rectal surgery. New York: Springer Verlag; 2006; with kind permission of Springer Science and Business Media.)

Emergency surgery may be required for three cancer complications: colonic obstruction, bleeding, or perforation. The surgeon should endeavor to remove the cancer whenever possible, but the complication rate is higher and the quality of the resection is worse when this surgery is performed in an emergency situation. Restoration of gastrointestinal continuity is generally not feasible

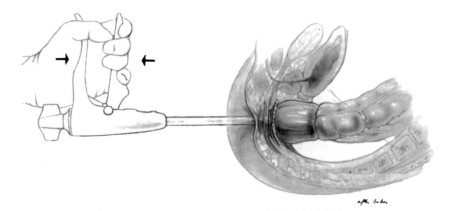

Fig. 6. Completion of stapled anastomosis after left colon resection by transanal insertion of a circular stapling device. (*From* Scott-Conner CEH, editor. Chassin's operative strategy in colon and rectal surgery. New York: Springer Verlag; 2006; with kind permission of Springer Science and Business Media.)

and the patient receives a colostomy. Preoperative marking of possible colostomy sites ensures proper placement of the stoma. With improvements in systemic therapy, many patients will survive for a significant time, and a functional stoma can positively impact on their quality of life.

Obstruction is the most common indication for emergency surgery. Surgery may be limited to a decompressive colostomy or may include resection of the cancer with creation of an end colostomy and distal blind pouch (Hartmann procedure). Primary anastomosis is ill advised because the proximal bowel is dilated and filled with feces. Temporizing endoscopic maneuvers (dilatation and stent placement) may permit colonic decompression without surgery that provides a period of time during which the medical condition can be optimized and the diagnosis confirmed. Elective resection may be performed thereafter under controlled conditions. Perforation of CRC is uncommon. It generally requires resection of the perforated colonic segment with creation of a proximal colostomy (Hartmann procedure). Bleeding that is sufficiently brisk to require surgery is rare.

The surgical treatment of an asymptomatic primary in the setting of advanced incurable cancer is uncertain. Fear of subsequent complications from the primary cancer needs to be balanced against delays in chemotherapy resulting from the surgery. Retrospective reviews demonstrate an acceptable complication rate, when the primary is left intact and untreated, of obstruction in 10% to 20%, bleeding in 4%, fistula formation in 4%, and perforation [6–8]. Bleeding, perforation and obstruction, though uncommon, can occur in up to 20% and 30% of patients who survive more than 2 years after such surgery with an "intact primary."

MANAGEMENT OF RECTAL CARCINOMA

Rectal adenocarcinoma was projected to afflict 41,400 Americans in the year 2007 [1]. Surgical and adjuvant therapies have recently evolved considerably to help preserve sphincter function and prevent pelvic recurrence. The traditional surgical treatment of rectal cancer of radical surgery had excessive local failure rates. The classic Miles procedure, first described in 1908, involved surgical removal of the distal rectum and perineum, including all radial margins out to the pelvic sidewall. This procedure, however, resulted in a permanent colostomy and frequent perineal wound complications [9]. Low anterior resection has therefore grown in favor as an alternative surgical technique, but local recurrence remains a problem. Improvements in surgical technique have not been limited to sphincter preservation. TME involves complete sharp surgical resection of all pelvic nodal tissue in conjunction with a rectal cancer. Using this technique, Heald and colleagues [10] reported a 5.0% local recurrence rate, which compared favorably to the best reported results of adjuvant studies conducted by the North Central Cancer Treatment Group (NCCTG) during the same period. The NCCTG reported a local recurrence rate of 25% using conventional surgery plus radiation, and a local recurrence rate of 13.5% using conventional surgery plus chemotherapy and radiation [11]. Although direct comparison of these results is not scientifically valid, the importance of TME cannot be ignored as a surgical technique for rectal cancer [12]. These surgical results, however, have not yet been duplicated. TME alone therefore is currently not a standard therapy for stage T3 with N+ disease; adjuvant therapy with fluoropyrimidines and radiation is a category 1 National Comprehensive Cancer Network recommendation [13].

Preoperative/neoadjuvant therapy for rectal cancer may provide potential benefits of downstaging of the lesion, increased margin clearance, possible sphincter preservation, decreased tumor spillage intraoperatively, and improved tissue oxygenation and hence radiation efficacy, aside from limiting small bowel radiation that may occur postoperatively. Generally, the pathologic CR rates with neoadjuvant therapy are 10% to 20% and the incidence of local recurrence is about 3% to 10%. This improvement is achieved at the expense of 15% to 25% grade 3 toxicity.

LAPAROSCOPIC COLON RESECTION

> There must be a final limit to the development of manipulative surgery. The knife cannot always have fresh fields for conquest....Very little remains for the boldest devise or the most dexterous to perform.
> —Sir John Erichsen, Introductory Address at University College, The Lancet, 1873;2:489-90

This quotation from the nineteenth century demonstrates how we often fail to anticipate what we cannot foresee. Minimally invasive surgery (MIS) is rapidly evolving throughout surgery. The modern trained general surgeon, surgical oncologist, and colorectal specialist are expanding the role of laparoscopy in the treatment of colorectal cancer. New indications and contraindications are emerging that may be modified with further experience. It is essential that cancer treatment is enhanced and not compromised by this new technique. Whether laparoscopy for colon cancer is ultimately embraced or rejected by the medical community is currently unknown. All clinicians involved in the diagnosis and treatment of colorectal cancer must understand how laparoscopy impacts on cancer care.

MIS slowly entered into colorectal surgery, possibly because of the technical complexity of colon surgery, which requires mobilization of large segments of bowel, dividing large blood vessels in the mesentery, and anastomosis of the enteric system, with inherent leak and infectious complications. Relative contraindications include: inadequate surgeon experience, prior surgery precluding safe dissection, and bowel obstruction that limits bowel mobility and intraperitoneal visualization. Certain situations entail more complex and difficult surgery. For example, obesity or rectal cancers seem to have the highest complication and conversion rates. There seem to be few absolute contraindications for laparoscopic surgery for colorectal cancer. With early cancer, curative MIS has been performed for all standard segmental colon resections with acceptable results. With advanced cancer, MIS may provide alternatives not usually considered, such as laparoscopic diversion of an obstructing rectal cancer, palliative resection, or bypass. When adequate cancer surgery cannot be performed for any reason, early conversion to open technique must be performed.

LAPAROSCOPIC EQUIPMENT AND TECHNIQUES

Successful laparoscopy requires adequate surgical training and adequate technical equipment. The equipment includes excellent video equipment; straight or zero-degree, angled or 30- or 45-degree laparoscopes of various diameters; specialized staplers; and other instruments. With better capture technology and brighter light sources, smaller-diameter laparoscopes can be used (from 10 mm down to 5 mm). Small (2 mm) scopes exist but these instruments may not be appropriate for oncologic colon resection. The video camera typically captures two-dimensional images that are directly in line with the lens using rigid instruments. Recent, exciting technical innovations include flexible laparoscopes and three-dimensional systems. With these innovations, the principles of dissection and anastomosis remain the same; most of these innovations have not significantly improved the basic technology for performing colon surgery.

Major improvements have been made in cutting and dissection instruments. Initially, laparoscopic surgeons divided the mesentery with electrocautery, ties, and metallic clip appliers. This technique was slow, and the clips had an unfortunate tendency to be dislodged during the procedure resulting in intraoperative hemorrhage. Recently developed instruments, such as ultrasonic shears (Harmonic scalpel) and vessel-sealing cautery shears (Ligasure), permit rapid, bloodless dissection. These instruments require little training and experience. New devices promise further improvements. Recently developed laparoscopic stapling devices that can be deployed through 12-mm ports come in a variety of thicknesses and lengths. They can be used on bowel or major vessels. Straight and circular staplers allow for many choices in anastomosis.

LAPAROSCOPIC RIGHT AND LEFT HEMICOLECTOMY

The preparation for laparoscopic colon resection is similar to that for conventional surgery. Several differences should be emphasized. Because the surgeon cannot palpate the colon, the cancer must be precisely localized preoperatively. Colonoscopic tattooing is recommended for small lesions because colonoscopic localization and colonic measurements are notoriously inaccurate when approached transperitoneally. External clues often suffice to localize large apple-core or serosally involved cancers. The operating surgeon should encircle the cancer from afar rather than palpate and manipulate the cancer. In selected cases, a radiographic contrast study, such as a contrast enema or CT scan, provides a roadmap. Intraoperative colonoscopy to localize a cancer is time consuming, fills the limited space within the peritoneal cavity with intraluminal gas, and renders it more difficult to manipulate the bowel and perform an anastomosis. The requirements for bowel cleansing and for general anesthesia are the same for laparoscopy as with open surgery. Epidural catheters are seldom required for postoperative pain management.

Laparoscopic right hemicolectomy is the simplest and easiest colonic MIS. The patient is positioned supine with the left arm tucked to increase the space for the surgeon and surgical assistant. In select cases lithotomy positioning may be used, but the perineum need not be prepped. Ports are placed and the colon is mobilized by gentle medial retraction of the lateral and inferior attachments. The transverse and ascending colon should become freely mobile to the midline. A 6-cm long incision is then made for specimen retrieval. Mesentery and bowel division can be performed extracorporeally with hand-sewn or stapled ileotransverse anastomosis. The mesenteric defect should be closed and the bowel returned to the abdominal cavity.

Laparoscopic left colon resection is somewhat different. The patient is positioned with the legs spread apart to allow access to the anus (Fig. 7). Ports are placed and the colon mobilized as described before (Fig. 8). The mesentery and distal colon are often divided with a linear stapler. A small incision is performed to remove the specimen. Intestinal continuity is restored by transanal insertion of a circular stapling device. The patient is left with several small incisions. Postoperative recovery is usually rapid.

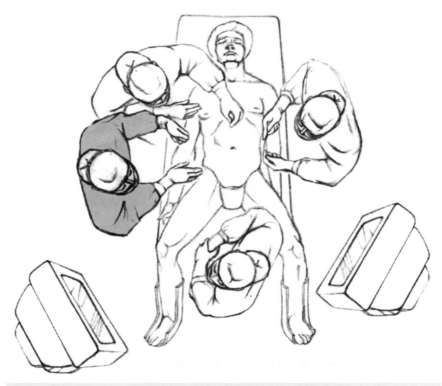

Fig. 7. Patient position and location of surgical team for laparoscopic left colon resection. (*From* Scott-Conner CEH, editor. Chassin's operative strategy in colon and rectal surgery. New York: Springer Verlag; 2006; with kind permission of Springer Science and Business Media.)

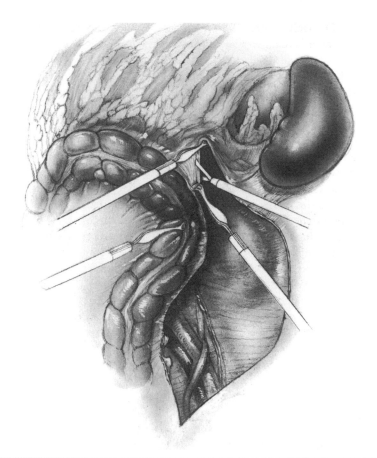

Fig. 8. Laparoscopic mobilization of splenic flexure during left colon resection. (*From* Scott-Conner CEH, editor. Chassin's operative strategy in colon and rectal surgery. New York: Springer Verlag; 2006; with kind permission of Springer Science and Business Media.)

TRAINING OF LAPAROSCOPIC SURGEONS

Laparoscopically assisted colectomy has evolved from a clinical experiment into an accepted procedure in selected surgical communities. Early reports demonstrated a long learning curve, associated with a technically demanding procedure. Fowler and colleagues [14] reported a 40% complication rate for the first 10 cases and a 0% complication rate for the next 30 cases. Bennett and colleagues [15] reported a less dramatic learning curve, but noted a complication rate of more than 10% until more than 39 cases have been performed. Generally, 30 cases are needed to become proficient in this technique. Conversion rates parallel the learning curve. They range from 0% to 42% (average 14%). MIS is converted to open surgery for multiple reasons. The conversion usually reflects sound surgical judgment. The benefits of MIS cannot come at the expense of adequate cancer surgery. Proper oncologic technique takes precedence over laparoscopic maneuvers. The well-trained surgeon should be able to convert to an open procedure when adequate laparoscopic resection cannot be achieved.

PORT SITE RECURRENCE

A working definition of port site recurrence is early cancer recurrence at a local incision after laparoscopy or thoracoscopy. This phenomenon is described in the literature using various terms, including metastasis, recurrence, and implant. Port site metastasis implies hematogenous or lymphatic spread and this term is often avoided for this reason. Implant and recurrence are equally good terms that are often used interchangeably. Soon after laparoscopic cholecystectomy became commonplace, cutaneous seeding of a port site was reported after laparoscopic resection of an unapparent gallbladder cancer [16]. Interestingly, this phenomenon is not specific to cancer. Endometrial implants have been reported following diagnostic laparoscopy for endometriosis [17]. Recurrence at the port site in benign and malignant diseases implies that the phenomenon is a local wound problem rather than a metastatic phenomenon.

Two main theories explain port site recurrence. First, indirect contamination, commonly called the "chimney effect," can occur when a pressure gradient between the pneumoperitoneum and ambient air drives cancer-contaminated fluid or air into subcutaneous tissue at the port site. Port site recurrences have occurred in gasless laparoscopy and thoracoscopy, however, where pressure gradients are unlikely. Second, direct contamination can occur when viable cancer cells are conveyed into the subcutaneous tissue by way of surgical instruments or during cancer extraction. Recurrences have been reported at ports sites that were not used for cancer manipulation or cancer extraction, however. Presently, neither theory can completely explain all port site recurrences, but neither theory can be completely discounted.

Because trocar recurrence is rare, most clinical data on this subject come from case reports or retrospective series. In large MIS colon cancer series, the risk for local and trocar recurrence parallels the risk in open surgical series. The currently reported port site recurrence rate is 0.0% to 0.5% (see trials discussed later). This rate compares favorably with incisional recurrence rates in open colon cancer surgery.

LAPAROSCOPY AND IMMUNOSUPPRESSION

Surgical trauma causes temporary cell-mediated immunosuppression, which can be measured as a decline in lymphocyte and neutrophil chemotaxis and as impaired antigen presentation. Does the compromised immunity from an open laparotomy have a detrimental oncologic effect? Can MIS decrease the immunosuppression and improve cancer outcome? Several studies have compared the systemic stress response from MIS versus open surgery. Cytokine release (including interleukin 6 and 10, C-reactive protein, and granulocyte elastase) seems to be less pronounced in the MIS group [18]. Theoretically, decreasing surgical trauma by MIS may better preserve immune function and benefit the cancer patient.

LAPAROSCOPIC CLINICAL TRIALS

Laparoscopic resection of colon cancer remains investigational in many regions of the United States. Clinical experience ranges from case series to retrospective reviews, with randomized controlled trials only recently reported. After completing the learning curve, the laparoscopic approach seems to have benefits over the standard open technique in less frequent hernia formation or small bowel obstruction, but does not seem to lower the rates of anastomotic leaks and wound infections or reduce the amount of blood loss. Numerous clinical trials have shown equivalent surgical margins and lymph node retrieval rates. Laparoscopic surgery causes less postoperative pain and earlier return of bowel function. With experienced surgeons and excellent technical hospital support, MIS seems to have the same complication rate as conventional surgery. Unfortunately, during the learning curve dramatic and otherwise highly unusual complications have been reported, such as major vascular injuries, uncontrolled bowel perforations with gross contamination, and missed lesions.

With growing experience in early enteral feeding of MIS patients, surgeons have explored a more aggressive feeding strategy after conventional open surgery. Many surgical patients can tolerate feeding much earlier than appreciated. Early feeding following surgery may be possible for MIS and conventional surgery, thus negating this benefit of MIS.

Numerous large clinical series examine the long-term surgical safety of colorectal MIS. Two large retrospective case series have demonstrated equivalent survival with MIS compared with national surgical standards, including comparisons to the National Cancer Database and Surveillance, Epidemiology and End Results. Two recent, large, well-designed, multi-institutional, randomized clinical trials compared the disease-free interval and overall survival for MIS versus open surgery (872 patients in Clinical Outcomes of Surgical Therapy (COST) and 794 patients in Conventional verses Laparoscopic-Assisted Surgery In patients with Colorectal Cancer (CLASICC) trial) [19,20]. Both trials concluded that MIS oncologic surgery could be performed in experienced hands (Table 1) [21,22].

In conclusion, with improving surgical instruments and technology and further surgical experience, laparoscopy should become an increasingly viable surgical option for patients who have colon cancer.

Table 1
Surgical outcomes comparing MIS and open techniques

Trial	Technique	Disease-free survival	Overall survival	Port site recurrence
COST [21]	MIS	84%	86%	<1%
	Open	82% (P = NS)	85% (P = NS)	<1% (P = NS)
CLASICC [22]	MIS	66%	68%	2.5%
	Open	68% (P = NS)	67% (P = NS)	0.6% (P = NS)

Abbreviations: COST, clinical outcomes of surgical therapy; CLASSICC, Conventional verses laparoscopic-assisted surgery in patients with colorectal cancer.

References

[1] Jemal A, Siegel R, Ward E, et al. Cancer statistics, 2007. CA Cancer J Clin 2007;57(1): 43–66.

[2] Parkin DM, Bray F, Ferlay J, et al. Global Cancer Statistics, 2002. CA Cancer J Clin 2005;55:74–108.

[3] Wolmark N, Rockette H, Fisher B, et al. The benefit of leucovorin-modulated fluorouracil as postoperative adjuvant therapy for primary colon cancer: results from National Surgical Adjuvant Breast and Bowel Project protocol C-03. J Clin Oncol 1993;11:1879–87.

[4] Moertel CG, Fleming TR, Macdonald JS, et al. Fluorouracil plus levamisole as effective adjuvant therapy after resection of Stage III colon carcinoma: a final report. Ann Intern Med 1995;122:321–6.

[5] Greene FL, Page DL, Fleming ID, et al, editors. American Joint Committee on Cancer Staging manual. 6th edition. Philadelphia: Springer; 2002.

[6] Ruo L, Gougoutas C, Paty PB, et al. Elective bowel resection for incurable stage IV colorectal cancer: prognostic variables for asymptomatic patients. J Am Coll Surg 2003;196:722–8.

[7] Tebbutt NC, Norman AR, Cunningham D, et al. Intestinal complications after chemotherapy for patients with unresected primary colorectal cancer and synchronous metastases. Gut 2003;52:568–73.

[8] Scoggins CR, Meszoely IM, Blanke CD, et al. Nonoperative management of primary colorectal cancer in patients with stage IV disease. Ann Surg Oncol 1999;6:651–7.

[9] Yeatman TJ, Bland KI. Sphincter-saving procedures for distal carcinoma of the rectum. Ann Surg 1989;209(1):1–18.

[10] MacFarlane J, Ryall R, Heald R. Mesorectal excision for rectal cancer. Lancet 1993;341(8843):457–60.

[11] Krook J, Moertel C, Gunderson L, et al. Effective surgical adjuvant therapy for high risk rectal carcinoma. N Engl J Med 1991;324:709–15.

[12] Birbeck K, Macklin C, Tiffin N, et al. Rates of circumferential resection margin involvement vary between surgeons and predict outcomes in rectal cancer surgery. Ann Surg 2002;235(4):449–57.

[13] Colon Cancer Clinical Practice Guidelines in Oncology. NCCN practice guidelines. National Comprehensive Cancer Network 2003;1(1):54–63. Available at: http://www.nccn.org/professionals/physician_gls/PDF/colon.pdf. Accessed February 1, 2008.

[14] Fowler DL, White SA, Anderson CA. Laparoscopic colon resection: 60 cases. Surg Laparosc Endosc 1995;5(6):468–71.

[15] Bennett CL, Stryker SJ, Ferreira MR, et al. The learning curve for laparoscopic colorectal surgery. Preliminary results from a perspective analysis of 1194 laparoscopic-assisted colectomies. Arch Surg 1997;132(1):41–4 [discussion: 45].

[16] Drouard F, Delamarre J, Capron JP. Cutaneous seeding of gallbladder cancer after laparoscopic cholecystectomy. N Engl J Med 1991;325(18):1316.

[17] Healy JT, Wilkinson NW, Sawyer M. Abdominal wall endometrioma in a laparoscopic trocar tract: a case report. Am Surg 1995;61(11):962–3.

[18] Hildebrandt U, Kessler K, Plusczyk T, et al. Surg Endosc 2003;17(2):242–6 [Epub Oct 29, 2002].

[19] Patankar SK, Larach SW, Ferrara A, et al. Dis Colon Rectum 2003;46(5):601–11.

[20] Lujan HJ, Plasencia G, Jacobs M, et al. Dis Colon Rectum 2002;45(4):491–501.

[21] Clinical Outcomes of Surgical Therapy Study Group. A comparison of laparoscopically assisted and open colectomy for colon cancer. N Engl J Med 2004;350:2050–9.

[22] Guillou PJ, Quirke P, Thorpe H, et al. Short-term endpoints of conventional versus laparoscopic-assisted surgery in patients with colorectal cancer (MRC CLASICC trial): multicentre, randomised controlled trial. Lancet 2005;365:1718–26.

Gastroenterol Clin N Am 37 (2008) 269–285

The Role of Radiation Therapy for Colorectal Cancer

John M. Robertson, MD

Department of Radiation Oncology, William Beaumont Hospital, 3601 West Thirteen Mile Road, Royal Oak, MI 48073, USA

Radiation therapy (RT) has been used to treat cancers for more than a century. It damages cellular deoxyribonucleic acid (DNA), leading to aborted cellular reproduction and death of the daughter cells. Fractionated treatment (the administration of smaller doses 5 days per week for a number of weeks) was discovered empirically early in the development of RT to be beneficial because fractionation permitted a higher total dose of RT to be administered with improved therapeutic efficacy and less toxicity to adjacent normal tissue.

Modern RT uses X rays produced by a linear accelerator. Depth of penetration is controlled by the energy used to produce the X rays and multiple tungsten leaves are used to shape the irradiated volume. Under computer control, some common RT plans can use seven different beam directions, with nine different beam shapes per direction, for a total of up to 7×9 or 63 beams, an advance from the traditional administration of 2 to 4 RT beams. The unit dose is the Gray (Gy) which is the deposition of one joule of energy per kilogram of tissue equivalent water. One centigray (cGy) equals the previously used unit of one rad.

A course of RT administered for curative intent for solid malignancy typically lasts 6 to 8 weeks, depending on the cancer. Adjuvant RT is usually given for 5 to 6 weeks, whereas palliative treatment can be accomplished in from 1 day to 3 weeks. The standard fractionated RT dose administered each day for either primary or adjuvant treatment is typically 1.8 or 2 Gy (called standard course of RT herein). It is usually 1.8 Gy per day for 28 fractions (treatments) administered 5 days per week, for a total dose of 50.4 Gy when used adjuvantly for rectal cancer. When the dose per day is increased, the total number of days is correspondingly decreased to limit the risks for injury to normal tissue from the increasing dose per fraction. "Short-course" RT referred to in this article consists of 5 Gy per day for only 5 days for a total dose of 25 Gy.

E-mail address: jrobertson@beaumont.edu

0889-8553/08/$ – see front matter
doi:10.1016/j.gtc.2007.12.010

RECTAL CANCER

Adjuvant Postoperative Treatment

Postoperative chemotherapy and RT was the standard of care for a number of years in patients who had resected transmural (T3) or lymph node positive (N+) rectal cancer based on three pivotal trials. First, in the Gastrointestinal Tumor Study Group (GITSG), 227 patients were randomized to observation; postoperative RT alone; postoperative 5-fluorouracil (5-FU) and semustine chemotherapy alone; or postoperative RT, 5-FU, and semustine [1]. This trial found that disease-free and overall survival were significantly better in the group receiving combined postoperative RT and chemotherapy [2]. Second, in the National Surgical Adjuvant Breast and Bowel Project (NSABP), 555 patients who had T3 or N+ tumors were randomized to observation, postoperative RT, or postoperative 5-FU with semustine and vincristine [3]. This trial concluded that disease-free and overall survival were better with adjuvant chemotherapy, but that adjuvant RT was associated with only a lower locoregional recurrence rate. Third, in the North Central Cancer Treatment Group (NCCTG), 204 patients were randomized to postoperative RT alone or postoperative RT with 5-FU preceded by 5-FU and semustine [4]. Like the GITSG trial, the NCCTG study found a significant disease-free and survival benefit for adjuvant postoperative combined RT and chemotherapy. All three studies showed that adjuvant postoperative RT with chemotherapy produced the best 5-year survival (Table 1). Moreover, pelvic recurrence rates were the lowest in the adjuvant postoperative RT with chemotherapy arms (Table 2). These three studies prompted the National Institutes of Health (NIH) to recommend in 1990 adjuvant postoperative RT with chemotherapy for patients who have transmural or lymph node–positive rectal cancer, although semustine was recommended only in a research setting because of an increased risk for leukemia and chronic renal toxicity [5]. Indeed, a subsequent trial concluded that semustine was unnecessary [6].

Chemotherapy and radiation therapy

Since 1990, most prospective trials of postoperative therapy for transmural or lymph node–positive rectal cancer have focused on the method of 5-FU delivery during RT and the optimal chemotherapeutic combination before and after RT administration. 5-FU helps sensitize malignant cells to RT [7]. It is therefore logical to combine a 24-hour continuous infusion of 5-FU with RT, so that

Table 1

Five-year survival rates for the three key randomized trials supporting adjuvant postoperative radiation therapy with chemotherapy for T3 or N+ rectal cancer

Study	Observation	Adjuvant chemotherapy	Adjuvant RT	Adjuvant chemotherapy + RT
GITSG [1]	43%	56%	52%	59%
NSABP [3]	43%	53%	41%	—
NCCTG [4]	—	—	47%	58%

Table 2
Five-year pelvic recurrence rates for the three key randomized trials supporting adjuvant postoperative radiation therapy with chemotherapy for T3 or N+ rectal cancer

Study	Observation (%)	Adjuvant chemotherapy (%)	Adjuvant RT (%)	Adjuvant chemotherapy + RT (%)
GITSG [1]	25	27	20	11
NSABP [3]	25	21	16	—
NCCTG [4]	—	—	25	14

every dose of radiation would be sensitized as compared with bolus 5-FU infusion, in which RT would be sensitized only for the 10 days of a typical 28-day RT course during which 5-FU was administered. This concept was verified by a randomized trial that showed improved 4-year survival in the continuous infusion arm versus the bolus arm (70% versus 60%) [6]. The pattern of improvement suggested the benefit was due mostly to reduced metastases, however. As a result, another study tested bolus 5-FU infusion before and after continuous 5-FU infusion during RT against continuous infusion of 5-FU before, during, and after RT [8]. A third arm tested whether addition of the biomodulator leucovorin to bolus 5-FU before, during, and after RT could obviate the need for continuous 5-FU infusion. After a median follow-up of more than 5 years, there were no differences in disease-free or overall survival, but less hematologic toxicity in the continuous infusion arm of 5-FU. Biomodulation of 5-FU was also studied in a four-arm trial, using bolus 5-FU in each arm, in a study begun before release of the infusional data [9]. This trial demonstrated that addition of leucovorin, levamisole, or both was not superior to bolus 5 FU alone. On the basis of these randomized trials, the optimal postoperative therapy seemed to be bolus 5-FU infusion for four cycles with continuous infusion of 5-FU during the approximately 5- to 6-week long RT course.

The need for RT has not been definitively established, however, when at least four cycles of adjuvant chemotherapy are given. The original GITSG trial was relatively small: 58 patients were in the observation arm, 48 were in the chemotherapy-alone arm, and 46 were in the combined modality arm [1]. The NCCTG study tested RT only against RT with chemotherapy but did not incorporate a chemotherapy-alone arm [4]. This evidence led the NSABP to perform a randomized trial of postoperative chemotherapy, with or without RT, in 694 patients who had Dukes' stage B (N = 207) or stage C (N = 487) tumors [10]. Although the cumulative incidence at 5 years of locoregional recurrence was significantly lower in the RT group (8% versus 13%), there was no disease-free or overall survival benefit from the addition of RT, in contrast to earlier NIH recommendations [5]. Subgroup analysis provided support that RT benefited patients younger than 60 years old ($P = .007$ for overall survival) or patients undergoing abdominoperineal resection ($P = .007$ for relapse-free survival and $P = .07$ for overall survival) [10].

Adjuvant postoperative RT has been supported by two other recent randomized trials. In one trial, 218 patients who had resected transmural or lymph node–positive rectal cancer were randomized to receive either RT alone versus RT with concurrent 5-FU and levamisole followed by five additional cycles of chemotherapy [11]. Although this trial lacked a chemotherapy-only arm, the addition of concurrent chemotherapy to RT increased the relative risk for death by 33% ($P = .18$) compared with the RT-only arm [12]. Although this increase may have been related to the increased rate of severe enteritis in the concurrent chemotherapy plus RT arm (14% versus 5%; $P = .03$), there was only one chemotherapy-related death in the chemotherapy plus RT arm, suggesting that other factors were involved [11]. Another recent randomized trial supported use of adjuvant postoperative RT in 308 patients who had resected transmural or lymph node–positive disease who were randomized to chemotherapy (5-FU with leucovorin) plus RT with the RT either given early (during first cycle of chemotherapy) or late (during third cycle of chemotherapy) [13]. During a median follow-up of only 37 months, this study showed a significant increase in disease-free survival for the early RT arm (81% versus 70%) but did not show an overall survival difference. This finding implied that RT did make a difference and that delays in RT administration may negatively impact on efficacy.

Selection of appropriate stages for radiation therapy

Selected patients may not need adjuvant RT; this may explain discrepancies between trials. A retrospective review of 117 patients who had T3 N0 rectal cancer suggested that neither RT nor chemotherapy was needed in patients treated with resection alone, who had favorable histologic features (well or moderately well differentiated, invading less than 2 mm into the perirectal fat, without lymphatic or venous vessel involvement) [14]. The 25 such patients had 10-year rates of local control and recurrence-free survival of 95% and 87%, respectively, versus 71% and 55% for 88 patients who did not have these features [14]. Data combining 3791 patients from five large North American randomized postoperative trials support the conclusion that adjuvant RT provides no additional survival benefit over adjuvant chemotherapy alone in patients who have T1-2 N1 or T3 N0 rectal cancer (Table 3) [15].

Studies have shown that the more lymph nodes assessed in lymph node–negative patients, the better the 5-year relapse ($P = .003$) and survival rates ($P = .02$), with the highest 5-year survival rate (82%) in patients who had

Table 3
Five-year overall survival rates of patients who have selected stages treated in the five large postoperative randomized trials

Stage	# patients	Adjuvant chemotherapy (%)	Adjuvant chemotherapy + RT (%)
T1/2 N1	355	85	78–83
T3 N0	1060	84	74–80

Data from Gunderson LL, Sargent DJ, Tepper JE, et al. Impact of T and N stage and treatment on survival and relapse in adjuvant rectal cancer: a pooled analysis. J Clin Oncol 2004;22:1785–96.

more than 13 lymph nodes assessed [16]. This effect was likely not therapeutic, in that removing more lymph nodes impacted on survival, because there was no similar benefit in lymph node–positive patients. Likely an increased lymph node harvest reflected an improved ability to detect lymph node metastases. Patients who had more than 13 lymph nodes examined were thus much more likely to be truly lymph node–negative. It therefore seems reasonable to consider adjuvant chemotherapy without RT in patients who have T1-2 N1 or T3 N0 rectal cancer if more than 13 lymph nodes were assessed, especially if a total mesorectal excision was done. Prospective studies, however, would be best to test this important change in therapy.

General recommendation for postoperative therapy
Currently, the most common schedule of adjuvant postoperative chemotherapy with RT is to administer two cycles of 5-FU–based chemotherapy, initiate RT with the third cycle, and follow this with two additional cycles of 5-FU–based chemotherapy [6,8,9]. The National Comprehensive Cancer Network, an alliance of 21 National Cancer Institute designated Comprehensive Cancer Centers, recommends four different alternatives for the initial chemotherapy-only portion of treatment: 5-FU alone, 5-FU with leucovorin, 5-FU with leucovorin and oxaliplatin, or capecitabine, because of disagreements among panel members (Table 4) [17]. Nevertheless, all these choices involve a delay in RT for at least 6 weeks from the initiation of chemotherapy. Because of the above report that RT during the first cycle of chemotherapy, compared with the third cycle, improves disease-free survival [13], further investigation of advancing RT to the first cycle of chemotherapy is warranted. Adjuvant therapy may also need to be individually tailored according to specific surgical staging, intermediate-risk versus high-risk cancers [15], or according to gender [10]. Studies of postoperative RT have been overshadowed by recent developments in preoperative therapy.

Preoperative Treatment
The concept of preoperative RT for rectal cancer has existed and been tested for decades. The first randomized trial was initiated in 1963 (see [18] for a summary of the randomized trials). Preoperative RT has been given from as few as

Table 4
Commonly accepted regimens for adjuvant chemoradiotherapy

Sequence	Stage	RT dose (total/dose per fraction)	Reference
Preoperative	Resectable	25 Gy/5Gy	[23,30,38]
	uT3/4, cT4, or uN+[a]	45 to 50.4 Gy/1.8 Gy	[24,28,30,33]
Postoperative	pT3 N0 or pT1/2 N1	None or 50.4 Gy/1.8 Gy	[1,5,6,8,9,15]
	Any pN+	45 to 50.4 Gy/1.8 Gy	[1,5,6,8,9]

All radiation schedules other than the short-course (25 Gy in 5-Gy fractions) should preferentially be given with chemotherapy. Both bolus 5-FU with leucovorin and continuous infusional 5-FU have been shown beneficial in randomized trials. Capecitabine may be equivalent but has not been randomized.
[a]Treatment of uN+ preoperatively is controversial; see text.

one fraction of 5 Gy to as many as 28 fractions and a total dose 50.4 Gy, both with and without chemotherapy [18]. When multiple randomized trials of preoperative RT were reported as negative, enthusiasm waned, and research efforts became focused on the appropriate patient selection and the optimal schedule of treatment for postoperative therapy.

Conversion of unresectable disease

Preoperative RT, with or without chemotherapy, however, still had a role for patients who had unresectable disease, to render the tumor resectable. The data were not solid because the presence of unresectable disease is relatively subjective and cannot be objective without mandatory exploratory laparotomy before treatment. In two prospective studies of preoperative chemotherapy and RT for patients deemed unresectable, the ultimate rate of curative, margin-negative resection was reported to be 61% (17 of 30 patients) with RT and continuous infusion of 5-FU [19] versus 85% (17 of 20 patients) for RT with bolus 5-FU and leucovorin [20]. The need for chemotherapy with preoperative RT in this setting has not been established, because earlier reports of RT alone found a complete resection rate of 75% (26 of 33 patients) [21]. Despite this uncertainty, however, the obvious efficacy of converting unresectable disease to resectable disease provided evidence of treatment efficacy and justified continued analysis of preoperative treatment. Currently, with more accurate preoperative staging [22], the publication of the Swedish Rectal Cancer Trial (Swedish RCT) [23], and the successful completion of the German Rectal Cancer Study Group (German RCSG) trial [24], the standard of care has shifted to rational application of preoperative therapy [25].

Benefits of preoperative treatment

Tumor shrinkage. Preoperative treatment is traditionally believed to have three advantages [25]. First, the tumor shrinks, allowing less radical surgery to be done with consequent preservation of the anal sphincter and a better quality of life. Single institution prospective studies support this concept, with reported conversion rates of 40% to 89% [26,27]. As with the difficulty in establishing the conversion rate from unresectable to resectable disease, determination of conversion to a sphincter-sparing procedure is limited and would ideally require surgical exploration to definitively establish the need for an abdominoperineal resection (APR), a requirement that is impractical. Reported improvement in sphincter preservation could thus reflect patient selection bias or subjectivity by the referring surgeon rather than a true treatment benefit. Other questions regarding the appropriate distal surgical margin, sphincter functionality, and quality of life of very low resections also remain to be answered.

Two published multi-institutional randomized trials of preoperative versus postoperative treatment required a surgical declaration of the intended procedure before randomization, but allowed that declaration to be changed during surgery. Although the NSABP R-03 study was not completed, the postoperative arm had 26 patients who had a pretreatment declaration that an APR was required and all 26 underwent the planned APR. In the preoperative arm, 22 had an APR planned, but only 16 required APR for a conversion rate of 27% [28]. The much larger, completed, German RCSG trial of preoperative versus postoperative treatment had 15 of 72 patients in the postoperative arm with a pretreatment declaration of APR requirement not undergoing APR, because 19% of patients had sphincter sparing based on improved evaluation with anesthetic relaxation of the pelvis [24]. The preoperative arm of the German RCSG study had 116 patients who had an APR planned, of whom 45 (39%) had a sphincter-sparing procedure after preoperative therapy. It thus appeared that the net conversion rate of patients from an APR to sphincter-sparing surgery because of preoperative treatment was 20% (derived from 39%−19%). It has traditionally been believed that short-course RT (25 Gy in 5 fractions), as given in the Swedish RCT [23], followed 1 week later by resection, did not allow enough time for an effect to permit sphincter-sparing surgery [29]. A randomized trial of preoperative short-course RT versus standard-course RT with chemotherapy found, despite significant downstaging, no evidence of increased sphincter sparing in the standard course group [30], in contrast to the German RCSG standard course experience [24]. This difference likely reflected subjective bias in that surgeons were reluctant to alter their planned procedure depending on tumor response [30].

Decreased toxicity. The second major potential benefit of preoperative compared with postoperative therapy is less acute toxicity, primarily less diarrhea [25]. Direct comparison of acute toxicity between studies is hampered by different toxicity criteria and selection bias inherent in nonrandomized trials. Studies of preoperative RT with chemotherapy have reported rates of severe diarrhea of 0%, 3%, or 11% [27,31,32]. These differences were likely partly attributable to the inclusion of chemotherapy and the variable chemotherapeutic agents used. For example, a randomized trial of preoperative RT alone compared with preoperative chemoradiotherapy found rates of severe diarrhea of 17% versus 34%, respectively, using a different toxicity scale than the above reports [33]. Studies of postoperative RT with chemotherapy have usually reported higher rates of severe diarrhea than studies of preoperative therapy, with a 14% to 35% incidence [4,6,9]. The rates also depend on the particular chemotherapeutic agent. When different studies using the same chemotherapy (bolus 5-FU with leucovorin) are compared, the rate of grade 3+ diarrhea was 11% for preoperative treatment [27] but 28% for postoperative treatment [9]. Most of the observed difference in clinical tolerability and diarrhea was attributable to inadvertent radiation of the small bowel during treatment. Based on this observation, routine use of a prone position and small bowel exclusion cradles for RT in rectal cancer is recommended [34]. Recent sophisticated three-dimensional analyses using multiple sets of CT scans in the treatment position during therapy have verified that preoperatively treated patients have significantly less irradiated small bowel than postoperatively treated patients [35].

The volume of small bowel irradiated is strongly correlated with the frequency of severe diarrhea [36].

Randomized trials of preoperative versus postoperative combined RT and chemotherapy have provided mixed results regarding diarrhea. Preliminary toxicity data from the NSABP R-03 trial on the first 116 enrolled patients showed that the incidence of grade 3 or worse diarrhea was much higher (23%) in the preoperative than the postoperative group (6%) [28]. The much larger, completed German RCSG study reported that grade 3 or worse diarrhea occurred in 12% of the preoperative group versus 18% of the postoperative group ($P = .04$) [24]. The same trial also found that the incidence of any grade 3 or worse acute toxicity was 27% for preoperatively treated patients versus 40% in postoperatively treated patients. Additionally, the incidence of any grade 3 or worse chronic toxicity was 14% in the preoperative group versus 24% in the postoperative group. When analyzing toxicity for all patients, however, including patients who for various reasons received no RT, there were no differences in either acute or chronic toxicity between the preoperative and postoperatively randomized groups [24].

Radiobiologic advantage. The third argument for preoperative treatment is that the presence of more radiation-sensitive oxygenated cells may be biologically advantageous [25] and may result in reduced tumor seeding, manifesting as lower pelvic and distant recurrence rates and improved survival. This concept is supported by the Swedish RCT [23]. In this study, 1168 patients younger than 80 years old who had resectable rectal cancer were randomized to short-course RT (25 Gy in 5 fractions) followed by surgery within 1 week versus surgery alone. After 5 years of follow-up, the local recurrence rate (11% versus 27%), cancer-specific survival (74% versus 65%), and overall survival (58% versus 48%) were all statistically significantly better in the preoperative RT group compared with the surgery-alone group [23]. Although this result disagreed with previous randomized trials, the Swedish RCT was the largest preoperative trial ever performed and was sufficiently powered to detect a 10% survival difference. Also, the Swedish RCT included more than 50% of eligible patients within Sweden during the enrollment period and was likely to be more generalizable than all other cancer trials [37]. In a meta-analysis, a particular dose of RT, used in both the Swedish RCT and in other trials, of a standard course of 46 Gy in 23 fractions, was associated with a 43% reduction in pelvic recurrence and a 22% reduction in rectal cancer mortality [18].

Total mesorectal excision (TME) instead of traditional blunt pelvic dissection may, however, obviate the observed survival benefit from short-course preoperative RT. In a large randomized study from the Dutch Colorectal Cancer Group (Dutch CCG), more than 1800 patients who had resectable rectal cancer were randomized to preoperative short-course RT, as in the Swedish RCT study, followed by TME versus TME alone with a median follow-up of nearly 5 years [38]. An update of this study reported in 2007 that overall survival rates were identical (64% versus 64%), although local recurrence rates were slightly different (6% with RT versus 11% without) [39]. Nevertheless, this same study group concluded that if the reduced local recurrence rate led to a survival advantage, short-course preoperative RT was therapeutically efficacious and cost-effective [40]. Another factor that may obviate the need for preoperative RT is selective application of postoperative RT with chemotherapy. The only trial that analyzed this issue was the German RCSG study of preoperative RT for 28 fractions (50.4 Gy) with concurrent chemotherapy compared with the same regimen given postoperatively, both of which were followed by four cycles of chemotherapy alone [24]. In this study, the overall 5-year survival was 76% for preoperative treatment versus 74% for postoperative treatment, although the incidence of local relapse was different at 6% versus 13%, respectively.

Overall preoperative experience. In summary, sphincter-sparing surgery was possible in an additional 20% of patients because of preoperative RT with chemotherapy. Toxicity was decreased, with a 6% lower rate of severe diarrhea, a 13% lower incidence of any grade 3+ acute toxicity, and a 10% lower incidence of any grade 3 or greater chronic toxicity [24]. The argument for a biologic advantage was substantiated by a 7% lower pelvic recurrence rate in preoperatively irradiated patients [24], although survival was equivalent for short-course preoperative RT when a TME was performed [38] and for standard-course preoperative RT with chemotherapy when postoperative RT with chemotherapy was given [24]. Commonly accepted regimens for preoperative therapy are shown in Table 4, although the short course (25 Gy in five fractions) is not in widespread use in North America.

Drawbacks of preoperative treatment
The primary drawback in routine preoperative treatment is overstaging leading to overtreatment. There is no controversy regarding patients who have fixed tumors because preoperative treatment has a well-established role in converting unresectable to resectable tumors. For other patients, clinical staging is usually accomplished by endorectal ultrasound. Preoperative treatment is offered to patients who have ultrasound-staged transmural extension (uT3) or lymph node involvement (uN+) [41]. Endorectal ultrasound is relatively accurate (80% accuracy) for T staging and N staging [22]. A pooled analysis of 11 studies, including T stage in 873 patients and N stage in 571 patients, reported that endorectal ultrasound was very accurate for T stage but only moderately accurate for N stage [42]. In this study, only 11% of uT3 patients, who would be offered preoperative treatment, were pathologically pT1 or pT2. The risk for overtreatment based on endorectal ultrasound for T staging was thus only about 10%, because 15% of pT2 patients would be expected to be eligible for postoperative therapy based on lymph node involvement. Overstaging of lymph node status was a potential issue, because 24% of uN+ patients ultimately were pathologically N0 [42]. The risk for overstaging the T stage at endorectal ultrasound may be much higher than 11%. In the largest single institution experience involving 545 patients, 28% of patients who were uT3

were pathologic T2 and 48% of patients who were uN+ were pathologic N0 [43]. This finding was not because of a learning curve: 88% of the endorectal ultrasounds were performed by colorectal surgeons highly experienced in rectal ultrasonography. If 15% of patients who were pT2 actually had lymph node involvement, as many as 25% of patients could be overtreated because of overstaging. The clinical experience in the German RCSG trial was intermediate between the 11% and 25% rates, with an overstaging incidence of 18% in the postoperative arm using the best available clinical staging [24].

Decision making for preoperative therapy

These data lead to a dilemma for physicians and patients in deciding between preoperative versus postoperative therapy. Does a 10% to 15% reduction in toxicity, a 20% improvement in sphincter sparing, and a 7% improvement in pelvic control justify a 20% chance that the patient is overstaged and overtreated? This question becomes even more problematic if one accepts that patients who are T3 N0 treated with a TME with an acceptable lymph node harvest may not need irradiation [15,16], and that preoperatively irradiated patients have the same survival as postoperatively irradiated patients [24]. Aside from overstaged uT3 patients, accurately staged uT3 patients who ultimately will be N0 need to be added to the overtreated group, likely around 28% [43], leading to a total of up to 50% of all patients who are uT3 who will be overtreated with RT, although they will still need chemotherapy. This issue should be investigated using sophisticated analysis, but this investigation seems unlikely given the difficulty in recruiting patients in the preoperative versus postoperative studies that led to failure to complete two of the three trials. The issue currently seems to be settled based on the German RSCG and Dutch CCG preoperative trials [24,38].

Surgery and Radiation Therapy

Surgical developments have impacted on the role of RT, especially the lower local recurrence rate reported with TME [24,38]. The Dutch CCG trial of short-course preoperative RT [38] and the German RCSG trial of preoperative versus postoperative standard-course RT with chemotherapy [24] required use of TME and found that local recurrence rates were improved by about 5% when preoperative treatment was used (Table 5). The ultimate rate of local recurrence may actually be higher, depending on the length of follow-up and the stage of disease. In the Swedish RCT study, the local recurrence curve did not plateau until after 7 years [23]. In the German RCSG trial, local recurrences were observed 5 years after treatment [24]. Aside from length of follow-up, the patient stage was also related to local recurrence rate, with N0 patients and N+ patients in the Swedish RCT exhibiting a 13% and a 20% lower local recurrence rate with RT, respectively [23]. An 11% benefit in N+ patients was also found in the Dutch CCG trial, with an overall 15% rate of local recurrence in the N+ group randomized to surgery only [38,39].

The contribution of TME to local control rates is not entirely clear. In one surgeon's personal experience of 532 resections done with diathermy or

Table 5
Local recurrence rates in selected studies

Study	TME used	RT course	Chemotherapy	Local recurrence rate (%)
Swedish RCT [23]	No	No	No	27
	No	25 Gy preop	No	11
Dutch CCG [38,39]	Yes	No	No	11
	Yes	25 Gy preop	No	6
German RCSG [24]	Yes	50.4 Gy preop	Yes	6
	Yes	55.8 Gy postop	Yes	13

Abbreviations: postop, postoperative treatment; preop, preoperative treatment; TME, total mesorectal excision.

scissors, without the sharp dissection required for TME, the 5-year local recurrence rate was only 7% [44]. With such a large sample size, adjuvant RT in only 33 patients (6%) and adjuvant chemotherapy in only 1 patient, the results likely reflected the surgical procedure itself. As with TME studies, there was a relationship between nodal positivity and local recurrence, with a local recurrence rate of 17% in the 190 lymph node–positive patients.

Assessment of pelvic control
Local recurrence rates may reflect symptomatic pelvic recurrences and may therefore understate the true pelvic failure rate. None of the prospective randomized trials required periodic CT assessment of the asymptomatic pelvis [8,9,23,24,38]. Instead, follow up always included clinical evaluation, with [9,24] or without [23] blood chemistries. Because abnormal liver function tests lead to evaluation of the asymptomatic liver, a direct comparison of distant failure rates to pelvic failure rates essentially compares rates of asymptomatic distant failure with symptomatic pelvic failure. Frankly, if comparisons of pelvic failure rates are used to compare effectiveness of therapies, then pelvic assessment should be optimized, or comparisons should be strictly limited to straightforward survival comparisons. A reasonable remedy would be to require pelvic assessment in prospective trials when either distant failure or pelvic symptoms were observed. Use of PET scans may remedy this problem because distant and pelvic failure can be assessed with this single study.

Complete clinical response to preoperative treatment
The appropriate surgical management of patients who have a complete clinical response to preoperative treatment is unknown. Because studies have reported residual microscopic disease in 70 of 93 patients who have a clinical complete response [45], radical surgery is still usually recommended. This approach is unproved, however. Some clinical data suggest, contrariwise, that complete pathologic response in the primary is associated with no lymph node metastases [46]. For example, a randomized trial of preoperative standard-course RT with chemotherapy found that patients who had a pathologic complete response or a partial response to a T1 tumor had a low rate of lymph node

metastases on radical resection (5% and 8%, respectively) [47]. In one prospective clinical study of 71 patients who had a complete clinical response, including a negative biopsy during proctoscopy 8 weeks after treatment, patients not undergoing radical surgery had a 5-year survival rate of 100% (92% disease-free survival), which was comparable to the 88% 5-year survival (83% disease-free survival) of 22 patients who had an incomplete clinical response, but a pathologic complete response in the specimen [48]. Alternatively, local excision after preoperative therapy is supported by retrospective evidence in responding T3 tumors [49] and by preliminary data from a prospective study of uT2 tumors [50]. More clinical studies are necessary before this can be recommended, even if the concept is attractive.

Radiation therapy after wide local excision
It is unknown whether postoperative RT with chemotherapy can replace radical resection in patients who have T2 tumors undergoing wide local excision. No randomized trials are available, but two prospective multi-institutional, non-randomized trials are relevant. In the first trial, patients were randomized to observation or one of two treatment arms combining RT with chemotherapy, depending on the presence of several adverse pathologic features [51]. The pelvic failure rate in T2 patients was 4 of 25 (16%) and in T3 patients was 3 of 13 (23%) during a median follow-up of 6 years. The second trial registered 51 patients who had T2 tumors treated with RT and bolus 5-FU chemotherapy [52]. With a median follow-up of 4 years, 7 patients (14%) who had T2 tumors had pelvic failure. This failure rate was higher than that reported for radical surgery, especially TME (see Table 5). These data raise concerns that this approach may increase the risk for local failure in some patients. Some data suggest that radical surgery is more appropriate even for T1 tumors. A single-institution, retrospective study reported that in T1 tumors with similar risk profiles, the estimated local recurrence rate at 5 years was 15% for patients treated with local excision alone versus 3% for radical surgery [53]. Nevertheless, the availability of a sphincter-preserving option for patients who have selected distal rectal tumors and the success of surgical salvage [51,52] has to be integrated into the clinical decision.

Functional Outcome and Quality of Life
Because survival outcomes were equivalent [24], comparisons of preoperative to postoperative therapy and strategies of downstaging to less radical surgical procedures depend on the functionality of the retained sphincter and impact on quality of life (QOL). The reported results of overall long-term bowel function in irradiated patients are mixed. Acceptable bowel complication rates were reported in the German RCSG randomized trial of preoperative standard course treatment versus postoperative treatment [24]. This landmark trial found long-term gastrointestinal side effects in 9% of the preoperatively treated group versus 15% of the postoperatively treated group, including a 2% and 1% rate of reoperation, respectively. The incidence of anastomotic strictures was markedly different, with 9% in the preoperative group versus 15% in the

postoperative group. Although these differences favor preoperative treatment, the rate of long-term effects was essentially identical when all patients were included, including those not eligible for postoperative treatment because of the pathologic findings [24]. Similarly, the randomized trial examining all four possible combinations of preoperative versus postoperative treatment with RT or chemotherapy found no significant differences in the incidence of late side effects among the four treatment groups [33]. In both trials, however, all patients received some form of RT.

Other studies have reported higher rates of long-term bowel dysfunction in irradiated versus unirradiated patients. Using a telephone questionnaire approximately 3.5 years after surgery, patients who had been irradiated reported a median of seven bowel movements per day versus two for patients who had not been irradiated, with occasional incontinence in 39% versus 7%, respectively [54]. In a mailed questionnaire to 400 patients who did not have recurrent or metastatic disease in the national rectal cancer database for Norway (80% questionnaire completion rate) patients who had been irradiated who had an anterior resection had a significantly higher median number of bowel movements per day than patients who had not been irradiated (6 versus 2.5), more incontinence, and reduced well-being [55]. Similar findings were reported in the Swedish RCT study and the Dutch CCG studies of short-course preoperative RT [56,57]. Thirty percent of patients who had been irradiated reported that they had an impaired social life because of bowel dysfunction versus 10% in the surgery-alone group [56]. This difference may not affect a person's overall health-related QOL, however, which was reported to be equivalent between the preoperative RT and surgery-only arms of the Dutch CCG study [58].

These reports are subject to limitations. Selection bias is always present in surveys, given that some questionnaires are not returned and patients who have complaints are more likely to return the questionnaires than patients who feel well. Another source of bias is that assessment of QOL was done in patients free of disease. Ideally, a comparison of different therapeutic strategies would include simultaneous assessment of QOL in patients who have disease recurrence to determine whether the negative QOL aspects of treatment are counterbalanced by the positive QOL aspects of disease control.

Objective data using anorectal manometry have been inconclusive. In one study of 21 patients irradiated with short-course preoperative RT versus 43 treated with surgery alone, the irradiated patients had significantly lower resting and squeeze pressures and evidence of anal sphincter scarring [59]. Another study using anorectal manometry before and after treatment found no significant difference in resting or squeeze pressures among 20 patients treated with standard course preoperative RT [60].

COLON CANCER

In retrospective reviews, adherence or invasion of colon cancer to adjacent structures and involvement of the resected margin are associated with high rates of local cancer treatment failure. In a large single institution review, patients who had resected T4 N0 and T4 N1 colon cancer had local failure rates of 31% and 53% with surgery alone, which was reduced to only 7% and 28%, respectively, with the addition of adjuvant RT [61]. The only randomized study of this issue closed after recruitment of only 187 of 700 planned patients, but did report identical local recurrence rates of 19% with or without RT [62]. Aside from early study closure, another confounding issue in this trial is optional use of abdominopelvic CT scans, so that the actual incidence of local failure may have been higher in both groups. Nevertheless, survival was equivalent between arms during a median follow-up of more than 6 years, suggesting that any potential benefit of improved local control was unassociated with improved survival.

SUMMARY

Postoperative RT with chemotherapy has been the standard of care for a number of years for transmural or lymph node–positive rectal cancer. The use of postoperative treatment has been overshadowed by recent research results in preoperative RT with chemotherapy. Preoperative RT with chemotherapy can downstage low rectal cancer, allowing more frequent sphincter-sparing surgery, reducing toxicity, and possibly improving pelvic control. Recent developments in surgery with TME and chemotherapy may require reevaluation of this strategy, however. Studies in colon cancer have also led to questioning of routine RT for T3 or T4 tumors because of no evident survival advantage, although the optimal use remains to be defined in T4 or margin-positive colon cancer.

Acknowledgments

The author wishes to acknowledge Maria M. Hardy, RN, MSN, for editing and proofreading assistance.

References

[1] Gastrointestinal Tumor Study Group. Prolongation of the disease-free interval in surgically treated rectal carcinoma. N Engl J Med 1985;312:1465–72.

[2] Thomas PRM, Lindblad AS. Adjuvant postoperative radiotherapy and chemotherapy in rectal carcinoma: a review of the Gastrointestinal Tumor Study Group experience. Radiother Oncol 1988;13:245–52.

[3] Fisher B, Wolmark N, Rockette H, et al. Postoperative adjuvant chemotherapy or radiation therapy for rectal cancer: results from NSABP protocol R-01. J Natl Cancer Inst 1988;80: 21–9.

[4] Krook JE, Moertel CG, Gunderson LL, et al. Effective surgical adjuvant therapy for high-risk rectal carcinoma. N Engl J Med 1991;324:709–15.

[5] NIH consensus conference on adjuvant therapy for patients with colon and rectal cancer. J Am Med Assoc 1990;264:1444–50.

[6] O'Connell MJ, Martenson JA, Wieand HS, et al. Improving adjuvant therapy for rectal cancer by combining protracted-infusion fluorouracil with radiation therapy after curative surgery. N Engl J Med 1994;331:502–7.

[7] Lawrence TS, Maybaum J. Fluoropyrimidines as radiation sensitizers. Semin Radiat Oncol 1993;3:20–8.

[8] Smalley SR, Benedetti JK, Williamson SK, et al. Phase III trial of fluorouracil-based chemotherapy regimens plus radiotherapy in postoperative adjuvant rectal cancer: GI INT 0144. J Clin Oncol 2006;24:3542–7.

[9] Tepper JE, O'Connell MJ, Petroni GR, et al. Adjuvant postoperative fluorouracil-modulated chemotherapy combined with pelvic radiation therapy for rectal cancer: initial results of Intergroup 0114. J Clin Oncol 1997;15:2030–9.

[10] Wolmark N, Wieand HS, Hyams DM, et al. Randomized trial of postoperative adjuvant chemotherapy with or without radiotherapy for carcinoma of the rectum: national surgical adjuvant breast and bowel project protocol R-02. J Natl Cancer Inst 2000;92:388–96.

[11] Cafiero F, Gipponi M, Peressini A, et al. Preliminary analysis of a randomized clinical trial of adjuvant postoperative RT vs. postoperative RT plus 5-FU and levamisole in patients with TNM stage II-III resectable rectal cancer. J Surg Oncol 2000;75:80–8.

[12] Cafiero F, Gipponi M, Lionetto R, et al. Randomised clinical trial of adjuvant postoperative RT vs. sequential postoperative RT plus 5-FU and levamisole in patients with stage II-III resectable rectal cancer: a final report. J Surg Oncol 2003;83:140–6.

[13] Lee J-H, Lee J-H, Ahn J-H, et al. Randomized trial of postoperative adjuvant therapy in stage II and III rectal cancer to define the optimal sequence of chemotherapy and radiotherapy: a preliminary report. J Clin Oncol 2002;20:1751–8.

[14] Willett CG, Badizadegan K, Ancukiewicz M, et al. Prognostic factors in stage T3N0 rectal cancer. Do all patients require postoperative pelvic irradiation and chemotherapy? Dis Colon Rectum 1999;42:167–73.

[15] Gunderson LL, Sargent DJ, Tepper JE, et al. Impact of T and N stage and treatment on survival and relapse in adjuvant rectal cancer: a pooled analysis. J Clin Oncol 2004;22:1785–96.

[16] Tepper JE, O'Connell MJ, Niedzwiecki D, et al. Impact of number of nodes retrieved on outcome in patients with rectal cancer. J Clin Oncol 2001;19:157–63.

[17] Engstrom PF, Benson AB III. Rectal cancer. Available at:http://www.nccn.org/professionals/physician_gls/PDF/rectal.pdf. Accessed January 29, 2008.

[18] Colorectal Cancer Collaborative Group. Adjuvant radiotherapy for rectal cancer: a systematic overview of 8507 patients from 22 randomised trials. Lancet 2001;358:1291–304.

[19] Rodel C, Grabenbauer GG, Matzel KE, et al. Extensive surgery after high-dose preoperative chemoradiotherapy for locally advanced recurrent rectal cancer. Dis Colon Rectum 2000;43:312–9.

[20] Minsky BD, Kemeny N, Cohen AM, et al. Preoperative high-dose leucovorin/5-fluorouracil and radiation therapy for unresectable rectal cancer. Cancer 1991;67:2859–66.

[21] Emami B, Pilepich M, Willett C, et al. Effect of preoperative irradiation on resectability of colorectal carcinomas. Int J Radiat Oncol Biol Phys 1982;8:1295–9.

[22] Heriot AG, Grundy A, Kumar D. Preoperative staging of rectal carcinoma. Br J Surg 1999;86:17–28.

[23] Swedish Rectal Cancer Trial. Improved survival with preoperative radiotherapy in resectable rectal cancer. N Engl J Med 1997;336:980–7.

[24] Sauer R, Becker H, Hohenberger W, et al. Preoperative versus postoperative chemoradiotherapy for rectal cancer. N Engl J Med 2004;351:1731–40.

[25] Minsky BD. Adjuvant therapy of resectable rectal cancer. Cancer Treat Rev 2002;28:181–8.

[26] Janjan NA, Khoo VS, Abbruzzese J, et al. Tumor downstaging and sphincter preservation with preoperative chemoradiation in locally advanced rectal cancer: the M.D. Anderson Cancer Center experience. Int J Radiat Oncol Biol Phys 1999;44:1027–38.

[27] Grann A, Feng C, Wong D, et al. Preoperative combined modality therapy for clinically resectable uT3 rectal adenocarcinoma. Int J Radiat Oncol Biol Phys 2001;49:987–95.

[28] Hyams DM, Mamounas EP, Petrelli N, et al. A clinical trial to evaluate the worth of preoperative multimodality therapy in patients with operable carcinoma of the rectum. A progress

report of the National Surgical Adjuvant Breast and Bowel Project protocol R-03. Dis Colon Rectum 1997;40:131–9.

[29] Marijnen CAM, Nagtegaal ID, Klein Kranenbarg E, et al. No downstaging after short-term preoperative radiotherapy in rectal cancer patients. J Clin Oncol 2001;19:1976–84.

[30] Bujko K, Nowacki MP, Nasierowska-Guttmejer A, et al. Sphincter preservation following preoperative radiotherapy for rectal cancer: report of a randomised trial comparing short-term radiotherapy vs. conventionally fractionated radiochemotherapy. Radiother Oncol 2004;72:15–24.

[31] Minsky BD, Cohen AM, Enker WE, et al. Sphincter preservation with preoperative radiation therapy and coloanal anastomosis. Int J Radiat Oncol Biol Phys 1995;31:553–9.

[32] Rullier E, Goffre B, Bonnel C, et al. Preoperative radiochemotherapy and sphincter-saving resection for T3 carcinomas of the lower third of the rectum. Ann Surg 2001;234:633–40.

[33] Bosset JF, Calais G, Daban A, et al. Preoperative chemoradiotherapy versus preoperative radiotherapy in rectal cancer patients: assessment of acute toxicity and treatment compliance. Report of the 22921 randomised trial conducted by the EORTC Radiotherapy Group. Eur J Cancer 2004;40:219–24.

[34] Willett CG. Technical advances in the treatment of patients with rectal cancer. Int J Radiat Oncol Biol Phys 1999;45:1107–8.

[35] Nuyttens JJ, Robertson JM, Yan D, et al. The position and volume of the small bowel during adjuvant radiation therapy for rectal cancer. Int J Radiat Oncol Biol Phys 2001;51:1271–80.

[36] Robertson JM, Lockman D, Yan D, et al. The dose-volume relationship of small bowel irradiation and acute grade 3 diarrhea during chemoradiotherapy for rectal cancer. Int J Radiat Oncol Biol Phys 2008;70:413–8.

[37] Dahlberg M, Glimelius B, Pahlman L. Improved survival and reduction in local failure rates after preoperative radiotherapy. Evidence for the generalizability of the results of Swedish Rectal Cancer Trial. Ann Surg 1999;229:493–7.

[38] Kapiteijn E, Marijnen CAM, Nagtegaal ID, et al. Preoperative radiotherapy combined with total mesorectal excision for resectable rectal cancer. N Engl J Med 2001;345:638–46.

[39] Peeters KCMJ, Marijnen CAM, Nagtegaal ID, et al. The TME trial after a median follow-up of 6 years. Increased local control but no survival benefit in irradiated patients with resectable rectal carcinoma. Ann Surg 2007;346:693–701.

[40] van den Brink M, van den Hout WB, Stiggelbout AM, et al. Cost-utility analysis of preoperative radiotherapy in patients with rectal cancer undergoing total mesorectal excision: a study of the Dutch Colorectal Cancer Group. J Clin Oncol 2004;22:244–53.

[41] Sauer R, Fietkau R, Wittekind C, et al. Adjuvant versus neoadjuvant radiochemotherapy for locally advanced rectal cancer. Strahlenther Onkol 2001;177:173–81.

[42] Solomon MJ, McLeod RS. Endoluminal transrectal ultrasonography: accuracy, reliability, and validity. Dis Colon Rectum 1993;36:200–5.

[43] Garcia-Aguilar J, Pollack J, Lee S-H, et al. Accuracy of endorectal ultrasonography in preoperative staging of rectal tumors. Dis Colon Rectum 2002;45:10–5.

[44] Killingback M, Barron P, Dent OF. Local recurrence after curative resection of cancer of the rectum without total mesorectal excision. Dis Colon Rectum 2001;44:473–86.

[45] Hiotis SP, Weber SM, Cohen AM, et al. Assessing the predictive value of clinical complete response to neoadjuvant therapy for rectal cancer: an analysis of 488 patients. J Am Coll Surg 2002;194:131–6.

[46] Tulchinsky H, Rabau M, Shacham-Shemueli E, et al. Can rectal cancers with pathologic T0 after neoadjuvant chemoradiation (ypT0) be treated by transanal excision alone? Ann Surg Oncol 2006;13:347–52.

[47] Bujko K, Nowacki MP, Nasierowska-Guttmejer A, et al. Prediction of mesorectal nodal metastases after chemoradiation for rectal cancer: results of a randomised trial. Implication for subsequent local excision. Radiother Oncol 2005;76:234–40.

[48] Habr-Gama A, Perez RO, Nadalin W, et al. Operative versus nonoperative treatment for stage 0 distal rectal cancer following chemoradiation therapy. Long-term results. Ann Surg 2004;240:711–8.

[49] Bonnen M, Crane C, Vauthey J-N, et al. Long-term results using local excision after preoperative chemoradiation among selected T3 rectal cancer patients. Int J Radiat Oncol Biol Phys 2004;60:1098–1105.

[50] Ota DM, Nelson H. Local excision of rectal cancer revisited: ACOSOG protocol Z6041. Ann Surg Oncol 2006;14:271.

[51] Russell AH, Harris J, Rosenberg PJ, et al. Anal sphincter conservation for patients with adenocarcinoma of the distal rectum: long-term results of Radiation Therapy Oncology Group protocol 89–02. Int J Radiat Oncol Biol Phys 2000;46:313–22.

[52] Steele GD Jr, Herndon JE, Bleday R, et al. Sphincter-sparing treatment for distal rectal adenocarcinoma. Ann Surg Oncol 1999;6:433–41.

[53] Bentrem DJ, Okabe S, Wong WD, et al. T1 adenocarcinoma of the rectum. Transanal excision or radical surgery? Ann Surg 2005;242:472–9.

[54] Kollmorgen CF, Meagher AP, Wolff BG, et al. The long-term effect of adjuvant postoperative chemoradiotherapy for rectal carcinoma on bowel function. Ann Surg 1994;220:676–82.

[55] Guren MG, Eriksen MT, Wiig JN, et al. Quality of life and functional outcome following anterior or abdominoperineal resection for rectal cancer. Eur J Surg Oncol 2005;31:735–42.

[56] Dahlberg M, Glimelius B, Graf W, et al. Preoperative irradiation affects functional results after surgery for rectal cancer: results from a randomized study. Dis Colon Rectum 1998;41:543–51.

[57] Peeters KCMJ, van de Velde CJH, Leer JWH, et al. Late side effects of short-course preoperative radiotherapy combined with total mesorectal excision for rectal cancer: increased bowel dysfunction in irradiated patients—a Dutch Colorectal Cancer Group study. J Clin Oncol 2005;23:6199–206.

[58] Marijnen CAM, van de Velde CJH, Putter H, et al. Impact of short-term preoperative radiotherapy on health-related quality of life and sexual functioning in primary rectal cancer: report of a multicenter randomized trial. J Clin Oncol 2005;23:1847–58.

[59] Pollack J, Holm T, Cedermark B, et al. Long-term effect of preoperative radiation therapy on anorectal function. Dis Colon Rectum 2006;49:345–52.

[60] Birnbaum EH, Myerson RJ, Fry RD, et al. Chronic effects of pelvic radiation therapy on anorectal function. Dis Colon Rectum 1994;37:909–15.

[61] Willett CG, Fung CY, Kaufman DS, et al. Postoperative radiation therapy for high-risk colon carcinoma. J Clin Oncol 1993;11:1112–7.

[62] Martenson JA Jr, Willett CG, Sargent DJ, et al. Phase III study of adjuvant chemotherapy and radiation therapy compared with chemotherapy alone in the surgical adjuvant treatment of colon cancer: results of Intergroup protocol 0130. J Clin Oncol 2004;22:3277–83.

Gastroenterol Clin N Am 37 (2008) 287–295

GASTROENTEROLOGY CLINICS
OF NORTH AMERICA

Systemic Therapy for Colon Cancer

Timothy R. Asmis, MD[a], Leonard Saltz, MD[a,b],*

[a]Gastrointestinal Oncology, Memorial Sloan Kettering Cancer Center, 1275 York Avenue,
New York, NY 10021, USA
[b]Weill Medical College of Cornell University, New York, USA

C olorectal cancer (CRC) is a common and frequently fatal disease in
North America. In the United States, 106,680 new cases of colon cancer
and 41,930 new cases of rectal cancer were reported in 2006, with an
estimated 55,170 deaths attributed to CRC [1]. In Canada, there were approximately 20,000 new cases of CRC, with an estimated 8500 deaths in 2006 [2].

RISK FACTORS
Many environmental and hereditary factors are associated with an increased
risk for developing CRC. There are multiple genetic predispositions to
CRC. The genetic condition associated with the highest risk for developing
CRC is familial adenomatous polyposis (FAP) caused by germline mutation
of the tumor-suppressor adenomatous polyposis coli (APC) gene. FAP is transmitted in an autosomal dominant fashion. Individuals who have FAP virtually
always develop CRC by the age of 40 years if not treated by prophylactic removal of the colon and rectum [3].

A more common genetic disorder that increases the risk for CRC is hereditary non-polyposis colorectal cancer (HNPCC), characterized by dysfunction
in DNA mismatch repair genes. HNPCC is inherited in an autosomal dominant manner [4]. It is associated with an early age of colon cancer diagnosis
and right-sided colon cancer. The diagnosis of HNPCC is suspected by either
the Amsterdam or the more recent and more liberal Bethesda Criteria, which
identify individuals who have a strong likelihood of mismatch repair gene
mutation. Such individuals should be referred for genetic counseling and
evaluation.

Other individual risk factors for CRC include a personal history of adenomatous polyps, a personal or family history of colon cancer, and a personal history of ulcerative colitis, especially pancolitis for more than 10 years. Protective
factors that may reduce the risk include a diet high in fruits and vegetables [5]
and low in animal fat and red meat [6]. Other suggested protective factors
include dietary calcium, nonsteroidal antiinflammatory drugs, and frequent

*Corresponding author. E-mail address: saltzl@mskcc.org (L. Saltz).

0889-8553/08/$ – see front matter
doi:10.1016/j.gtc.2007.12.005

physical activity. Postmenopausal women administered hormone replacement therapy have a decreased incidence of CRC [7].

Screening the general population for CRC reduces disease morbidity and mortality [8]. Various screening tools have been recommended, including colonoscopy, double contrast barium enemas, sigmoidoscopy, annual fecal occult blood test (FOBT), and CT virtual colonoscopy. Of these screening tests, colonoscopy is considered the gold standard because it directly visualizes the entire colon, provides biopsy capability, and is therapeutic in the removal of precancerous polyps. The American Cancer Society (ACS) recommends that all asymptomatic individuals undergo initial screening colonoscopy at age 50. Individuals at a higher-than-average risk, on the basis of family history, genetic screening, or other risk factors, should begin screening before age 50. Routine screening colonoscopies should be repeated every 10 years in asymptomatic individuals who have a negative index colonoscopy.

Patients who have first-degree relatives who had CRC should undergo CRC screening beginning at age 40, or 10 years earlier than the age of onset of the CRC in their first-degree relative [9]. Our practice is to initiate colonoscopic screening at either age 40, or 20 years younger than the index case, whichever occurs sooner.

Despite the established benefit and clear guidelines for screening, the North American population is underscreened. More than 70 million people in the United States are 50 years of age or older and thus eligible for screening. Yet as of 2004, only 28.3 million (40.4%) have been screened for CRC, including 21.6 million by colonoscopy and 6.7 million by FOBT [10]. In Canada, only about 20% of individuals aged 50 to 59 years have been screened for CRC [11] by any screening method, with a mere 4% of the screen-eligible population aged 50 to 74 years undergoing screening colonoscopy in 2001 [12].

PRESENTATION AND EVALUATION

Patients typically present with nonspecific symptoms, including abdominal pain, change in bowel habits, melena, hematochezia, or fatigue. Patients frequently are anemic. Approximately 20% of patients initially present with metastatic disease. Preoperative staging routinely includes an abdominal and pelvic CT scan. The role of preoperative chest roentgenogram versus chest CT is controversial. The current American Society of Clinical Oncology (ASCO) surveillance guidelines, however, recommend chest CT [13]. Because of the emerging role of metastasectomy for liver metastasis and the increasing role of neoadjuvant systemic therapy, a baseline chest CT is reasonable. Measurement of a carcinoembryonic antigen (CEA) level is recommended preoperatively.

NUTRITIONAL STATUS

Optimizing the nutritional status of the patient who has CRC is an important concern of the surgeon, gastroenterologist, and medical and radiation oncologist. Many solid tumors, including CRC, are associated with obesity and the metabolic syndrome of hyperglycemia and insulin resistance [14].

Paradoxically, malignancy and its various treatment modalities induce a catabolic state and impair the function of the GI tract, resulting in weight loss. These metabolic abnormalities increase surgical complication rates, including impaired wound healing and thromboembolism. An increased body mass index (BMI) also presents challenges to the medical and radiation oncologist when calculating the ideal dose of therapy. Patients who have CRC should work with their physicians and dietitians to develop a customized dietary plan to maintain an ideal BMI. Patients who have CRC who consume a diet high in fruits, vegetables, and non-red meats have an improved outcome when compared with those who consume a traditional Western diet high in red meat and refined grains [15].

SURGERY

The primary curative therapy is surgery, either by traditional open colectomy or, most recently, laparoscopically assisted colonic resection. These two techniques were reported as equivalent in efficacy in a large randomized trial performed by experienced surgeons [16]. Surgical resection optimally includes complete resection of the primary tumor and sampling of at least 12 regional lymph nodes. The surgeon should also inspect the entire abdominal cavity, palpate for evidence of metastatic disease, and obtain biopsies should a questionable metastatic lesion be encountered.

The optimal locoregional management of rectal cancer is more complex and anatomically more difficult than that for colon cancer because of its location within the bony pelvis, as opposed to the abdomen, and its location below the peritoneal reflection. Endorectal ultrasound or pelvic MRI should be standardly performed preoperatively. Tumors that are imaged as non–full thickness (T1–2, N0) should undergo initial surgical resection. If the final pathology remains non–full thickness and node-negative, no further therapy is routinely indicated. If the final pathology demonstrates full thickness, or if lymph nodes contain cancer, then postoperative chemoradiotherapy is indicated. If the initial endorectal evaluation indicates a full-thickness tumor (T3–4), preoperative chemoradiotherapy should be administered. Appropriate surgical treatment includes total mesorectal excision.

Metastasectomy is well established. Single or few metastatic lesions confined to either lung, liver, or ovary are potentially curable and should be considered for resection. A dedicated hepatic surgeon can aggressively resect liver metastases. Patients who have liver-only metastases deserve evaluation by a hepatic surgeon unless there is multifocal spread to all hepatic lobes. In patients who have surgically resectable hepatic metastases, 5-year survival approaches 40% [17].

Postoperative Management of Stage II and III Disease

Postoperative, or adjuvant, systemic therapy has become routine and standard for stage III colon cancer. Adjuvant therapy should also be strongly considered in stage II patients. It is generally recommended for any medically fit patient who has stage II cancer with unfavorable factors, including colonic perforation, unfavorable histology, colonic obstruction, or lymphovascular invasion. The optimal choice of adjuvant chemotherapy has recently changed from a 6-month course of 5-fluorouracil (5FU)-based chemotherapy alone to a 6-month course of infusional 5FU plus leucovorin (LV) and oxaliplatin (FOLFOX) based on

Table 1
Systemic therapy for colorectal cancer

Therapy	Mechanism of action	Indications	Potential common toxicities
5-Fluorouracil (5-FU)	Blocks the enzyme thymidylate synthase, which is essential for DNA synthesis	Multiple uses in combination with other agents in the adjuvant (postoperative) and palliative settings	Nausea, diarrhea Myelosuppression Fatigue
Capecitabine	Blocks thymidylate synthase (orally administered prodrug converted to 5-FU)	Multiple uses in combination with other agents in the adjuvant (postoperative) and metastatic setting	Nausea, diarrhea Myelosuppression Fatigue Palmar-plantar syndrome (hand-foot syndrome)
Oxaliplatin	Inhibits DNA replication and transcription by forming inter- and intra-strand DNA adducts/cross-links	Used in combination with 5FU, LV (FOLFOX) in the adjuvant (postoperative) and metastatic setting	Peripheral neuropathy Nausea, diarrhea Fatigue Myelosuppression Hypersensitivity
Irinotecan	Inhibits topoisomerase I, an enzyme that facilitates the uncoiling and recoiling of DNA during replication	Used alone or in combination with 5FU, LV (FOLFIRI) in the metastatic setting	Cholinergic (acute diarrhea) Nausea, late diarrhea Fatigue Myelosuppression Alopecia
Bevacizumab	Monoclonal antibody that binds to VEGF ligand	Used in combination with either FOLFOX or FOLFIRI in the metastatic setting	Hypertension Arterial thrombotic events Impaired wound healing Gastrointestinal perforation
Cetuximab	Monoclonal antibody to EGFR (chimeric) that blocks the ligand-binding site	Used with irinotecan or as a single agent in the metastatic setting	Acneform rash Hypersensitivity Hypomagnesemia Fatigue
Panitumumab	Monoclonal antibody to EGFR (fully humanized) that blocks the ligand-binding site	Used as a single agent in the metastatic setting	Acneform rash Hypomagnesemia Fatigue

Abbreviations: EGFR, epidermal growth factor receptor; VEGF, vascular endothelial growth factor.

a large trial of adjuvant systemic therapy for resected stage II or III colon cancer (Table 1) [18]. This trial demonstrated an increase in disease-free survival at 3 years from 72.9% to 78.2% ($P = .002$) with addition of oxaliplatin to FU/LV. Toxicities were comparable between the two groups, with the exception that oxaliplatin is associated with a much higher rate of paresthesia: 12.4% versus 0.2% grade 3 (serious) toxicity. This neurotoxicity persisted at a grade 3 level in 1.1% of treated patients at 1 year of follow-up.

In addition to adjuvant chemotherapy, patients should undergo follow-up for recurrent disease and metachronous cancer. Follow-up guidelines are somewhat controversial. A typical approach used at Memorial Sloan Kettering, and endorsed by ASCO, is to examine the patient every 3 to 4 months for the first several years postoperatively, with CEA monitoring at each visit, and annual CT scans of the chest, abdomen, and pelvis for the first 3 years. Full colonoscopy should be performed at 1, then 3, and then every 5 years after resection, unless colonoscopic findings or other factors necessitate more frequent colonoscopy.

CHEMOTHERAPY FOR METASTATIC DISEASE

Approximately 20% or more of patients who have CRC initially present with metastatic disease (mCRC). Approximately 35% of patients who present with stage III, 20% of patients with stage II, and 5% to 10% of patients with stage I cancer eventually relapse and subsequently die from mCRC. The most common sites of metastases are the liver, lung, peritoneum, and retroperitoneum.

Many advances have occurred recently in the treatment of mCRC. Active agents, in addition to the original 5FU, that have been approved by the US Food and Drug Administration (FDA) for mCRC include irinotecan, capecitabine, oxaliplatin, bevacizumab, cetuximab, and panitumumab. The goals of systemic therapy of mCRC include palliation of symptoms, prolongation of life, and, in selected cases of liver-only metastases, tumor regression to facilitate surgical resection of these metastases. The median survival of a patient who has mCRC has improved during the last decade from less than 1 year (with only 5FU-based therapy) to approximately 2 years (with multiagent systemic therapy).

Several factors help guide the selection of the appropriate first-line therapy for mCRC. The efficacy of systemic therapy is usually established in patients who have a good "performance status," or general medical status, at therapy initiation. A patient who has good performance status can provide for his or her own care and is active for most of the day. A patient who spends more than half of waking hours confined to a bed or chair has a poor performance status. Clinical trials for efficacy of chemotherapy and other systemic agents are restricted to patients who have a good performance status. The benefit of systemic therapy in patients who have poor performance status has not been well established and therefore should not be assumed. In patients who have poor performance status, initial efforts should focus on improvement of performance status through ambulation, nutrition, pain control, and medical treatment of underlying conditions, to render the patient a better candidate for chemotherapy. Patients receiving chemotherapy should also have adequate liver, kidney, and bone marrow function, or dose modifications may be required.

To determine the efficacy of chemotherapy for metastatic cancer, several measures are used. The definition of a response to therapy is a reduction, usually by at least some prespecified percentage, in cancer size. Reduction in the serum level of a tumor marker, such as CEA, can be confirmatory, but is an inadequate criterion. A partial response is defined as a 30% decrease in the longest dimension of each measurable tumor deposit, using unidimensional, or response evaluation criteria in solid tumors (RECIST), criteria [19]. A complete response is complete disappearance of all clinically detectable disease. The response rate (RR) is the percentage of patients who meet either criterion. Measures used to determine the duration of benefit include: (1) progression-free survival, which is the time from the start of treatment to the date the disease worsens, and (2) overall survival, which is the length of time patients are alive after diagnosis.

5FU, often modified by LV, has been clinically used for half a century [20] as a standard agent for mCRC. It was the only available agent until 1996, when irinotecan was approved. Over the last decade, oxaliplatin, capecitabine, bevacizumab, cetuximab, and most recently panitumumab have also been approved. 5FU blocks the enzyme thymidylate synthase, which is essential for DNA synthesis. LV, also known as folinic acid, enhances the antineoplastic effects of 5FU. Both LV (FOL, folinic acid) and 5FU (F, fluorouracil) can be combined with irinotecan (IRI) or oxaliplatin (OX) with the treatment acronyms FOLFIRI or FOLFOX, respectively. These alternative treatments consist of administration of a bolus of 5FU, LV, and either oxaliplatin or irinotecan. The patient is then sent home with a 2-day infusion of low-dose 5FU, administered by a small, lightweight, portable pump, usually worn on a belt or shoulder strap, infused through a centrally placed catheter. The patient or health care provider can simply disconnect the catheter after the 2-day infusion. Capecitabine is an oral fluoropyrimidine with a similar mechanism of action and similar efficacy as 5FU.

Irinotecan is a derivative of camptothecin, found in *Camptotheca acuminata*, a plant native to China. It potently inhibits topoisomerase I, an enzyme that facilitates the uncoiling and recoiling of DNA during replication by cleaving one strand and subsequently reattaching that strand. Oxaliplatin is a platinum chemotherapy that inhibits DNA replication and transcription by forming inter- and intra-strand DNA adducts/cross-links.

In patients who have mCRC, optimal chemotherapy consists of initial administration of a fluoropyrimidine and oxaliplatin or irinotecan (eg, FOLFOX or FOLFIRI). Tournigand and colleagues [21] and Colucci and colleagues [22] performed randomized trials in which patients received either FOLFIRI followed by FOLFOX, or vice versa. In the Tournigand and colleagues study, FOLIRI was found to have an RR of 56% and an 8.5-month median progression-free survival (mPFS), whereas FOLFOX had an RR of 54% and an mPFS of 8 months. Colucci and colleagues found that FOLFIRI had an RR of 31%

and FOLFOX had an RR of 34%. Both regimens had an mPFS of 7 months. Both investigators concluded that the regimens had similar efficacy when used as first-line therapy. Either FOLFOX or FOLFIRI can therefore be considered standard options for first-line treatment of mCRC. These regimens are typically given with bevacizumab.

Bevacizumab is a monoclonal antibody that binds to vascular endothelial growth factor ligand to inhibit angiogenesis. Its antineoplastic effect is ascribed to regression of microvascular density, inhibition of neovascularization, and normalization of grossly abnormal tumor vasculature that permits more effective chemotherapy delivery to the tumor. The FDA recently approved bevacizumab in combination with 5FU-based chemotherapy for mCRC based on findings that addition of bevacizumab to irinotecan, FU, and LV for mCRC improved progression-free survival from 6.2 months to 10.6 months, improved the response rate from 35% to 45% [23], and improved overall survival from 15.6 to 20.3 months. Most recently, Saltz and colleagues [24] reported on a randomized trial that found that the addition of bevacizumab to oxaliplatin-based chemotherapy significantly improved progression-free survival from 8.0 to 9.4 months. The addition of bevacizumab did not improve the response rate, however.

In 2004, the FDA approved cetuximab, the chimeric (human/mouse) monoclonal antibody targeting epidermal growth factor receptor (EGFR), for treatment of mCRC with irinotecan and as a single agent for patients intolerant of irinotecan-based therapy. In a single-arm, nonrandomized trial, cetuximab as a single agent had a 9% RR and a 35% rate of minor response or disease stability for at least 12 weeks [25]. When cetuximab was combined with irinotecan, the response rate was 22.9% versus 10.8% for irinotecan alone [26]. Cetuximab causes an acneform rash on the face and upper body in more than 80% of patients. The rash is associated with RR. Although the FDA approved cetuximab for use in EGFR-expressing mCRC, there is no evidence that the presence or absence of EGFR expression influences RR, and routine testing for this is unnecessary.

In 2006, the FDA approved panitumumab, a monoclonal antibody to EGFR, that unlike cetuximab is fully humanized (not chimeric). It is indicated for patients who have mCRC that has progressed on or following 5FU, oxaliplatin, and irinotecan-containing regimens. In a large randomized trial of panitumumab versus best supportive care for mCRC, a response rate of 8% was found [27]. Like cetuximab, panitumumab causes an acneform skin rash. As a fully human monoclonal antibody, panitumumab entails a lower risk for serious infusion reactions than the 3% rate observed with cetuximab. The relative activity of cetuximab versus panitumumab and the relative activity of panitumumab when given with chemotherapy are currently unknown.

SUMMARY

The prevention, treatment, and posttreatment care of colorectal cancer is a multidisciplinary process that involves surgeons, radiation therapists, and medical oncologists, along with gastroenterologists, radiologists, pathologists, and primary care physicians. The care of patients who have colorectal cancer is rapidly evolving. Despite numerous recent advances, the gains have been modest and incremental; CRC still remains the number two cause of cancer mortality in the United States. The mortality and morbidity from CRC can be dramatically reduced with effective implementation of universal screening. Further advances in medical oncology will result from better understanding of tumor genetics and biology and of host response to cancer that will allow therapy tailored to critical tumor-specific molecular targets while minimizing toxicity to normal tissue. With these advances it is hoped that CRC will become a rare disease, presenting in a small unscreened segment of the population, but treatable with highly effective, low-toxicity medical treatments.

References

[1] Jemal A, Siegel R, Ward E, et al. Cancer statistics, 2006. CA Cancer J Clin 2006;56(2): 106–30.

[2] Canadian cancer statistics. Ottawa (Ontario): Health Statistics Division, Stastics. Canada; 2006. Available at: http://www.cancer.ca/ccs/internet/standard/0,3182,3596_316704__langId-en,00.html. Accessed January 22, 2008.

[3] Guillem JG, Wood WC, Moley JF, et al. ASCO/SSO review of current role of risk-reducing surgery in common hereditary cancer syndromes. J Clin Oncol 2006;24(28):4642–60.

[4] Peltomaki P. Role of DNA mismatch repair defects in the pathogenesis of human cancer. J Clin Oncol 2003;21(6):1174–9.

[5] Terry P, Giovannucci E, Michels KB, et al. Fruit, vegetables, dietary fiber, and risk of colorectal cancer. J Natl Cancer Inst 2001;93(7):525–33.

[6] Chao A, Thun MJ, Connell CJ, et al. Meat consumption and risk of colorectal cancer. JAMA 2005;293(2):172–82.

[7] Chlebowski RT, Wactawski-Wende J, Ritenbaugh C, et al. Estrogen plus progestin and colorectal cancer in postmenopausal women. N Engl J Med 2004;350(10):991–1004.

[8] Winawer SJ, Zauber AG, Ho MN, et al. Prevention of colorectal cancer by colonoscopic polypectomy. The National Polyp Study Workgroup. N Engl J Med 1993;329(27): 1977–81.

[9] Winawer S, Fletcher R, Rex D, et al. Colorectal cancer screening and surveillance: clinical guidelines and rationale—update based on new evidence. Gastroenterology 2003; 124(2):544–60.

[10] Seeff LC, Manninen DL, Dong FB, et al. Is there endoscopic capacity to provide colorectal cancer screening to the unscreened population in the United States? Gastroenterology 2004;127(6):1661–9.

[11] Rabeneck L, Paszat LF. A population-based estimate of the extent of colorectal cancer screening in Ontario. Am J Gastroenterol 2004;99(6):1141–4.

[12] Vinden C, Schultz S, Rabeneck L. Use of large bowel procedures in Ontario: an ICES Research atlas. Institute for clinical evaluative sciences; 2004. Available at: http://www.ices.on.ca/webpage.cfm?site_id=1&org_id=67&morg_id=0&gsec_id=0&item_id=1947&type=atlas.

[13] Desch CE, Benson AB III, Somerfield MR, et al. Colorectal cancer surveillance: 2005 update of an American Society of Clinical Oncology practice guideline. J Clin Oncol 2005;23(33): 8512–9.

[14] Giovannucci E, Michaud D. The role of obesity and related metabolic disturbances in cancers of the colon, prostate, and pancreas. Gastroenterology 2007;132(6):2208–25.

[15] Meyerhardt JA, Niedzwiecki D, Hollis D, et al. The impact of dietary patterns on cancer recurrence and survival in patients with stage III colon cancer: findings from CALGB

89803. [abstract 4019]. Presented at the ASCO Annual Meeting. Chicago; June 1–4, 2007.

[16] Tinmouth J, Tomlinson G, Dalibon N, et al. A comparison of laparoscopically assisted and open colectomy for colon cancer. N Engl J Med 2004;350(20):2050–9.

[17] Fong Y, Cohen AM, Fortner JG, et al. Liver resection for colorectal metastases. J Clin Oncol 1997;15(3):938–46.

[18] Andre T, Boni C, Mounedji-Boudiaf L, et al. Oxaliplatin, fluorouracil, and leucovorin as adjuvant treatment for colon cancer. N Engl J Med 2004;350(23):2343–51.

[19] Therasse P, Arbuck SG, Eisenhauer EA, et al. New guidelines to evaluate the response to treatment in solid tumors. European Organization for Research and Treatment of Cancer, National Cancer Institute of the United States, National Cancer Institute of Canada. J Natl Cancer Inst 2000;92(3):205–16.

[20] Krueger GM, Alexander LL, Whippen DA, et al. Arnoldus Goudsmit, MD, PhD: chemotherapist, visionary, founder of the American Society of Clinical Oncology, 1909–2005. J Clin Oncol 2006;24(24):4033–6.

[21] Tournigand C, Andre T, Achille E, et al. FOLFIRI followed by FOLFOX6 or the reverse sequence in advanced colorectal cancer: a randomized GERCOR study. J Clin Oncol 2004;22(2):229–37.

[22] Colucci G, Gebbia V, Paoletti G, et al. Phase III randomized trial of FOLFIRI versus FOLFOX4 in the treatment of advanced colorectal cancer: a multicenter study of the Gruppo Oncologico Dell'Italia Meridionale. J Clin Oncol 2005;23(22):4866–75.

[23] Hurwitz H, Fehrenbacher L, Novotny W, et al. Bevacizumab plus irinotecan, fluorouracil, and leucovorin for metastatic colorectal cancer. N Engl J Med 2004;350(23):2335–42.

[24] Saltz L, Clarke S, Diaz-Rubio E, et al. Bevacizumab (Bev) in combination with XELOX or FOLFOX4: efficacy results from XELOX-1/NO16966, a randomized phase III trial in the first-line treatment of metastatic colorectal cancer (MCRC). Gastrointestinal Cancers Symposium. Orlando: ASCO; 2007.

[25] Saltz LB, Meropol NJ, Loehrer PJ Sr, et al. Phase II trial of cetuximab in patients with refractory colorectal cancer that expresses the epidermal growth factor receptor. J Clin Oncol 2004;22(7):1201–8.

[26] Cunningham D, Humblet Y, Siena S, et al. Cetuximab monotherapy and cetuximab plus irinotecan in irinotecan-refractory metastatic colorectal cancer. N Engl J Med 2004;351(4): 337–45.

[27] Van Cutsem E, Peeters M, Siena S, et al. Open-label phase III trial of panitumumab plus best supportive care compared with best supportive care alone in patients with chemotherapy-refractory metastatic colorectal cancer. J Clin Oncol 2007;25:1658–64.

Gastroenterol Clin N Am 37 (2008) 297–305

GASTROENTEROLOGY CLINICS
OF NORTH AMERICA

INDEX

Note: Page numbers of article titles are in **boldface** type.

0889-8553/08/$ – see front matter
doi:10.1016/S0889-8553(08)00009-5